Praise for *Taking Turns: Stories from HIV/AIDS Care Unit 371*

"MK Czerwiec's tales of her nursing work on an AIDS unit chart a remarkable episode in the history of medicine. . . . Through the lives and deaths of individual patients, written and drawn in documentary detail, we see the power dynamic between doctor and patient begin to shift. When cure is not an option, care takes on a new meaning."
—Alison Bechdel, author of *Fun Home*

"Rather than the usual medical tales of professional-minded strangers treating faceless victims, Czerwiec's vignettes become about bonding intimately over suffering and death, watching the community be decimated at the same time as mutual nursing was building connections. Some of the pages are heart-wrenching, and the story has the potential to be supremely depressing, but Czerwiec wrings hope from the honesty of her simple, cheerful cartooning style."
—*Publishers Weekly*

"With simple, even amateur panels and wise words, Czerwiec reveals a hospital at the heart of the AIDS crisis. Working as a nurse on a unit for AIDS patients, she and her colleagues helped patients die, celebrated life, and strove to combat the poorly understood disease. Cathartic and clinical, often simultaneously."
—Emilia Packard, *Library Journal*

"[Czerwiec's] chronicle reminds us that the era was marked as much by courage and compassion as it was by the tragedy of lives lost too soon."
—Gordon Flagg, *Booklist*

"It is not likely that c[...] medical scientific p[...] brought to tears ov[...]
—Adrian Bussone, 7[...]

D0851465

"Whatever role we play in the health care system, this moving memoir reminds us to look beyond our institutional affiliations and find our place in the wider human community."
—*JAMA*

"For health care providers, the years that followed [the first official reporting of what would become the AIDS epidemic] were a time of tremendous loss, requiring a new type of caregiving in the face of a disease with no cure. MK Czerwiec, a nurse and the artist-in-residence at Northwestern University's Feinberg School of Medicine, captures this tragic time with great reverence and attention to detail."
—Jessica Bylander, *Health Affairs*

"A reminder of the need for love, compassion, acceptance, and human connectivity when providing care to some of society's most vulnerable and often ostracized patient populations."
—*Doody's Review Service*

"Among the takeaways one has after reading MK Czerwiec's graphic novel *Taking Turns* is that even in the form of sequential art, the story of the early days of the HIV epidemic is a visceral and heart-wrenching experience."
—Savas Abadsidis, *Advocate / HIV Plus*

"*Taking Turns* chronicles [Czerwiec's] experiences on the evening shift at Unit 371 with patients and other caregivers, often told through voices other than her own, some of the stories funny, some very touching, especially the stories about patients with whom she became close before they died."
—Hank Trout, *A&U Magazine: America's AIDS Magazine*

"The emotional honesty of the comic book is quintessential to the visceral experience of *Taking Turns*—funny, terrifying and heartbreaking. As much as it informs the reader about the devastation of HIV/AIDS, the book allows the reader to see the disease through the eyes of a person who is literally on the front lines."
—Gretchen Rachel Hammond, *Windy City Times*

"The author's deft handling of the multiplicity of relationships involved in patient care is the strength of the book, and they are all represented throughout the narrative. Czerwiec does an excellent job of showing how Unit 371's commitment to care facilitated a depth of intimacy between provider and patient not often found in today's productivity-driven medical care."
—Dr. Devlyn McCreight, *Graphic Medicine*

"Czerwiec's role as a writer and illustrator of graphic medicine texts as well as one of the primary theorists and advocates of the genre means that this, her first single-author entry into the form she helped establish, is, like its author, doing the work of defining and practicing this new and compelling literary and artistic form."
—Ajuan Mance, *Women's Review of Books*

"Czerwiec . . . does much more than just provide younger readers with a history lesson. For example, she thoughtfully explores what it means to be a healthcare provider. Czerwiec also explores the role of boundaries between healthcare providers and their patients and the need for empathy. These topics, I believe, would resonate with and be useful to students interested in medical or allied health careers. Instructors can use the book as a way to begin these conversations."
—David R. Wessner, *Journal of Microbiology & Biology Education*

"A valuable reflection on and historical portrait of the AIDS hysteria of the eighties and nineties in America. Combining [Czerwiec's] memories of that era with her contemporary perspective shows, and makes it seem unbelievable, that a group of people suffered so greatly because of their outsider status as patients with a transmittable, incurable, deadly disease. *Taking Turns* shows us the cost."
—*The Oral History Review*

"*Taking Turns* bears important witness to a specific moment in the history of HIV/AIDS through the testimony of caregivers, patients, and volunteers. MK Czerwiec's story also issues a gracious challenge: knowing that we all live in vulnerable bodies, knowing that we will all 'take turns' needing others and being needed, how can we make this one life we have meaningful? This luminous graphic novel models how we can start: through creativity, community, generosity, and vulnerability."
—Ann Fox, Davidson College

"An important work that takes the field of graphic medicine in new directions, both in terms of its object—the philosophy and practices of a clinical unit dedicated to the care of people with AIDS in a particular place and historical moment—and its approach—drawing on the comic artist's own experience as a nurse on the unit as well as her interviews with other practitioners and patients."
—Lisa Diedrich, author of *Indirect Action: Schizophrenia, Epilepsy, AIDS, and the Course of Health Activism*

Taking Turns

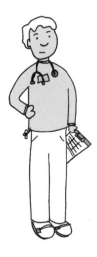

MK Czerwiec

Taking Turns

Stories from HIV/AIDS
Care Unit 371

graphic mundi

Dedicated to the patients, friends, families, and staff of Unit 371
and to Lorraine, who taught me how to be a good nurse.

Preface

It was well after the closing of HIV/AIDS Care Unit 371 in Chicago that I created this book, originally published in 2017. I assumed, wrongly, that any sort of global epidemic or pandemic I would see in my lifetime was in the past. The virus that caused AIDS finally had drugs to keep it in check, and it was time, now, to create a graphic novel to share some of the experiences and insights I had gained working as a nurse in a very special HIV/AIDS care unit at the height of the epidemic. In March 2020—three years after the first publication of *Taking Turns*, and as COVID-19 was becoming a clear global threat—I was no longer working as a nurse. Nonetheless, as the COVID virus spread throughout the world, drawings and comics about the pandemic started showing up in my social media feeds and email inbox in a sudden and eerie reminder of what I had seen working on the front lines of the HIV/AIDS crisis.

When I saw these comics, I flashed back to images of full-body PPE used during the early days of the AIDS crisis, to frontline caregivers standing in as family members at the bedside of those dying from the virus. I flashed back to political scapegoating and marginalized communities bearing the disproportionate burden of the crisis. I flashed back to the intense contrast between life inside the hospital, where every shift felt like barely managed chaos, and outside the hospital, where resistance to accepting that we were in any kind of crisis ran rampant. I flashed back to health care systems motivated by profit instead of patient well-being, money over lives. And I flashed back to the idea of "taking turns being sick," as caregivers again became patients in their own care units.

If the many images of COVID that emerged in comic form in 2020 reminded me of this painful past public health crisis, they also revealed profound differences between the two viral outbreaks. With COVID-19, the route of infection was much more immediate and the spread much more swift than with HIV. And this new pandemic felt like all of those agonizing years of the AIDS crisis compressed into a traumatizing fraction of the time.

As I share in this book, I started making comics as a way to cope with the pressures of being a nurse on HIV/AIDS Care Unit 371. I made my first comic in a moment of desperation, and that first comic helped me find hope. Comics can be like that. Because making comics worked for me, I kept making them. When Unit 371 closed in 2000, I was of course joyful that our patients finally had the medications that could help them recover, but I was also secretly bereft, because I never thought I would find work that was as rewarding—and a community of support as embracing. I was wrong. Comics have led me to pursue rewarding work as an educator, comics artist, and co-curator of Graphic Medicine (https://www.graphicmedicine.org), a website that explores the interaction between comics and health, illness, caregiving, and disability. I'm happy to be a member of these vital communities. Through our work, we lift one another up, and the success of one of us becomes the success of us all. Comics can be like that too.

The COVID-19 pandemic has shined a light on the essential value and fragility of frontline care workers like never before. The questions that inspired me to create this book, including all of the oral history research I conducted in the decade prior to drawing *Taking Turns*, are as important today as they were then: How do frontline workers recover from the intensity of caregiving during a pandemic? Could this time truly be both terrible and utterly formative? How can we metabolize all of this trauma? How can we learn to prioritize relief of suffering over all else? What can we learn from how we coped, or how we didn't? How has all of this changed us and our world? How do we resist the urge to pretend it didn't?

I hope this book will serve as a reminder of some of the hard-earned knowledge we've gained through both the AIDS epidemic and the COVID pandemic: the understanding that when we can't cure, we can still be present, and we can still care, and that hope lies in community action, strength in coming together to discover what good we can still do. As Dr. Walter Miller, the psychiatric liaison to Unit 371, tells us about the profound grief that comes with being a witness to someone's death, what matters is "who you become as a result of that."

MK Czerwiec
LAKESIDE, MICHIGAN
JUNE 2021

Acknowledgments

Thank you to my wife, Cindy Homan. Without your support, encouragement, and faith, this book would not exist.

Thank you to the narrators of Unit 371, for sharing your memories. Not explicitly included in this book, but who contributed interviews and insights, are Jo Kim, Michael Bauer, Bruce Campbell, Jim Ludwig, Tom Tunney, Rodney Anderson, and a very special couple who taught me some Yiddish on Unit 371. I also want to recognize Lori Schwartz, Staff Support Coordinator.

Thank you, Lynda Barry, for teaching me that comics can be good for the hard stuff. Thank you, Alice Dreger, for insisting that this project needed to go from an idea to reality. Thank you, Gretchen Case, for teaching me to do oral history and for your encouragement. Thank you to Cate Belling, Katie Watson, Kathryn Montgomery, Tod Chambers, and the Medical Humanities & Bioethics Program at Northwestern Feinberg School of Medicine for your encouragement, guidance, and support. I'm also grateful to the faculty of the Program in Narrative Medicine at Columbia University Medical Center.

Thank you to Mita Mahato and Sarah Leavitt for our blog and our friendships. Thanks to our many comrades in Graphic Medicine, specifically Ian Williams, Susan Squier, Michael Green, Brian Fies, Kimberly Myers, Peter Dunlap-Shohl, Linda and Marc Raphael, Muna Al-Jawad, America Waters, Katie Green, Paula Knight, Nicola Streeten, Sarah Lightman, David Small, Esther Saltzman, Sharon Rosenzweig, Aaron Freeman, Marsha Hurst, Lois Perlson-Gross, Philippa Perry, and Karrie Fransman. You have all taught, encouraged, and inspired me. Some of you even hosted me. Thanks also to Kendra Boileau for believing in the potential of Graphic Medicine.

For reviewing drafts of this project and sharing insights that helped shape it, thanks to several of you mentioned above and also Michael J. Hess, RL Hansen, Barbara Shomaker, Riva Lehrer, George Fitchett, MaryEllen Schneider,

Ann Fox, Lisa Diedrich, and Jim McDonough. Appreciation also goes to my mentor nurses from the American Society of Bioethics and Humanities, Anita Catlin and Joan Liaschenko.

For research and production assistance, special thanks to Kelli Lynch, Katie McMahon, Esther Block, Carrie Wagner, and the librarians at Illinois Masonic Medical Center.

To John, Karen, Maddie, and Jack, for being family and fans. A very special thank you to Maribel Lim for taking such amazing care of Mom that I could spend my days making comics. Thanks to Jim Fitzmaurice and Doug GeBraad. . . . for everything.

Thanks to Teresa Sullinger for encouragement and great haircuts that came with page deadlines. Thanks to Tim Sullivan, Mike Humphrey, Tom Dunn, Geordan Capes, Tim England, and the entire Michigan crew for weekends of fun that kept me going as I worked on this book.

I am grateful to those who encouraged this work who have died and I miss, especially Lorraine A. Czerwiec, mentor and Mom. I also owe a debt of gratitude to Brenda Skinner, Roger Goodman, Editha Peregrino, Dick Westley, Bob Williams, and Don and Mary Kennedy.

Podcasts were a lifeline as I worked on this book. Thanks to *Out on the Wire*, *Double X Gabfest*, *Pop Culture Happy Hour*, *Slate Culture Gabfest*, the *Sistah Speak* family, *Nerdette*, *Fresh Air*, *On Being*, the entire Maximum Fun Network, and *Invisibilia*. You fed the process and the product.

And finally, speaking of feeding, a warm thank you to Café Selmarie in Lincoln Square for your salmon club sandwich.

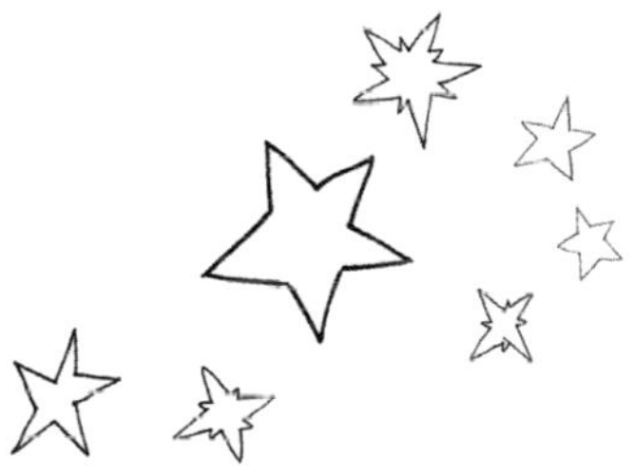

The unendurable happens. You know, people we love and we can't live without are going to die. We're going to die . . . it's unendurable. . . . Art holds that knowledge. All art holds the knowledge that we're both living and dying at the same time. Art can hold it.

—MARIE HOWE

1993

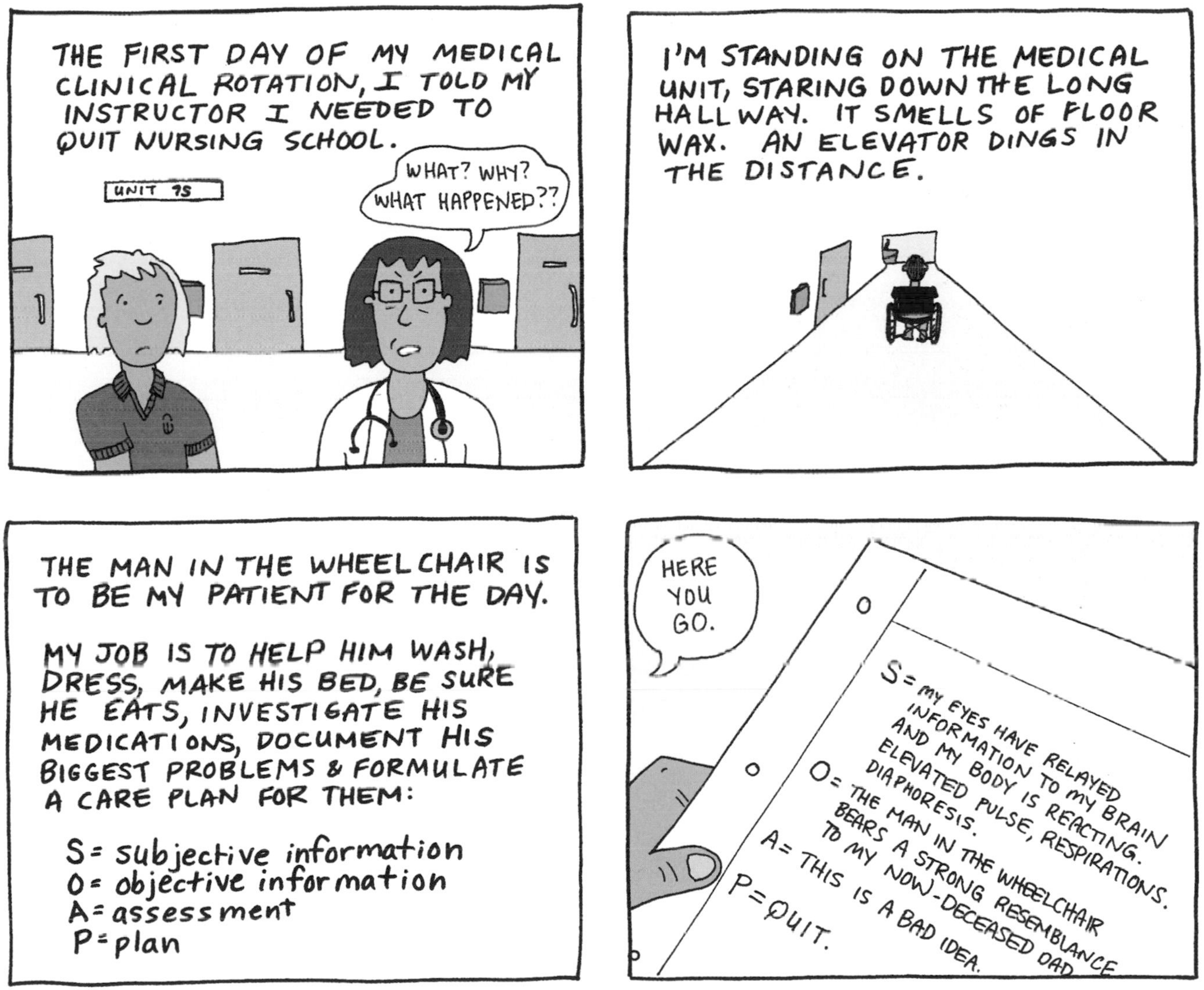
THE FIRST DAY OF MY MEDICAL CLINICAL ROTATION, I TOLD MY INSTRUCTOR I NEEDED TO QUIT NURSING SCHOOL.
UNIT 9S
WHAT? WHY? WHAT HAPPENED??
I'M STANDING ON THE MEDICAL UNIT, STARING DOWN THE LONG HALLWAY. IT SMELLS OF FLOOR WAX. AN ELEVATOR DINGS IN THE DISTANCE.
THE MAN IN THE WHEELCHAIR IS TO BE MY PATIENT FOR THE DAY.
MY JOB IS TO HELP HIM WASH, DRESS, MAKE HIS BED, BE SURE HE EATS, INVESTIGATE HIS MEDICATIONS, DOCUMENT HIS BIGGEST PROBLEMS & FORMULATE A CARE PLAN FOR THEM:
S= subjective information
O= objective information
A= assessment
P= plan
HERE YOU GO.
S= MY EYES HAVE RELAYED INFORMATION TO MY BRAIN AND MY BODY IS REACTING. ELEVATED PULSE, RESPIRATIONS. DIAPHORESIS.
O= THE MAN IN THE WHEELCHAIR BEARS A STRONG RESEMBLANCE TO MY NOW-DECEASED DAD
A= THIS IS A BAD IDEA.
P= QUIT.

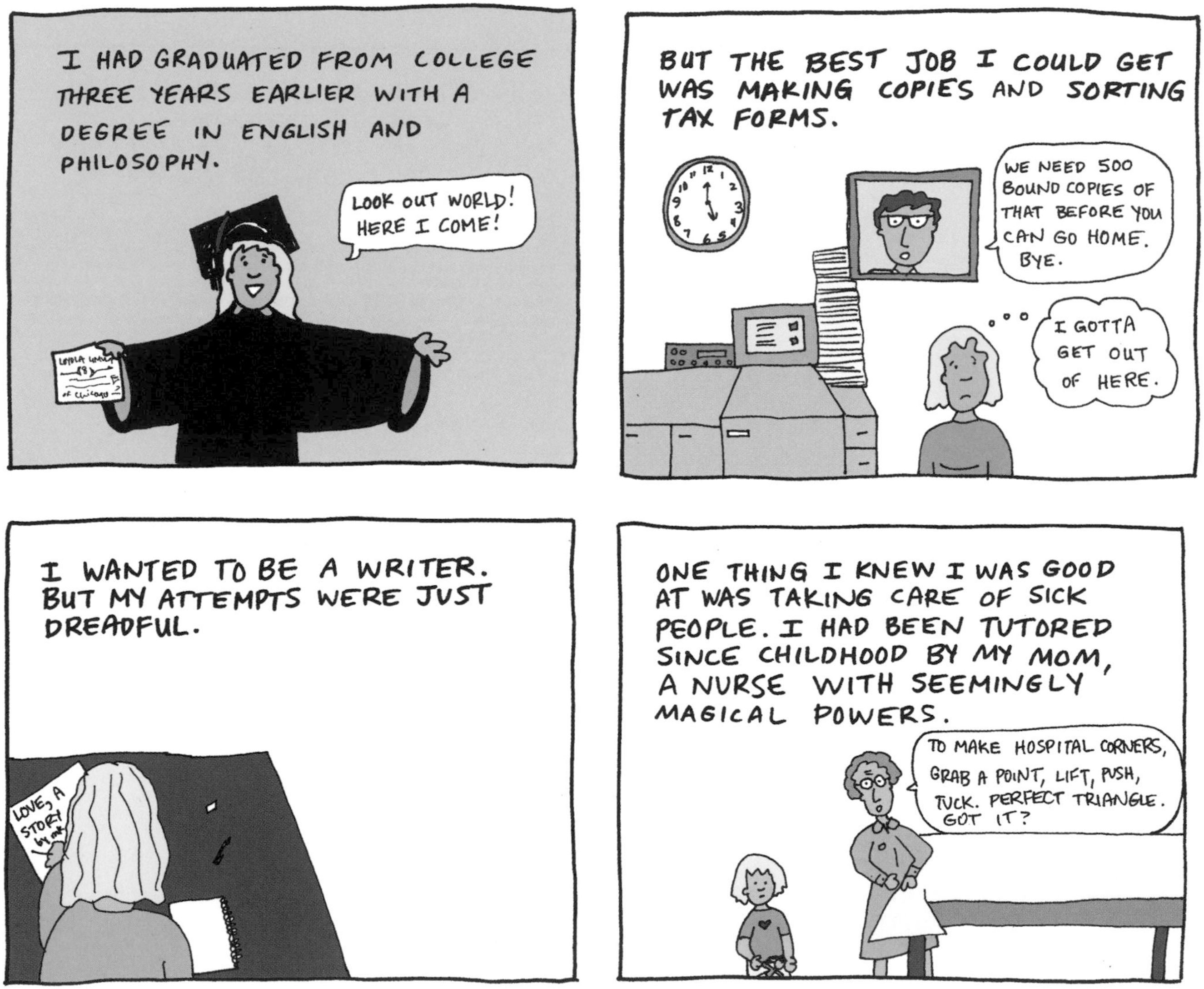
I HAD GRADUATED FROM COLLEGE THREE YEARS EARLIER WITH A DEGREE IN ENGLISH AND PHILOSOPHY.
LOOK OUT WORLD! HERE I COME!
BUT THE BEST JOB I COULD GET WAS MAKING COPIES AND SORTING TAX FORMS.
WE NEED 500 BOUND COPIES OF THAT BEFORE YOU CAN GO HOME. BYE.
I GOTTA GET OUT OF HERE.
I WANTED TO BE A WRITER. BUT MY ATTEMPTS WERE JUST DREADFUL.
LOVE, A STORY
ONE THING I KNEW I WAS GOOD AT WAS TAKING CARE OF SICK PEOPLE. I HAD BEEN TUTORED SINCE CHILDHOOD BY MY MOM, A NURSE WITH SEEMINGLY MAGICAL POWERS.
TO MAKE HOSPITAL CORNERS, GRAB A POINT, LIFT, PUSH, TUCK. PERFECT TRIANGLE. GOT IT?

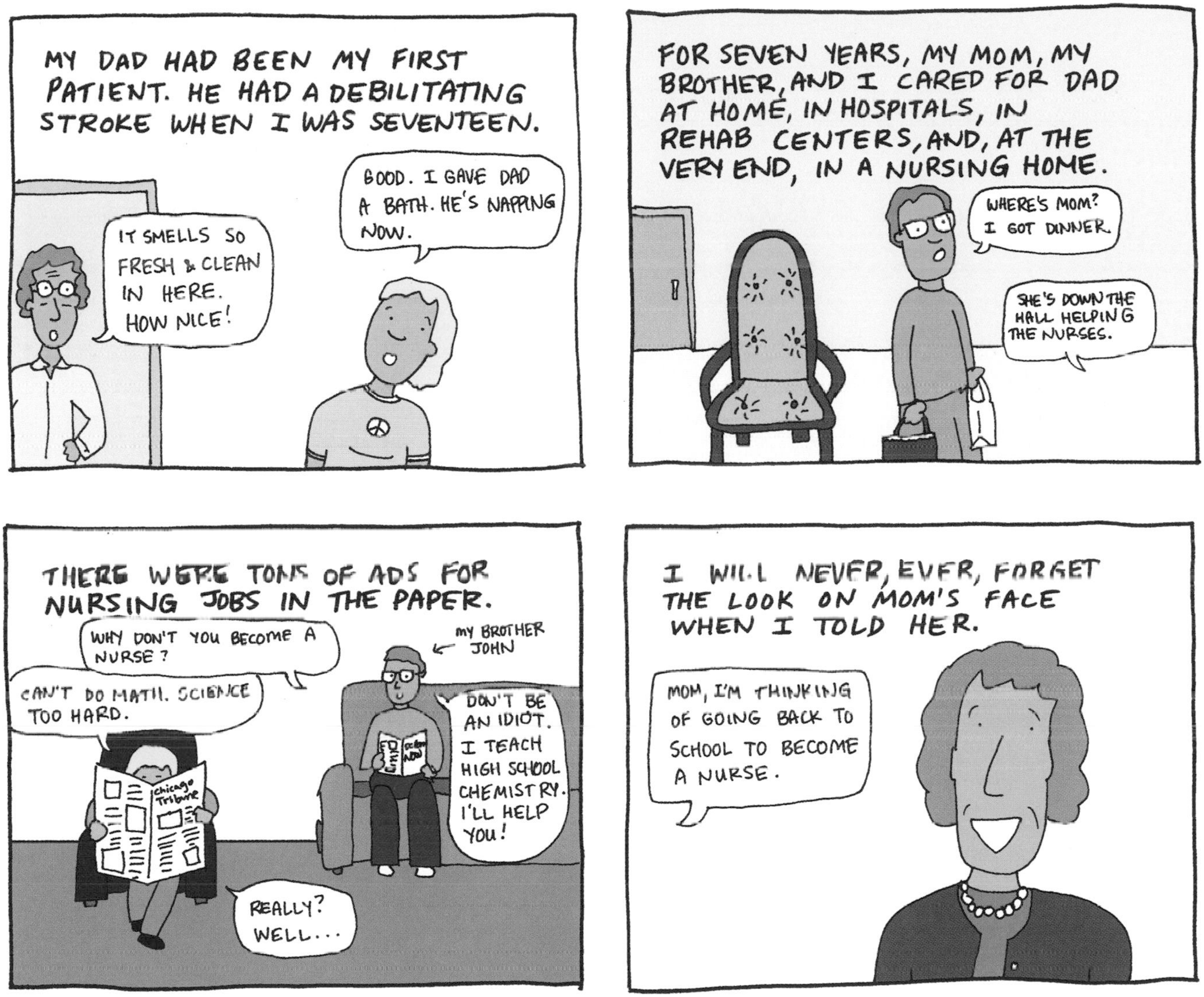
MY DAD HAD BEEN MY FIRST PATIENT. HE HAD A DEBILITATING STROKE WHEN I WAS SEVENTEEN.
GOOD. I GAVE DAD A BATH. HE'S NAPPING NOW.
IT SMELLS SO FRESH & CLEAN IN HERE. HOW NICE!
FOR SEVEN YEARS, MY MOM, MY BROTHER, AND I CARED FOR DAD AT HOME, IN HOSPITALS, IN REHAB CENTERS, AND, AT THE VERY END, IN A NURSING HOME.
WHERE'S MOM? I GOT DINNER.
SHE'S DOWN THE HALL HELPING THE NURSES.
THERE WERE TONS OF ADS FOR NURSING JOBS IN THE PAPER.
WHY DON'T YOU BECOME A NURSE?
my BROTHER JOHN
CAN'T DO MATH. SCIENCE TOO HARD.
DON'T BE AN IDIOT. I TEACH HIGH SCHOOL CHEMISTRY. I'LL HELP YOU!
Chicago Tribune
REALLY? WELL...
I WILL NEVER, EVER, FORGET THE LOOK ON MOM'S FACE WHEN I TOLD HER.
MOM, I'M THINKING OF GOING BACK TO SCHOOL TO BECOME A NURSE.

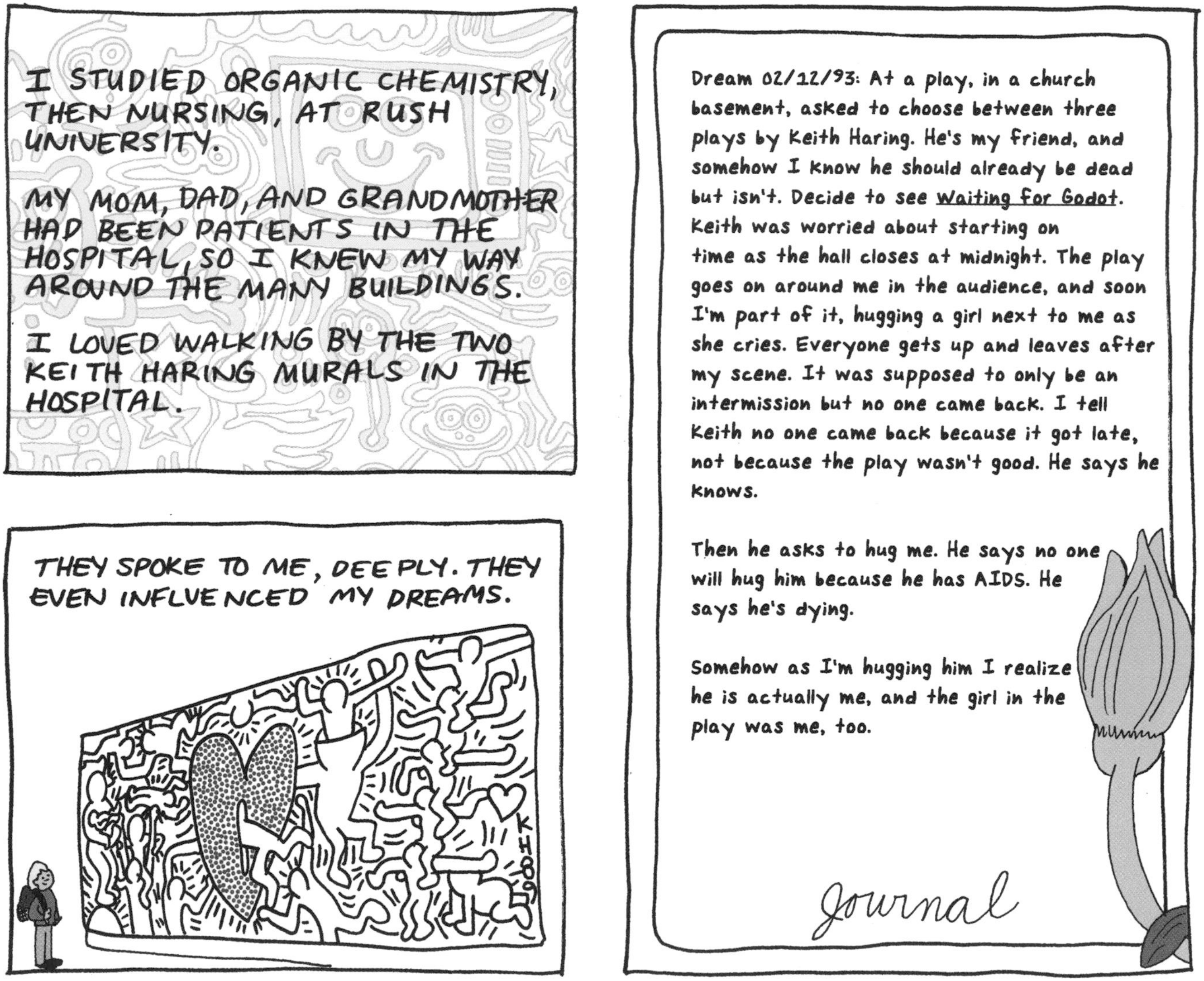
I STUDIED ORGANIC CHEMISTRY, THEN NURSING, AT RUSH UNIVERSITY.
MY MOM, DAD, AND GRANDMOTHER HAD BEEN PATIENTS IN THE HOSPITAL, SO I KNEW MY WAY AROUND THE MANY BUILDINGS.
I LOVED WALKING BY THE TWO KEITH HARING MURALS IN THE HOSPITAL.
THEY SPOKE TO ME, DEEPLY. THEY EVEN INFLUENCED MY DREAMS.
KH 89
Dream 02/12/93: At a play, in a church basement, asked to choose between three plays by Keith Haring. He's my friend, and somehow I know he should already be dead but isn't. Decide to see Waiting for Godot. Keith was worried about starting on time as the hall closes at midnight. The play goes on around me in the audience, and soon I'm part of it, hugging a girl next to me as she cries. Everyone gets up and leaves after my scene. It was supposed to only be an intermission but no one came back. I tell Keith no one came back because it got late, not because the play wasn't good. He says he knows.
Then he asks to hug me. He says no one will hug him because he has AIDS. He says he's dying.
Somehow as I'm hugging him I realize he is actually me, and the girl in the play was me, too.
Journal

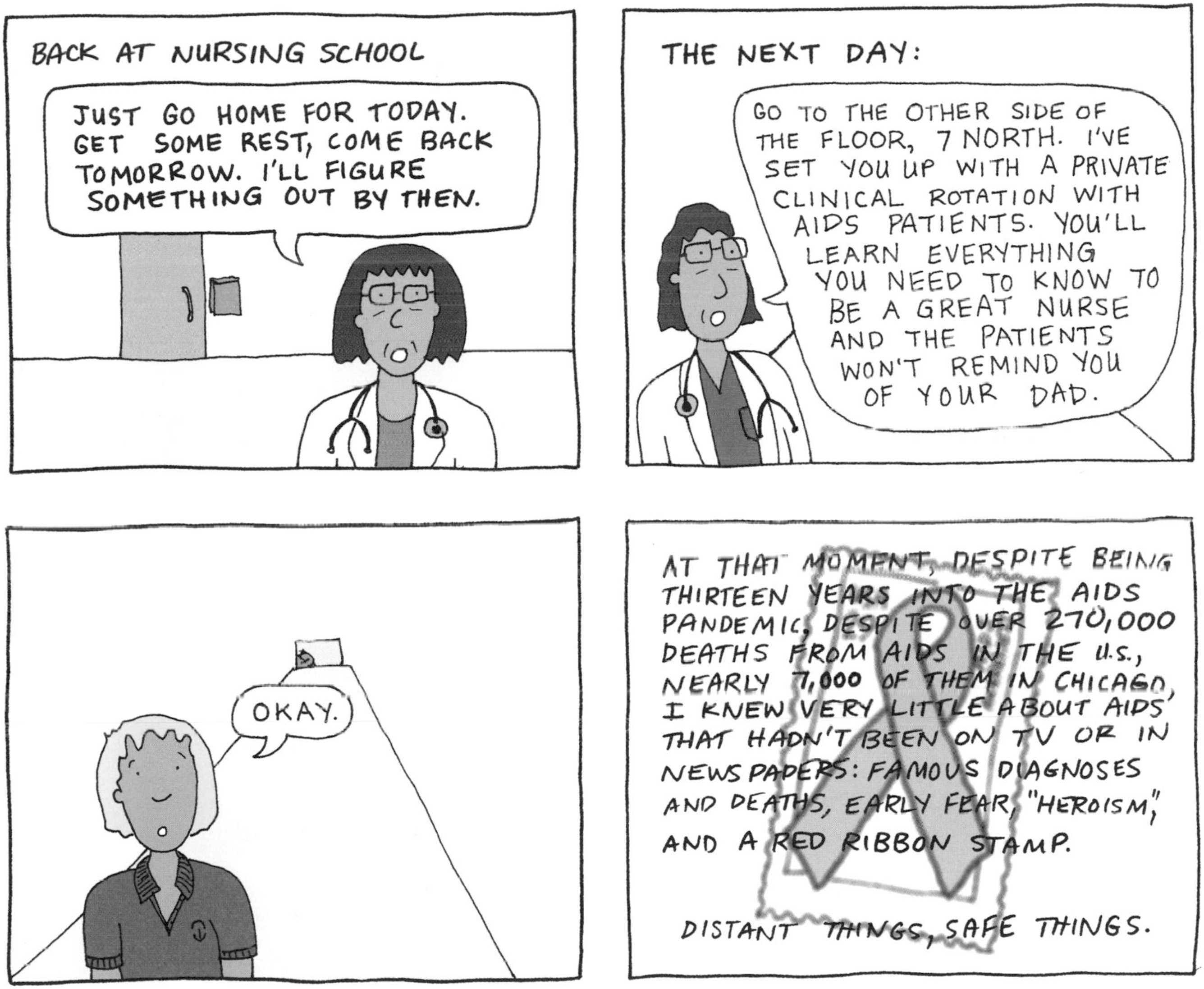
BACK AT NURSING SCHOOL
JUST GO HOME FOR TODAY. GET SOME REST, COME BACK TOMORROW. I'LL FIGURE SOMETHING OUT BY THEN.
THE NEXT DAY:
GO TO THE OTHER SIDE OF THE FLOOR, 7 NORTH. I'VE SET YOU UP WITH A PRIVATE CLINICAL ROTATION WITH AIDS PATIENTS. YOU'LL LEARN EVERYTHING YOU NEED TO KNOW TO BE A GREAT NURSE AND THE PATIENTS WON'T REMIND YOU OF YOUR DAD.
OKAY.
AT THAT MOMENT, DESPITE BEING THIRTEEN YEARS INTO THE AIDS PANDEMIC, DESPITE OVER 270,000 DEATHS FROM AIDS IN THE U.S., NEARLY 7,000 OF THEM IN CHICAGO, I KNEW VERY LITTLE ABOUT AIDS THAT HADN'T BEEN ON TV OR IN NEWSPAPERS: FAMOUS DIAGNOSES AND DEATHS, EARLY FEAR, "HEROISM," AND A RED RIBBON STAMP.
DISTANT THINGS, SAFE THINGS.

ACQUIRED IMMUNE DEFICIENCY SYNDROME IS CAUSED BY THE HUMAN IMMUNODEFICIENCY VIRUS, WHICH IS A SINGLE STRAND OF RIBONUCLEIC ACID IN A PROTEIN ENVELOPE. ONCE IN THE HUMAN BODY, IT LATCHES ON TO A CD4 T-CELL, A CRITICAL PIECE OF OUR IMMUNE SYSTEM. BEFORE DESTROYING THE T-CELL, HIV TURNS IT INTO A FACTORY FOR MAKING MORE HIV — A TOTALLY JERKY, BUT ALSO BRILLIANT, MOVE FOR THE HIV.

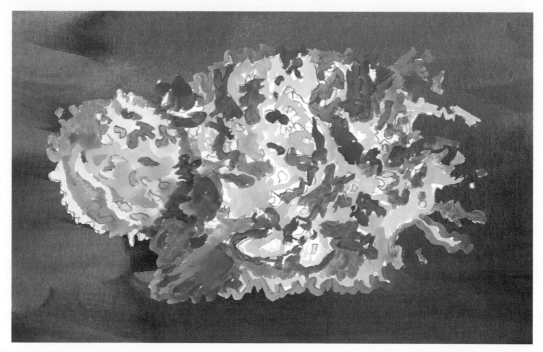

THE NEW VIRIONS HEAD OFF TO DO THE SAME TO OTHER T-CELLS, EVENTUALLY LEAVING NO MORE CD4 T-CELLS, AND BILLIONS OF HIV, IN THE BODY.

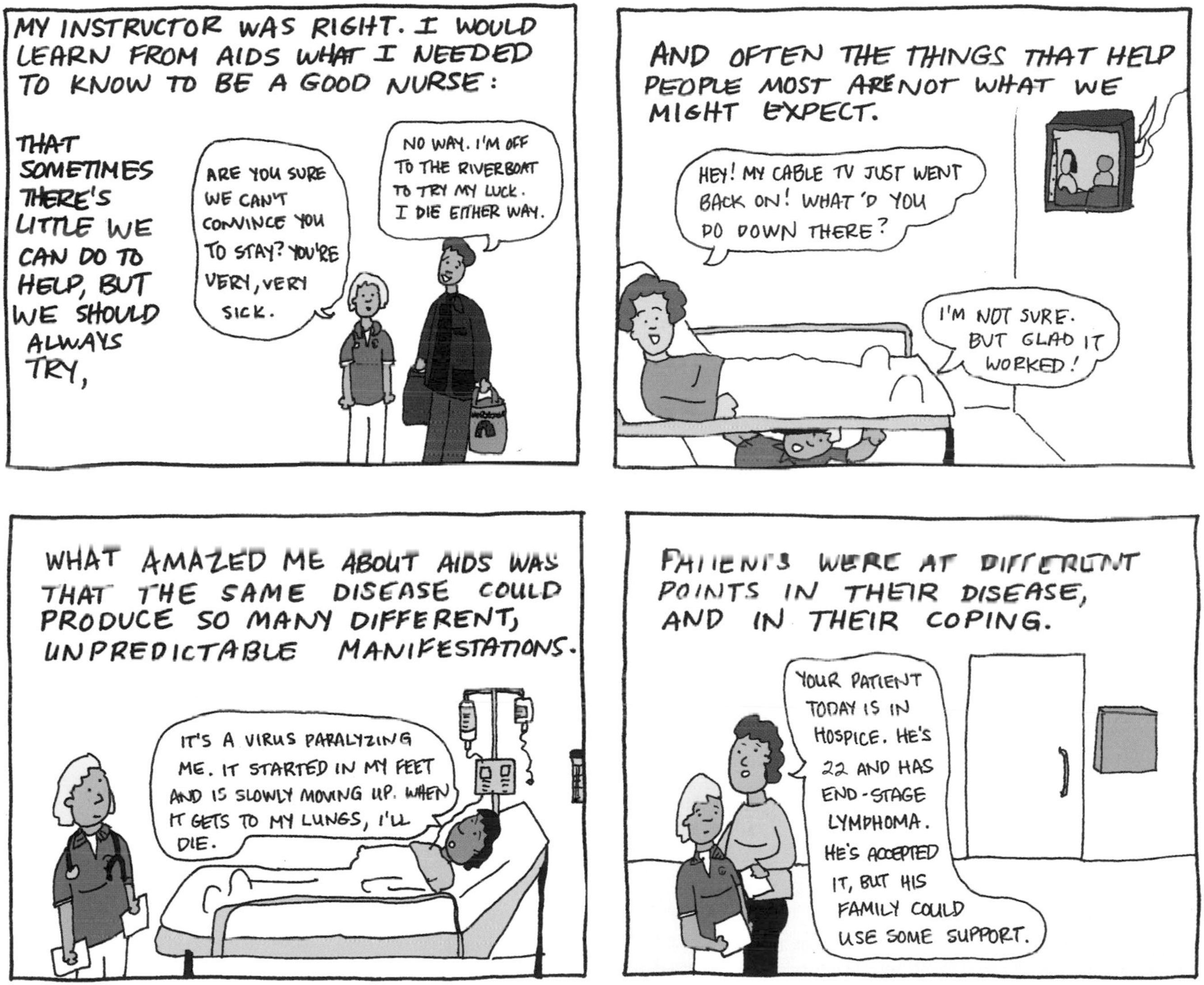
MY INSTRUCTOR WAS RIGHT. I WOULD LEARN FROM AIDS WHAT I NEEDED TO KNOW TO BE A GOOD NURSE:
THAT SOMETIMES THERE'S LITTLE WE CAN DO TO HELP, BUT WE SHOULD ALWAYS TRY,
ARE YOU SURE WE CAN'T CONVINCE YOU TO STAY? YOU'RE VERY, VERY SICK.
NO WAY. I'M OFF TO THE RIVERBOAT TO TRY MY LUCK. I DIE EITHER WAY.
AND OFTEN THE THINGS THAT HELP PEOPLE MOST ARE NOT WHAT WE MIGHT EXPECT.
HEY! MY CABLE TV JUST WENT BACK ON! WHAT'D YOU DO DOWN THERE?
I'M NOT SURE. BUT GLAD IT WORKED!
WHAT AMAZED ME ABOUT AIDS WAS THAT THE SAME DISEASE COULD PRODUCE SO MANY DIFFERENT, UNPREDICTABLE MANIFESTATIONS.
IT'S A VIRUS PARALYZING ME. IT STARTED IN MY FEET AND IS SLOWLY MOVING UP. WHEN IT GETS TO MY LUNGS, I'LL DIE.
PATIENTS WERE AT DIFFERENT POINTS IN THEIR DISEASE, AND IN THEIR COPING.
YOUR PATIENT TODAY IS IN HOSPICE. HE'S 22 AND HAS END-STAGE LYMPHOMA. HE'S ACCEPTED IT, BUT HIS FAMILY COULD USE SOME SUPPORT.

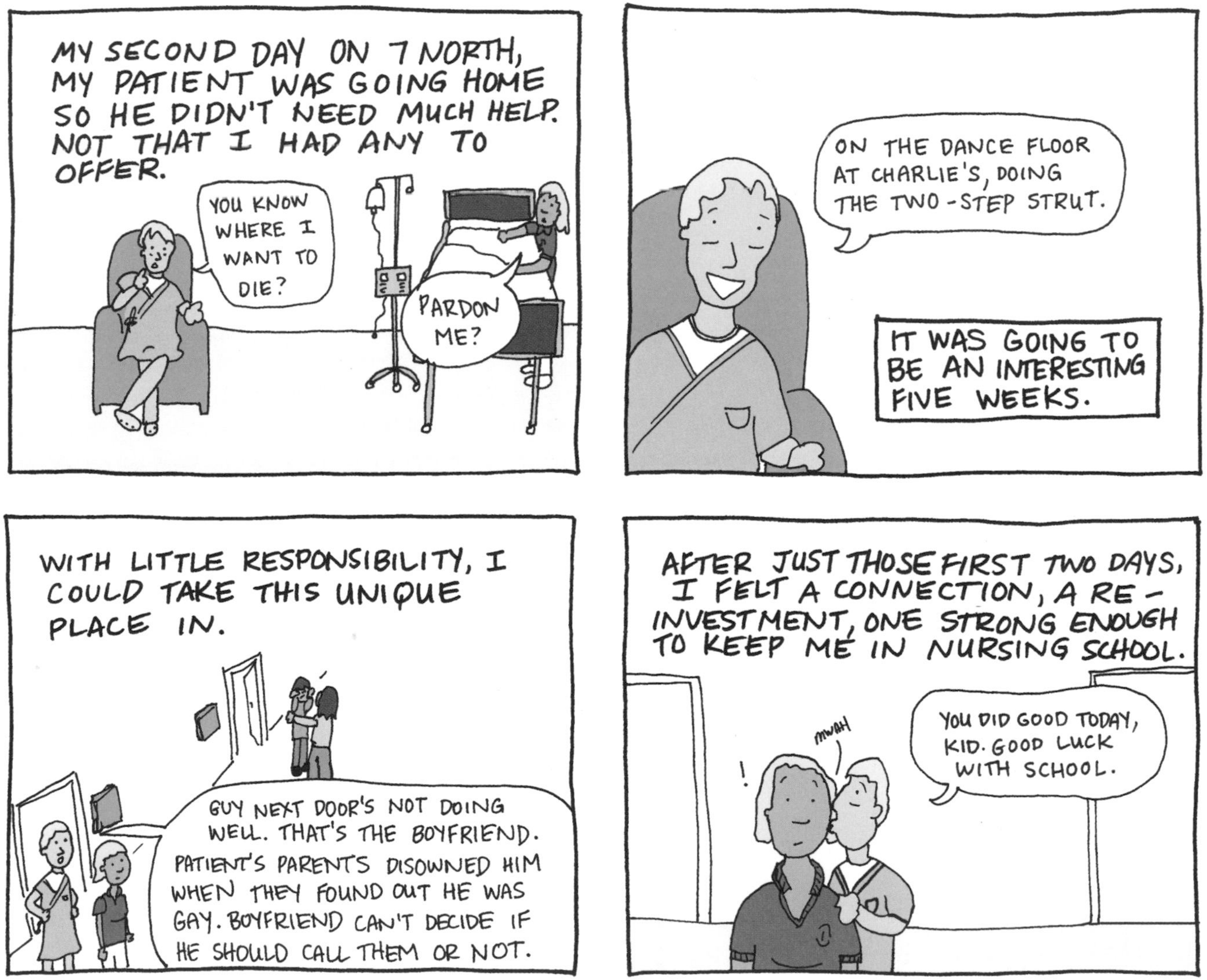
MY SECOND DAY ON 7 NORTH, MY PATIENT WAS GOING HOME SO HE DIDN'T NEED MUCH HELP. NOT THAT I HAD ANY TO OFFER.
YOU KNOW WHERE I WANT TO DIE?
PARDON ME?
ON THE DANCE FLOOR AT CHARLIE'S, DOING THE TWO-STEP STRUT.
IT WAS GOING TO BE AN INTERESTING FIVE WEEKS.
WITH LITTLE RESPONSIBILITY, I COULD TAKE THIS UNIQUE PLACE IN.
GUY NEXT DOOR'S NOT DOING WELL. THAT'S THE BOYFRIEND. PATIENT'S PARENTS DISOWNED HIM WHEN THEY FOUND OUT HE WAS GAY. BOYFRIEND CAN'T DECIDE IF HE SHOULD CALL THEM OR NOT.
AFTER JUST THOSE FIRST TWO DAYS, I FELT A CONNECTION, A RE-INVESTMENT, ONE STRONG ENOUGH TO KEEP ME IN NURSING SCHOOL.
MWAH
!
YOU DID GOOD TODAY, KID. GOOD LUCK WITH SCHOOL.

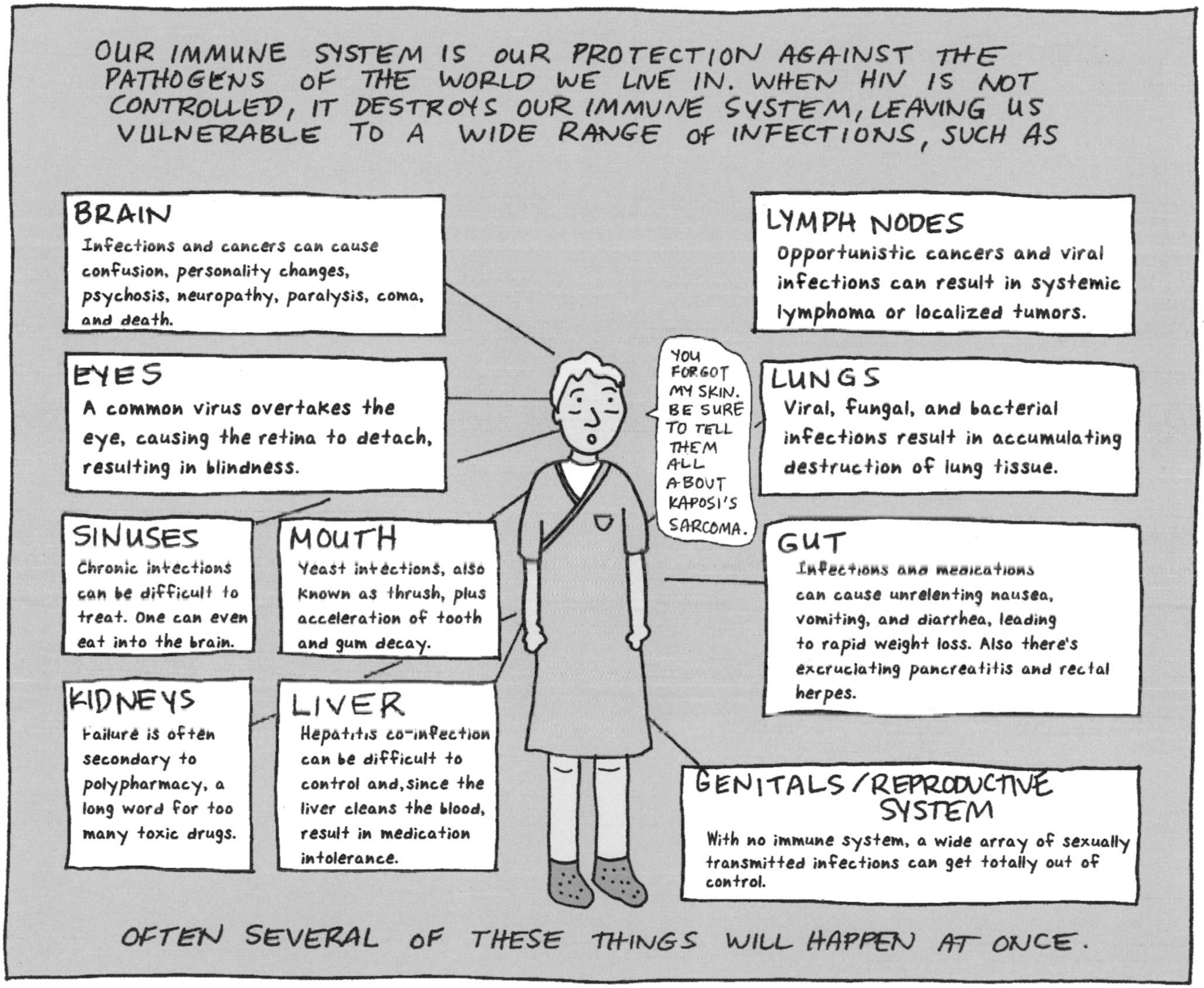
OUR IMMUNE SYSTEM IS OUR PROTECTION AGAINST THE PATHOGENS OF THE WORLD WE LIVE IN. WHEN HIV IS NOT CONTROLLED, IT DESTROYS OUR IMMUNE SYSTEM, LEAVING US VULNERABLE TO A WIDE RANGE OF INFECTIONS, SUCH AS
BRAIN
Infections and cancers can cause confusion, personality changes, psychosis, neuropathy, paralysis, coma, and death.
EYES
A common virus overtakes the eye, causing the retina to detach, resulting in blindness.
SINUSES
Chronic infections can be difficult to treat. One can even eat into the brain.
MOUTH
Yeast infections, also known as thrush, plus acceleration of tooth and gum decay.
KIDNEYS
Failure is often secondary to polypharmacy, a long word for too many toxic drugs.
LIVER
Hepatitis co-infection can be difficult to control and, since the liver cleans the blood, result in medication intolerance.
YOU FORGOT MY SKIN. BE SURE TO TELL THEM ALL ABOUT KAPOSI'S SARCOMA.
LYMPH NODES
Opportunistic cancers and viral infections can result in systemic lymphoma or localized tumors.
LUNGS
Viral, fungal, and bacterial infections result in accumulating destruction of lung tissue.
GUT
Infections and medications can cause unrelenting nausea, vomiting, and diarrhea, leading to rapid weight loss. Also there's excruciating pancreatitis and rectal herpes.
GENITALS/REPRODUCTIVE SYSTEM
With no immune system, a wide array of sexually transmitted infections can get totally out of control.
OFTEN SEVERAL OF THESE THINGS WILL HAPPEN AT ONCE.

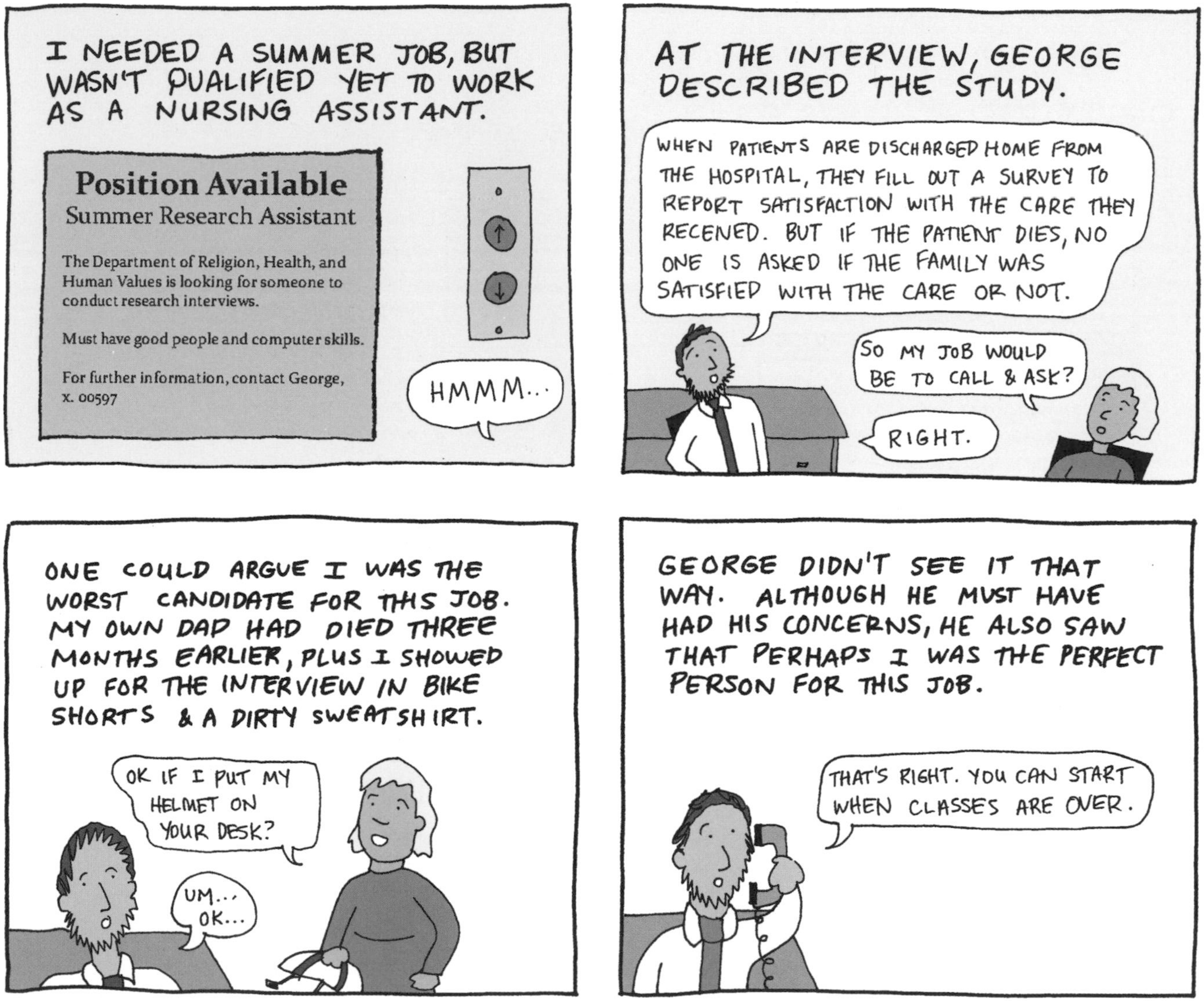

I NEEDED A SUMMER JOB, BUT WASN'T QUALIFIED YET TO WORK AS A NURSING ASSISTANT.

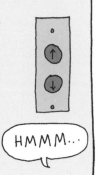

Position Available
Summer Research Assistant

The Department of Religion, Health, and Human Values is looking for someone to conduct research interviews.

Must have good people and computer skills.

For further information, contact George, x. 00597

HMMM...

AT THE INTERVIEW, GEORGE DESCRIBED THE STUDY.

WHEN PATIENTS ARE DISCHARGED HOME FROM THE HOSPITAL, THEY FILL OUT A SURVEY TO REPORT SATISFACTION WITH THE CARE THEY RECEIVED. BUT IF THE PATIENT DIES, NO ONE IS ASKED IF THE FAMILY WAS SATISFIED WITH THE CARE OR NOT.

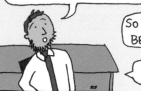

SO MY JOB WOULD BE TO CALL & ASK?

RIGHT.

ONE COULD ARGUE I WAS THE WORST CANDIDATE FOR THIS JOB. MY OWN DAD HAD DIED THREE MONTHS EARLIER, PLUS I SHOWED UP FOR THE INTERVIEW IN BIKE SHORTS & A DIRTY SWEATSHIRT.

OK IF I PUT MY HELMET ON YOUR DESK?

UM... OK...

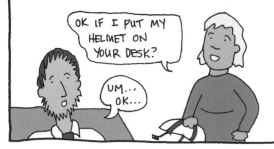

GEORGE DIDN'T SEE IT THAT WAY. ALTHOUGH HE MUST HAVE HAD HIS CONCERNS, HE ALSO SAW THAT PERHAPS I WAS THE PERFECT PERSON FOR THIS JOB.

THAT'S RIGHT. YOU CAN START WHEN CLASSES ARE OVER.

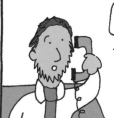

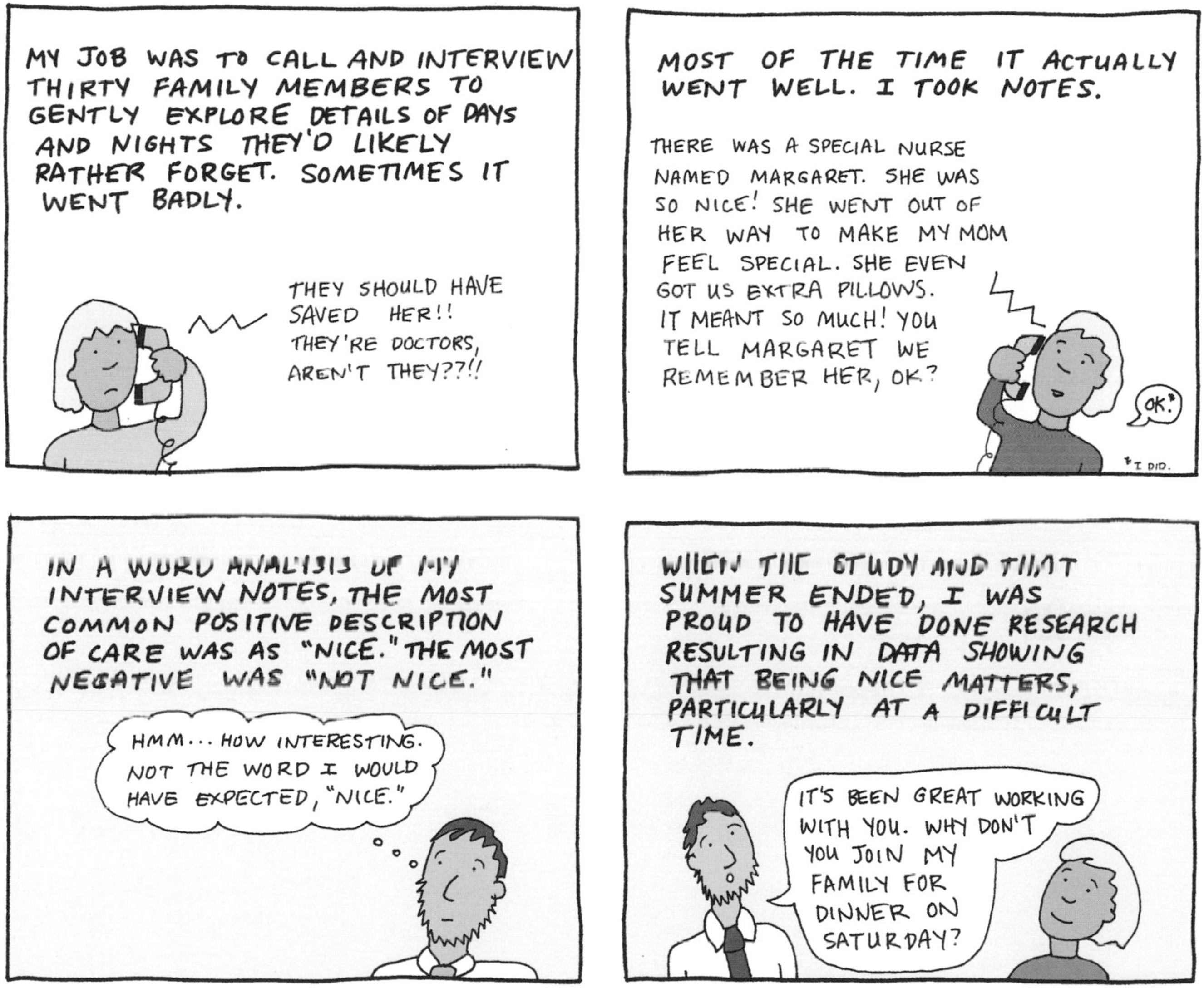
MY JOB WAS TO CALL AND INTERVIEW THIRTY FAMILY MEMBERS TO GENTLY EXPLORE DETAILS OF DAYS AND NIGHTS THEY'D LIKELY RATHER FORGET. SOMETIMES IT WENT BADLY.
THEY SHOULD HAVE SAVED HER!! THEY'RE DOCTORS, AREN'T THEY??!!
MOST OF THE TIME IT ACTUALLY WENT WELL. I TOOK NOTES.
THERE WAS A SPECIAL NURSE NAMED MARGARET. SHE WAS SO NICE! SHE WENT OUT OF HER WAY TO MAKE MY MOM FEEL SPECIAL. SHE EVEN GOT US EXTRA PILLOWS. IT MEANT SO MUCH! YOU TELL MARGARET WE REMEMBER HER, OK?
OK.*
*I DID.
IN A WORD ANALYSIS OF MY INTERVIEW NOTES, THE MOST COMMON POSITIVE DESCRIPTION OF CARE WAS AS "NICE." THE MOST NEGATIVE WAS "NOT NICE."
HMM... HOW INTERESTING. NOT THE WORD I WOULD HAVE EXPECTED, "NICE."
WHEN THE STUDY AND THAT SUMMER ENDED, I WAS PROUD TO HAVE DONE RESEARCH RESULTING IN DATA SHOWING THAT BEING NICE MATTERS, PARTICULARLY AT A DIFFICULT TIME.
IT'S BEEN GREAT WORKING WITH YOU. WHY DON'T YOU JOIN MY FAMILY FOR DINNER ON SATURDAY?

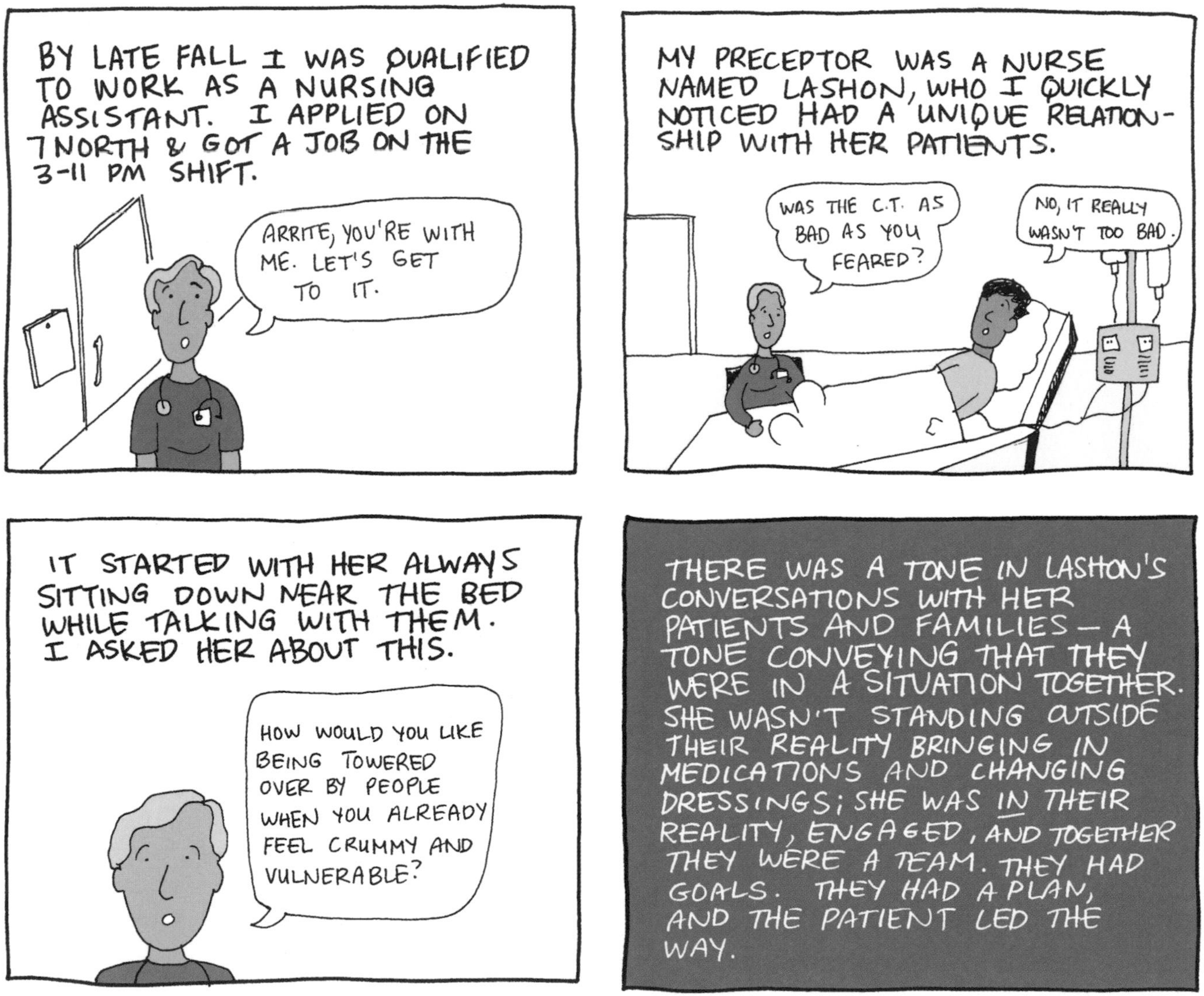
BY LATE FALL I WAS QUALIFIED TO WORK AS A NURSING ASSISTANT. I APPLIED ON 7 NORTH & GOT A JOB ON THE 3-11 PM SHIFT.
ARRITE, YOU'RE WITH ME. LET'S GET TO IT.
MY PRECEPTOR WAS A NURSE NAMED LASHON, WHO I QUICKLY NOTICED HAD A UNIQUE RELATIONSHIP WITH HER PATIENTS.
WAS THE C.T. AS BAD AS YOU FEARED?
NO, IT REALLY WASN'T TOO BAD.
IT STARTED WITH HER ALWAYS SITTING DOWN NEAR THE BED WHILE TALKING WITH THEM. I ASKED HER ABOUT THIS.
HOW WOULD YOU LIKE BEING TOWERED OVER BY PEOPLE WHEN YOU ALREADY FEEL CRUMMY AND VULNERABLE?
THERE WAS A TONE IN LASHON'S CONVERSATIONS WITH HER PATIENTS AND FAMILIES — A TONE CONVEYING THAT THEY WERE IN A SITUATION TOGETHER. SHE WASN'T STANDING OUTSIDE THEIR REALITY BRINGING IN MEDICATIONS AND CHANGING DRESSINGS; SHE WAS IN THEIR REALITY, ENGAGED, AND TOGETHER THEY WERE A TEAM. THEY HAD GOALS. THEY HAD A PLAN, AND THE PATIENT LED THE WAY.

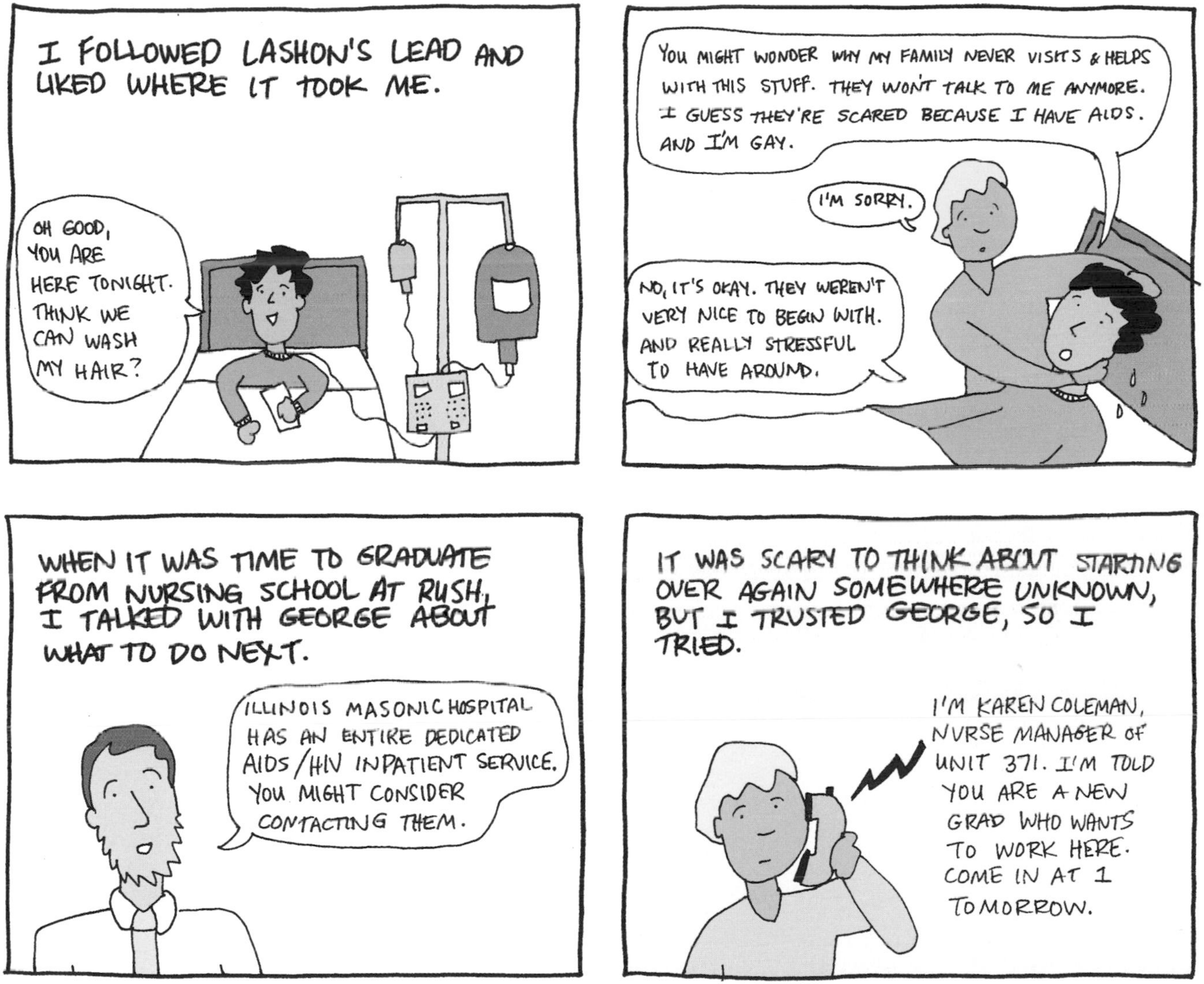
I FOLLOWED LASHON'S LEAD AND LIKED WHERE IT TOOK ME.
OH GOOD, YOU ARE HERE TONIGHT. THINK WE CAN WASH MY HAIR?
YOU MIGHT WONDER WHY MY FAMILY NEVER VISITS & HELPS WITH THIS STUFF. THEY WON'T TALK TO ME ANYMORE. I GUESS THEY'RE SCARED BECAUSE I HAVE AIDS. AND I'M GAY.
I'M SORRY.
NO, IT'S OKAY. THEY WEREN'T VERY NICE TO BEGIN WITH. AND REALLY STRESSFUL TO HAVE AROUND.
WHEN IT WAS TIME TO GRADUATE FROM NURSING SCHOOL AT RUSH, I TALKED WITH GEORGE ABOUT WHAT TO DO NEXT.
ILLINOIS MASONIC HOSPITAL HAS AN ENTIRE DEDICATED AIDS/HIV INPATIENT SERVICE. YOU MIGHT CONSIDER CONTACTING THEM.
IT WAS SCARY TO THINK ABOUT STARTING OVER AGAIN SOMEWHERE UNKNOWN, BUT I TRUSTED GEORGE, SO I TRIED.
I'M KAREN COLEMAN, NURSE MANAGER OF UNIT 371. I'M TOLD YOU ARE A NEW GRAD WHO WANTS TO WORK HERE. COME IN AT 1 TOMORROW.

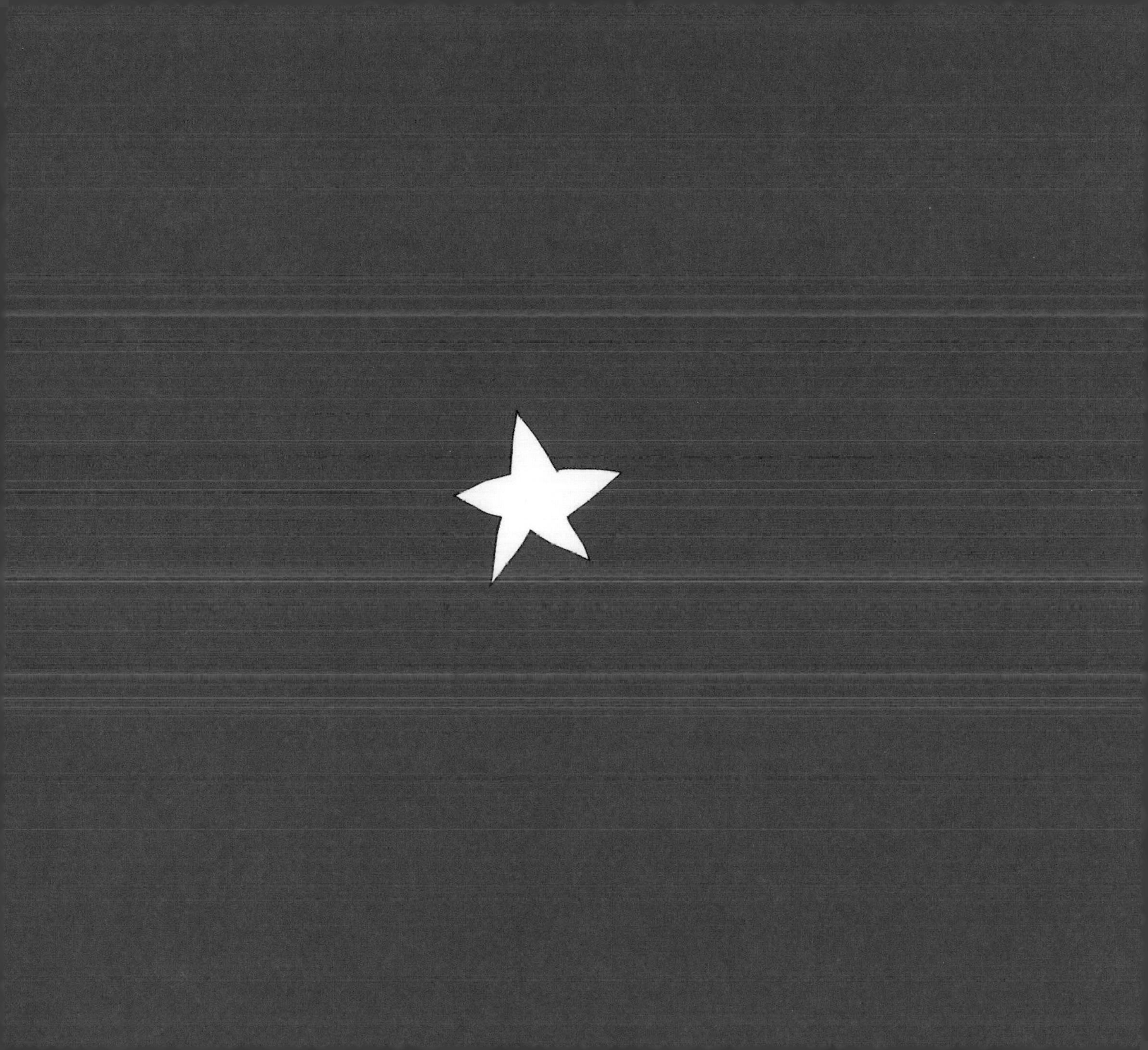

IN 1897 MEMBERS OF A BAPTIST SUNDAY SCHOOL CLASS FOUNDED CHICAGO UNION HOSPITAL ON WELLINGTON AVENUE NEAR HALSTED STREET ON CHICAGO'S NORTH SIDE.

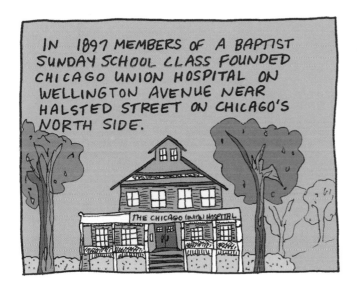

THE CHICAGO (UNION) HOSPITAL

FREEMASONS PURCHASED CHICAGO UNION HOSPITAL IN 1921 AND RENAMED IT ILLINOIS MASONIC.

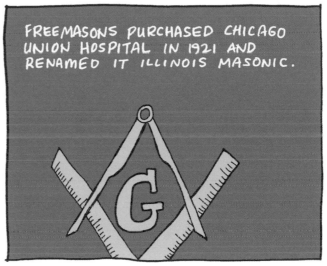

THE MISSION OF THE HOSPITAL WAS TO PROVIDE COMPASSIONATE CARE FOR THE COMMUNITY IT SERVED.

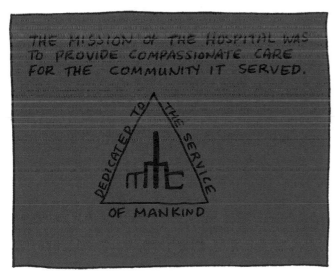

DEDICATED TO THE SERVICE OF MANKIND

IN 1970 THE FIRST CHICAGO GAY PRIDE PARADE MARCHED PAST ILLINOIS MASONIC. THE NEIGHBOR-HOOD HAD BECOME INFORMALLY KNOWN AS BOYSTOWN.

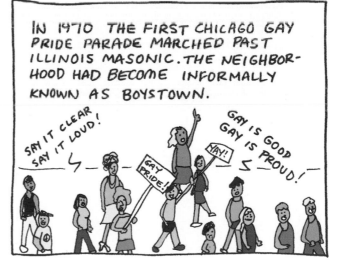

SAY IT CLEAR SAY IT LOUD!

GAY IS GOOD GAY IS PROUD!

GAY PRIDE!

YAY!

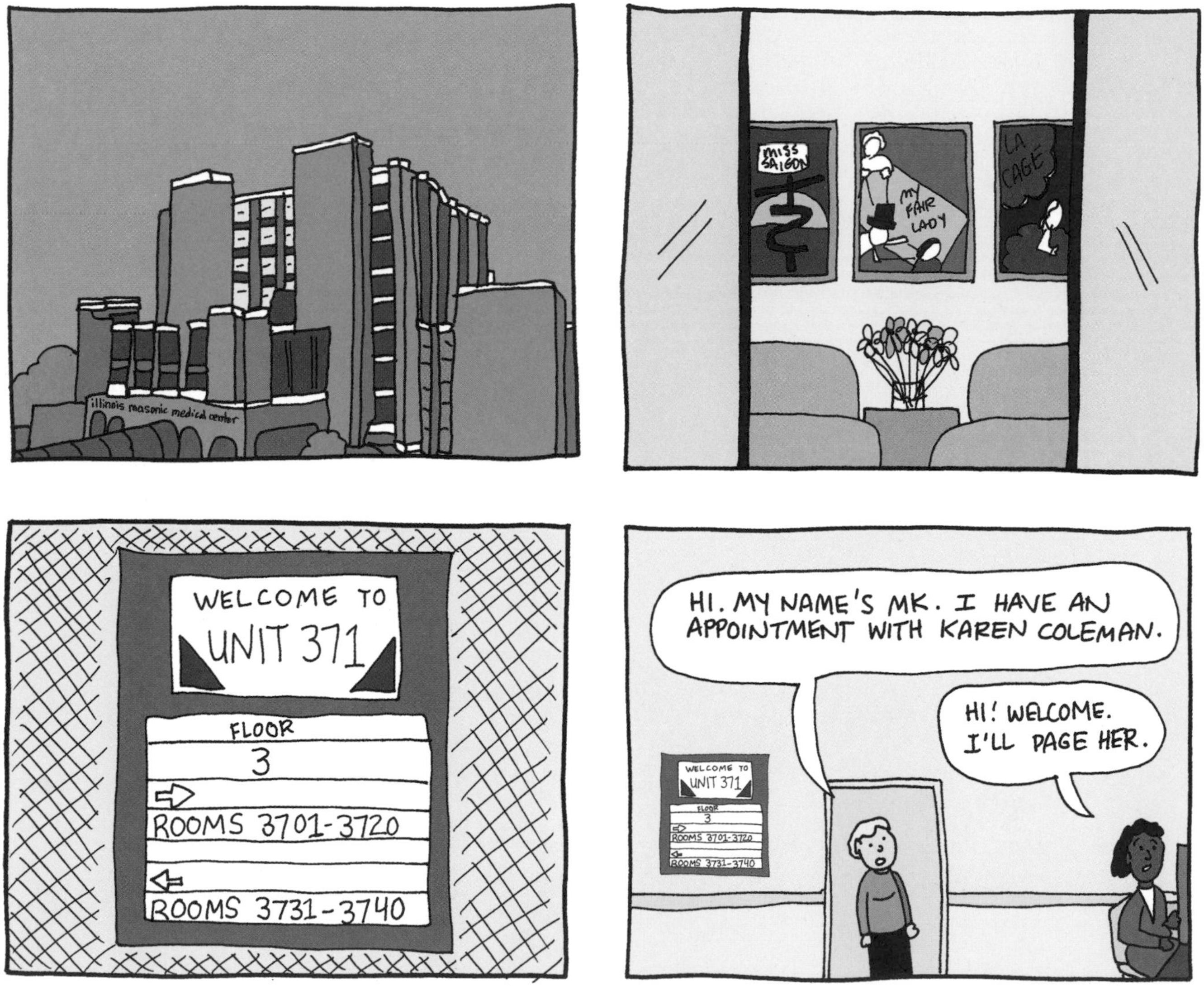
illinois masonic medical center
MISS SAIGON
MY FAIR LADY
LA CAGE
WELCOME TO
UNIT 371
FLOOR
3
ROOMS 3701-3720
ROOMS 3731-3740
HI. MY NAME'S MK. I HAVE AN APPOINTMENT WITH KAREN COLEMAN.
HI! WELCOME. I'LL PAGE HER.

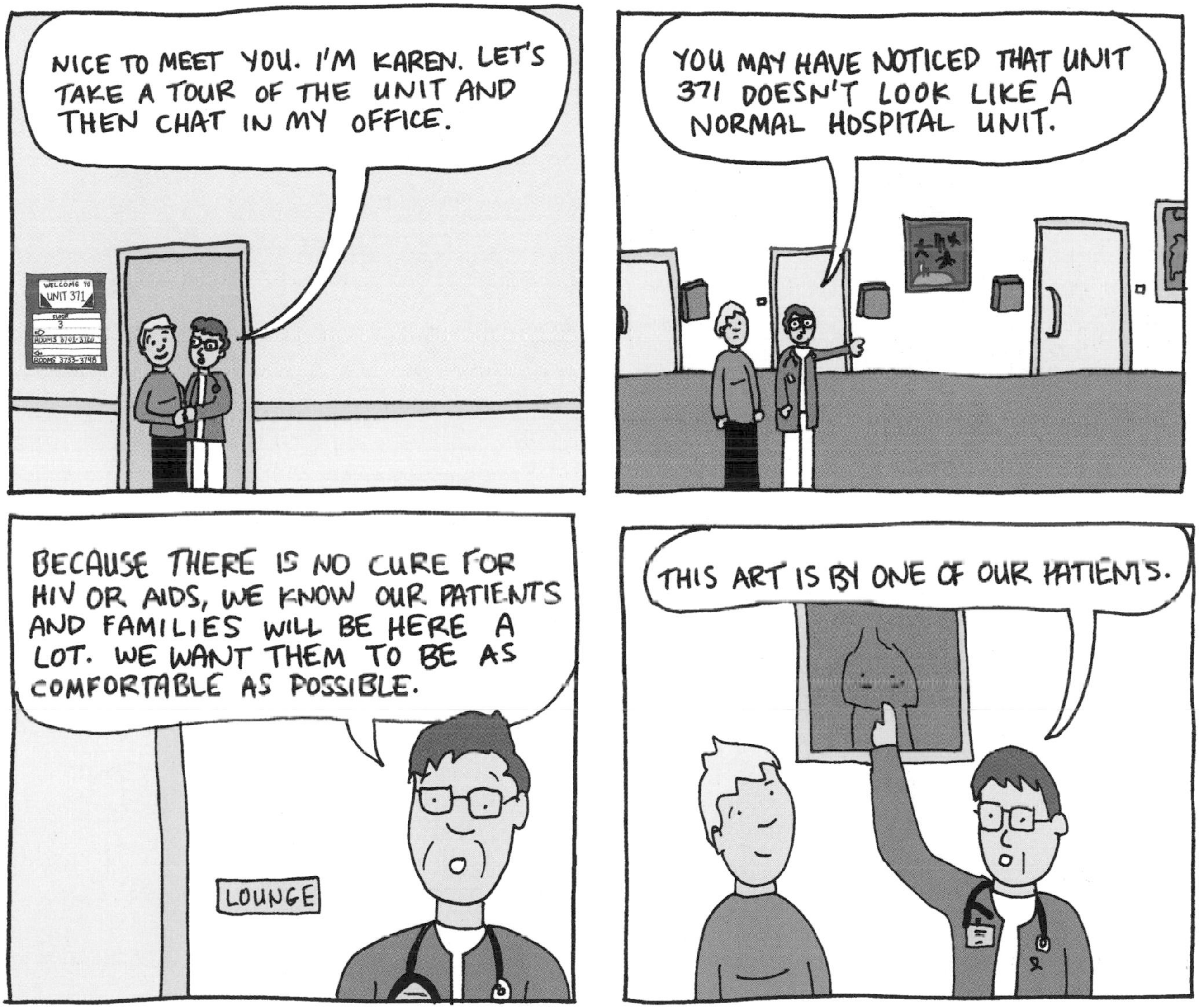
NICE TO MEET YOU. I'M KAREN. LET'S TAKE A TOUR OF THE UNIT AND THEN CHAT IN MY OFFICE.
WELCOME TO
UNIT 371
YOU MAY HAVE NOTICED THAT UNIT 371 DOESN'T LOOK LIKE A NORMAL HOSPITAL UNIT.
BECAUSE THERE IS NO CURE FOR HIV OR AIDS, WE KNOW OUR PATIENTS AND FAMILIES WILL BE HERE A LOT. WE WANT THEM TO BE AS COMFORTABLE AS POSSIBLE.
LOUNGE
THIS ART IS BY ONE OF OUR PATIENTS.

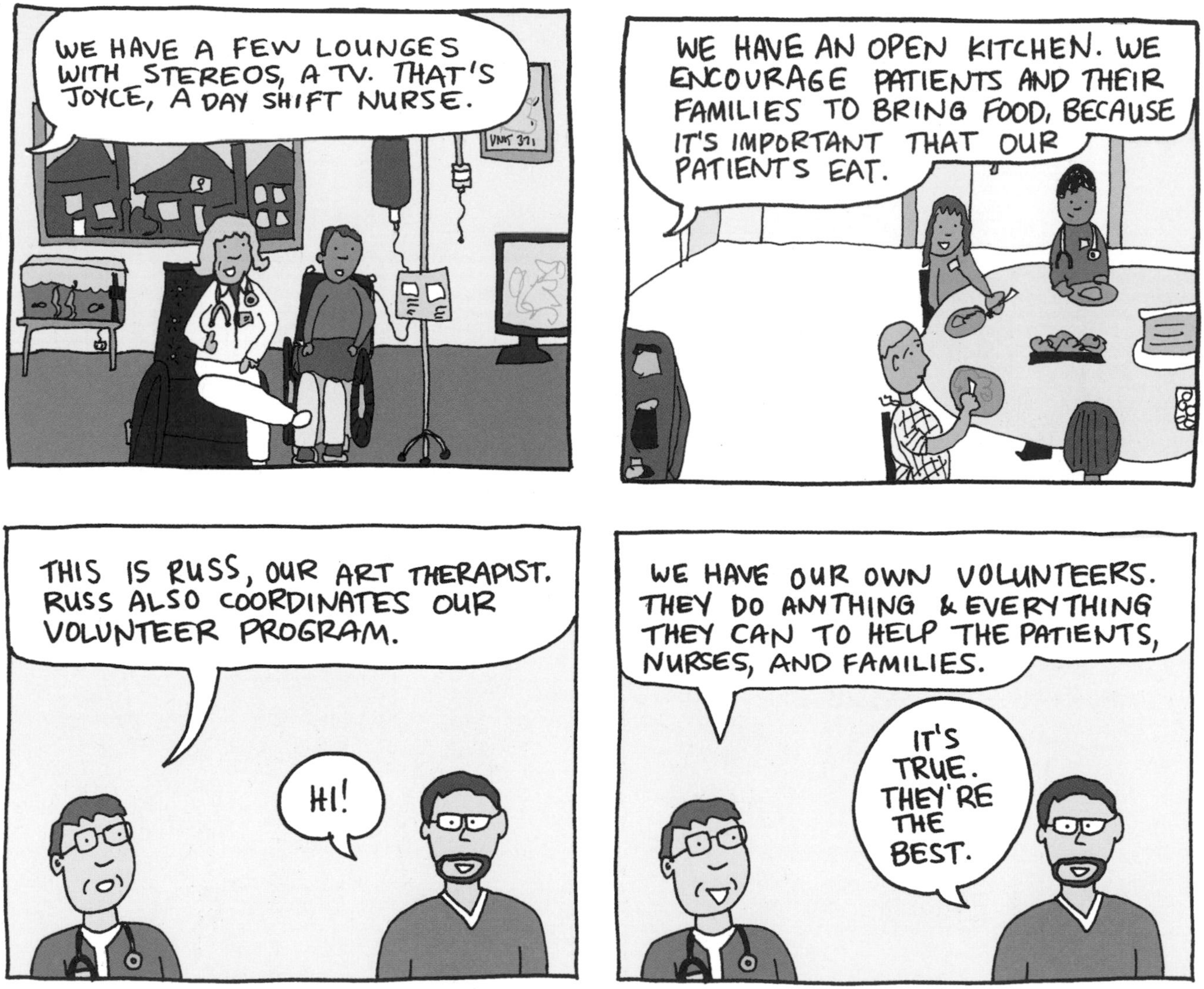
WE HAVE A FEW LOUNGES WITH STEREOS, A TV. THAT'S JOYCE, A DAY SHIFT NURSE.
WE HAVE AN OPEN KITCHEN. WE ENCOURAGE PATIENTS AND THEIR FAMILIES TO BRING FOOD, BECAUSE IT'S IMPORTANT THAT OUR PATIENTS EAT.
THIS IS RUSS, OUR ART THERAPIST. RUSS ALSO COORDINATES OUR VOLUNTEER PROGRAM.
HI!
WE HAVE OUR OWN VOLUNTEERS. THEY DO ANYTHING & EVERYTHING THEY CAN TO HELP THE PATIENTS, NURSES, AND FAMILIES.
IT'S TRUE. THEY'RE THE BEST.

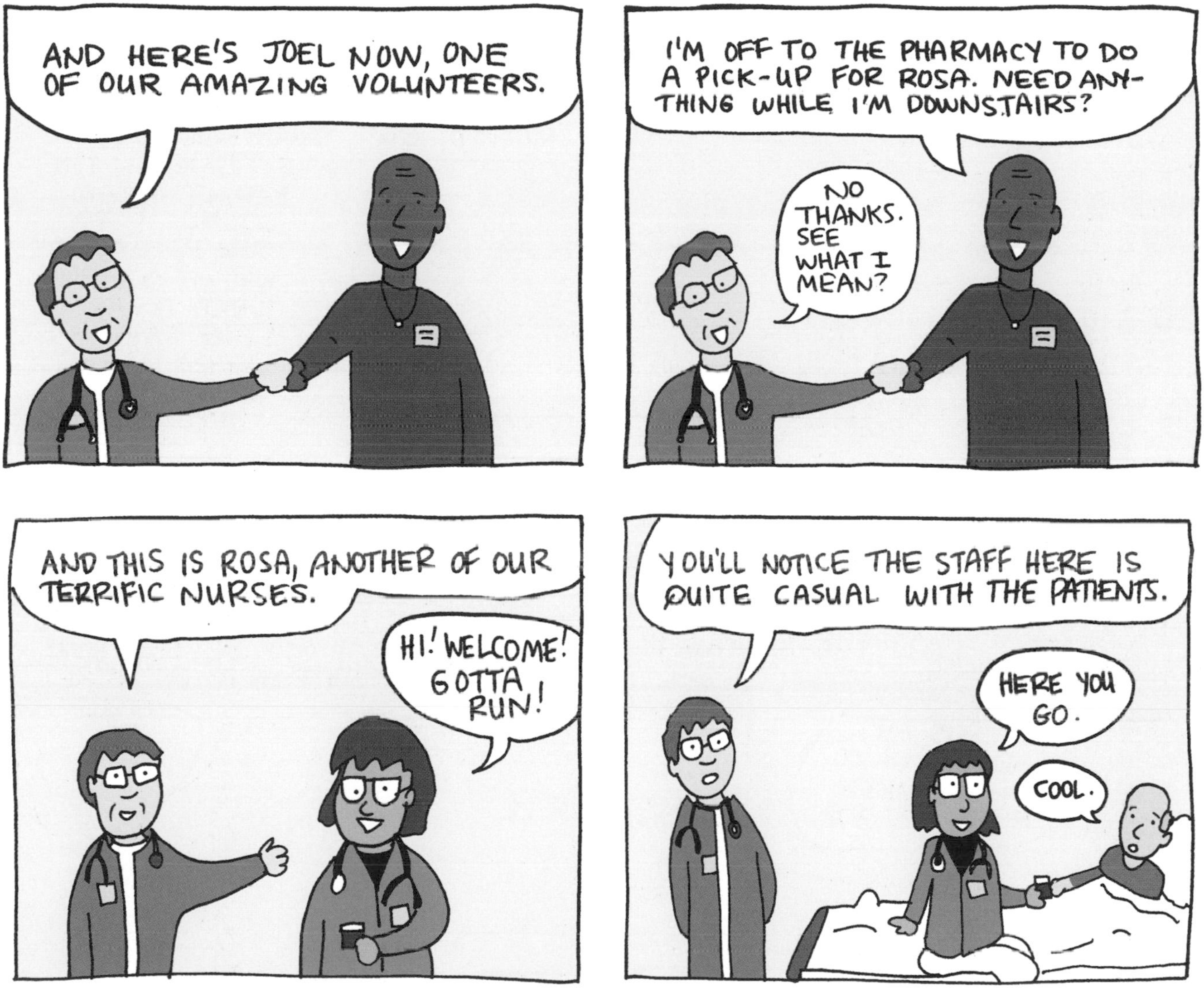
AND HERE'S JOEL NOW, ONE OF OUR AMAZING VOLUNTEERS.
I'M OFF TO THE PHARMACY TO DO A PICK-UP FOR ROSA. NEED ANY-THING WHILE I'M DOWNSTAIRS?
NO THANKS. SEE WHAT I MEAN?
AND THIS IS ROSA, ANOTHER OF OUR TERRIFIC NURSES.
HI! WELCOME! GOTTA RUN!
YOU'LL NOTICE THE STAFF HERE IS QUITE CASUAL WITH THE PATIENTS.
HERE YOU GO.
COOL.

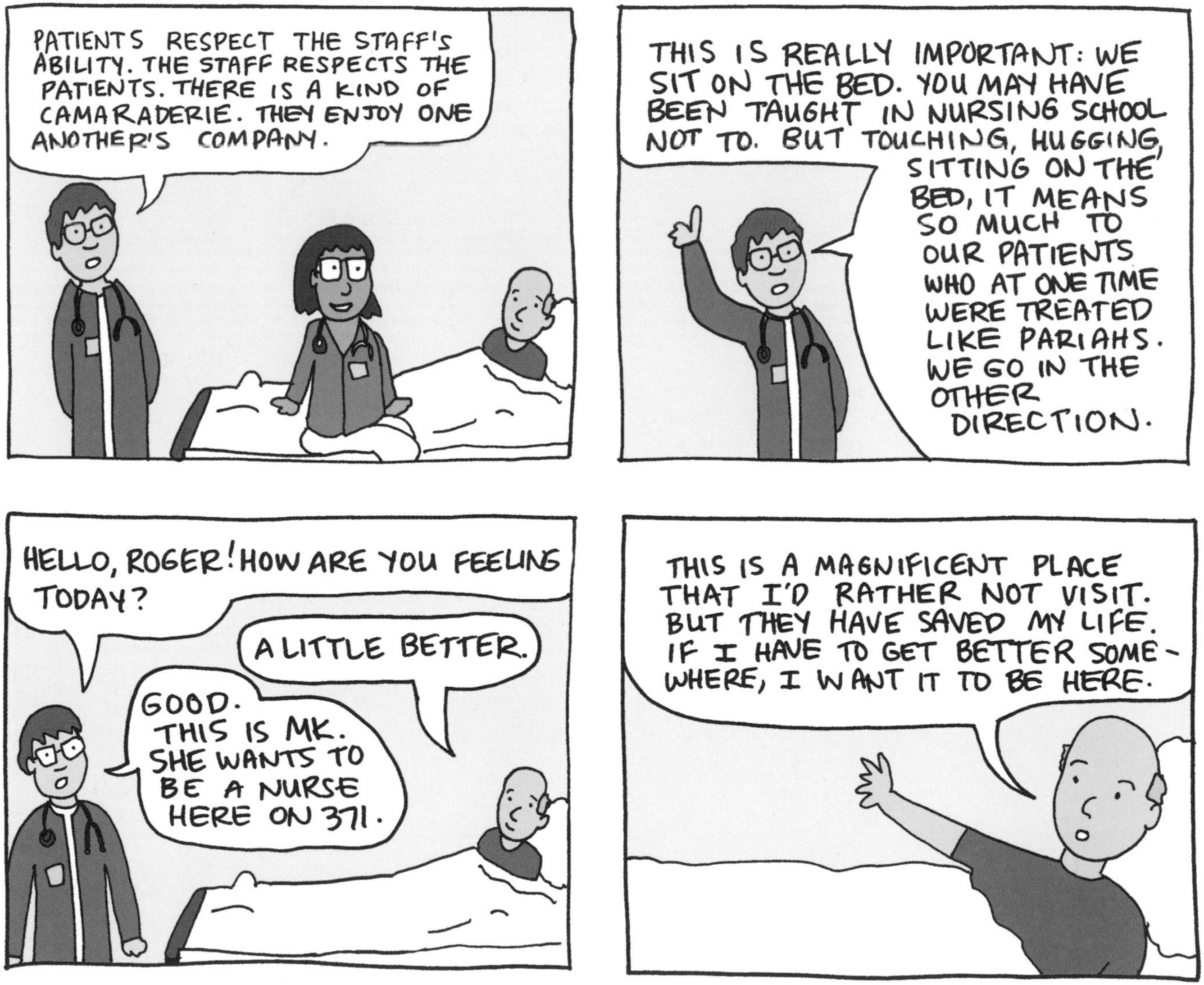
PATIENTS RESPECT THE STAFF'S ABILITY. THE STAFF RESPECTS THE PATIENTS. THERE IS A KIND OF CAMARADERIE. THEY ENJOY ONE ANOTHER'S COMPANY.
THIS IS REALLY IMPORTANT: WE SIT ON THE BED. YOU MAY HAVE BEEN TAUGHT IN NURSING SCHOOL NOT TO. BUT TOUCHING, HUGGING, SITTING ON THE BED, IT MEANS SO MUCH TO OUR PATIENTS WHO AT ONE TIME WERE TREATED LIKE PARIAHS. WE GO IN THE OTHER DIRECTION.
HELLO, ROGER! HOW ARE YOU FEELING TODAY?
A LITTLE BETTER.
GOOD. THIS IS MK. SHE WANTS TO BE A NURSE HERE ON 371.
THIS IS A MAGNIFICENT PLACE THAT I'D RATHER NOT VISIT. BUT THEY HAVE SAVED MY LIFE. IF I HAVE TO GET BETTER SOME-WHERE, I WANT IT TO BE HERE.

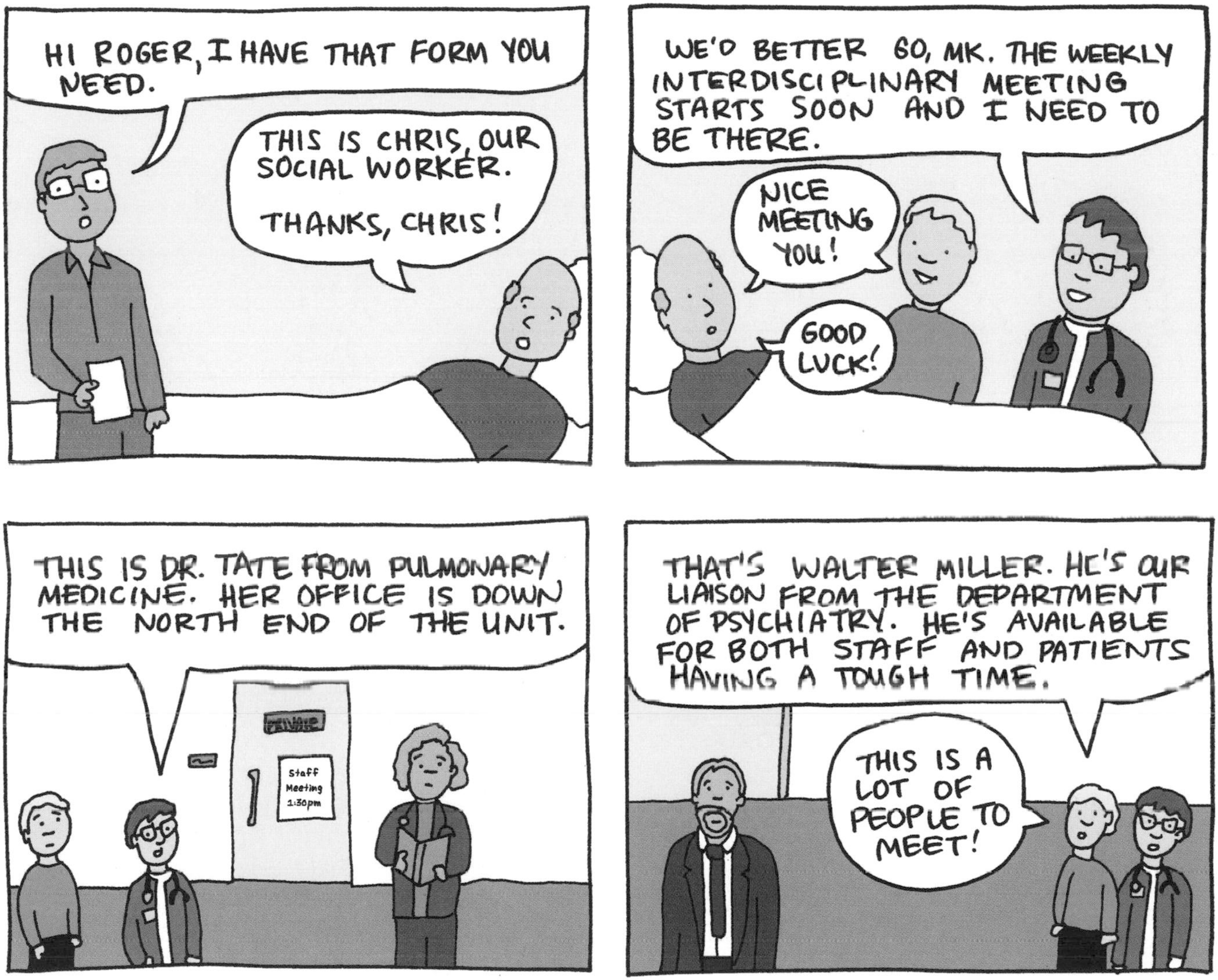
HI ROGER, I HAVE THAT FORM YOU NEED.
THIS IS CHRIS, OUR SOCIAL WORKER. THANKS, CHRIS!
WE'D BETTER GO, MK. THE WEEKLY INTERDISCIPLINARY MEETING STARTS SOON AND I NEED TO BE THERE.
NICE MEETING YOU!
GOOD LUCK!
THIS IS DR. TATE FROM PULMONARY MEDICINE. HER OFFICE IS DOWN THE NORTH END OF THE UNIT.
Staff Meeting 1:30pm
THAT'S WALTER MILLER. HE'S OUR LIAISON FROM THE DEPARTMENT OF PSYCHIATRY. HE'S AVAILABLE FOR BOTH STAFF AND PATIENTS HAVING A TOUGH TIME.
THIS IS A LOT OF PEOPLE TO MEET!

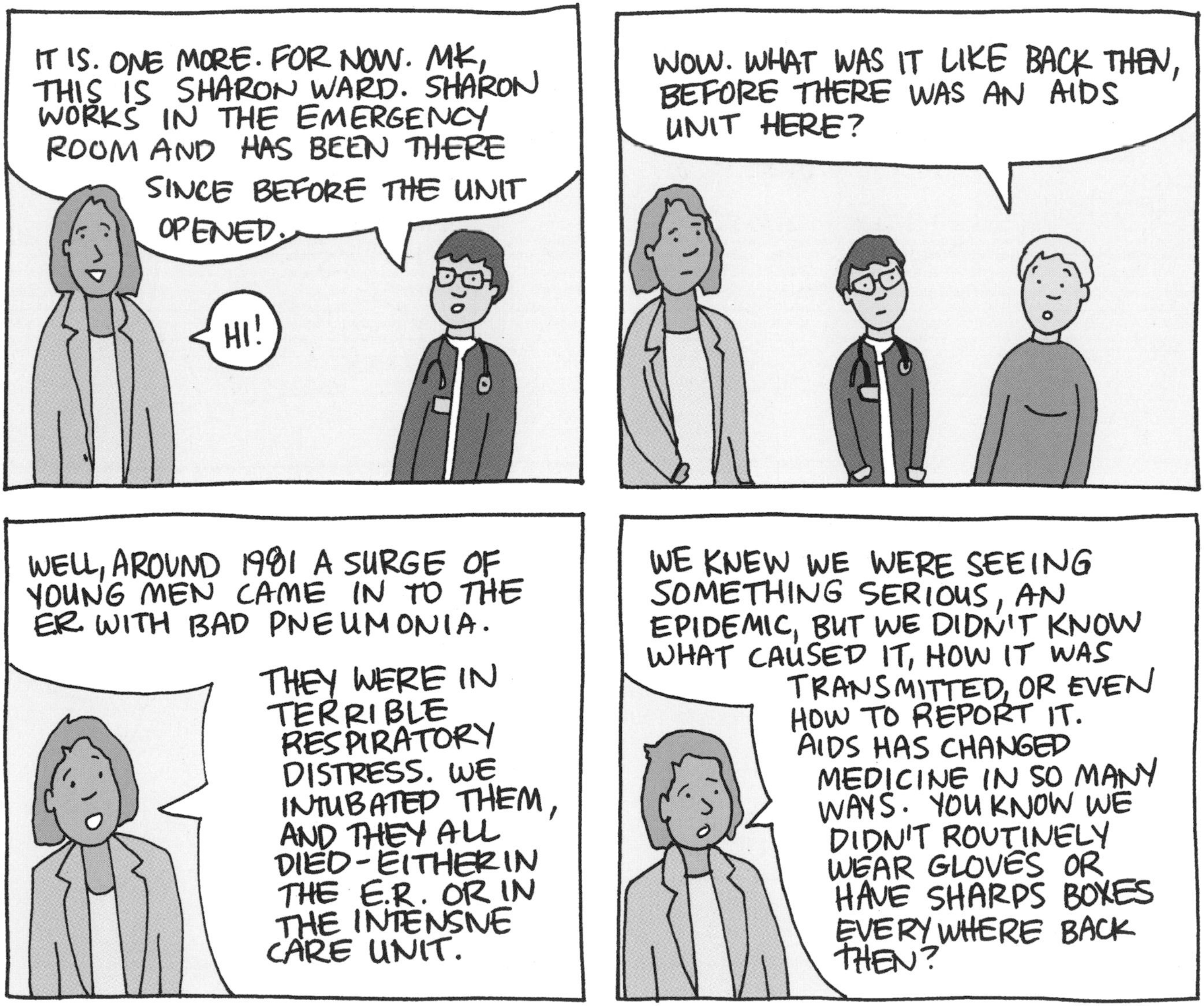
IT IS. ONE MORE. FOR NOW. MK, THIS IS SHARON WARD. SHARON WORKS IN THE EMERGENCY ROOM AND HAS BEEN THERE SINCE BEFORE THE UNIT OPENED.
HI!
WOW. WHAT WAS IT LIKE BACK THEN, BEFORE THERE WAS AN AIDS UNIT HERE?
WELL, AROUND 1981 A SURGE OF YOUNG MEN CAME IN TO THE ER WITH BAD PNEUMONIA.
THEY WERE IN TERRIBLE RESPIRATORY DISTRESS. WE INTUBATED THEM, AND THEY ALL DIED-EITHER IN THE E.R. OR IN THE INTENSIVE CARE UNIT.
WE KNEW WE WERE SEEING SOMETHING SERIOUS, AN EPIDEMIC, BUT WE DIDN'T KNOW WHAT CAUSED IT, HOW IT WAS TRANSMITTED, OR EVEN HOW TO REPORT IT. AIDS HAS CHANGED MEDICINE IN SO MANY WAYS. YOU KNOW WE DIDN'T ROUTINELY WEAR GLOVES OR HAVE SHARPS BOXES EVERYWHERE BACK THEN?

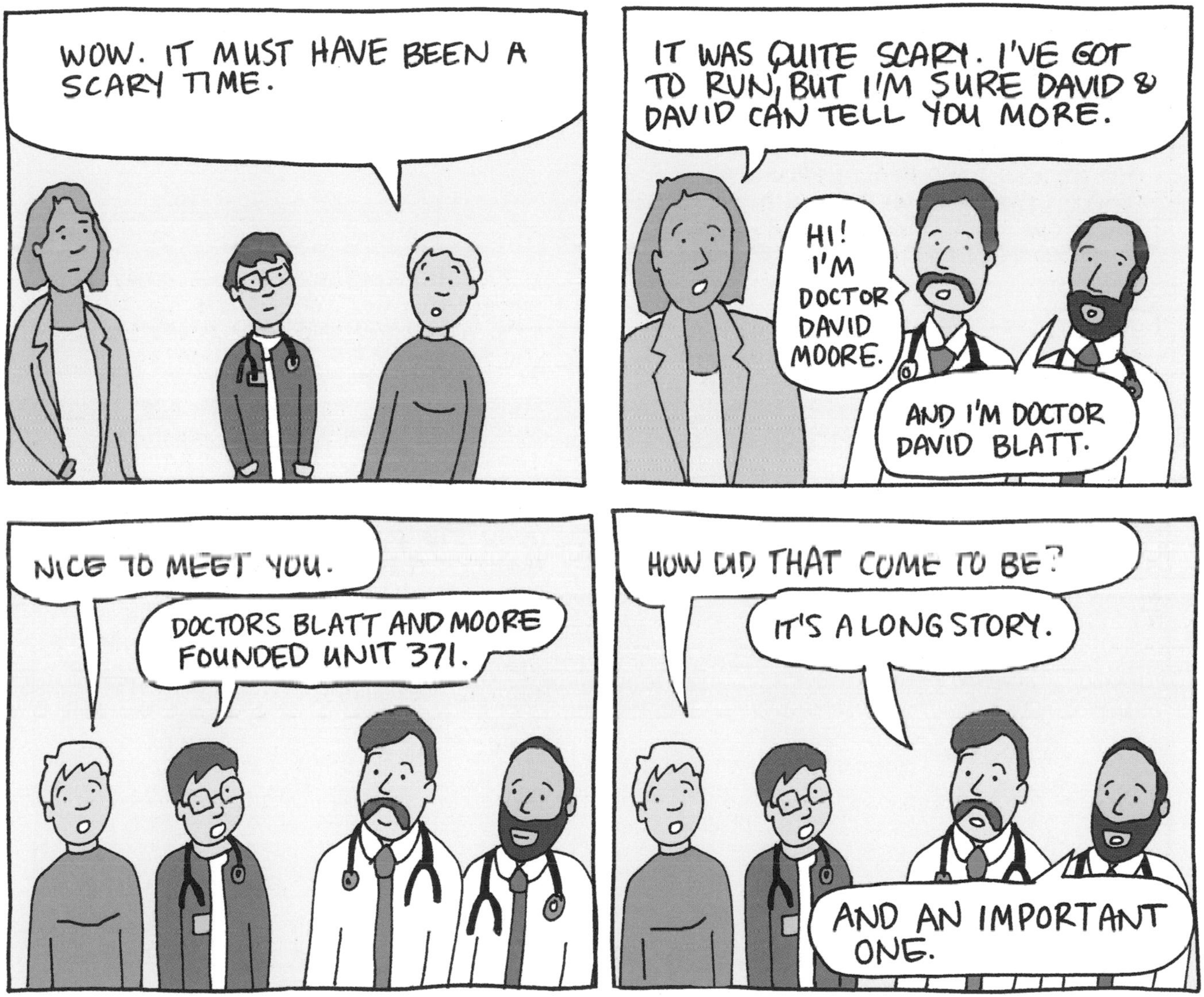
WOW. IT MUST HAVE BEEN A SCARY TIME.
IT WAS QUITE SCARY. I'VE GOT TO RUN, BUT I'M SURE DAVID & DAVID CAN TELL YOU MORE.
HI! I'M DOCTOR DAVID MOORE.
AND I'M DOCTOR DAVID BLATT.
NICE TO MEET YOU.
DOCTORS BLATT AND MOORE FOUNDED UNIT 371.
HOW DID THAT COME TO BE?
IT'S A LONG STORY.
AND AN IMPORTANT ONE.

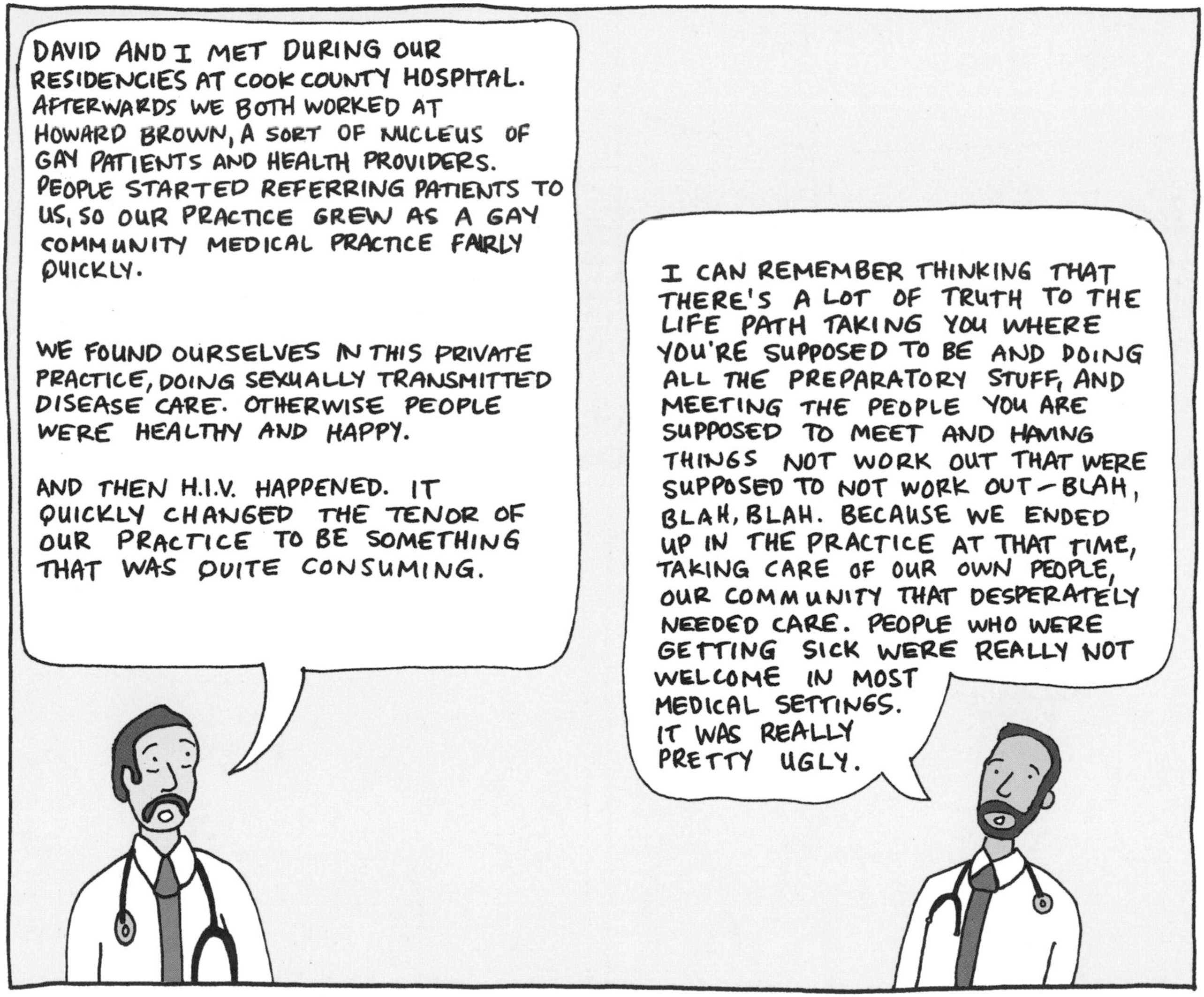
DAVID AND I MET DURING OUR RESIDENCIES AT COOK COUNTY HOSPITAL. AFTERWARDS WE BOTH WORKED AT HOWARD BROWN, A SORT OF NUCLEUS OF GAY PATIENTS AND HEALTH PROVIDERS. PEOPLE STARTED REFERRING PATIENTS TO US, SO OUR PRACTICE GREW AS A GAY COMMUNITY MEDICAL PRACTICE FAIRLY QUICKLY.
WE FOUND OURSELVES IN THIS PRIVATE PRACTICE, DOING SEXUALLY TRANSMITTED DISEASE CARE. OTHERWISE PEOPLE WERE HEALTHY AND HAPPY.
AND THEN H.I.V. HAPPENED. IT QUICKLY CHANGED THE TENOR OF OUR PRACTICE TO BE SOMETHING THAT WAS QUITE CONSUMING.
I CAN REMEMBER THINKING THAT THERE'S A LOT OF TRUTH TO THE LIFE PATH TAKING YOU WHERE YOU'RE SUPPOSED TO BE AND DOING ALL THE PREPARATORY STUFF, AND MEETING THE PEOPLE YOU ARE SUPPOSED TO MEET AND HAVING THINGS NOT WORK OUT THAT WERE SUPPOSED TO NOT WORK OUT—BLAH, BLAH, BLAH. BECAUSE WE ENDED UP IN THE PRACTICE AT THAT TIME, TAKING CARE OF OUR OWN PEOPLE, OUR COMMUNITY THAT DESPERATELY NEEDED CARE. PEOPLE WHO WERE GETTING SICK WERE REALLY NOT WELCOME IN MOST MEDICAL SETTINGS. IT WAS REALLY PRETTY UGLY.

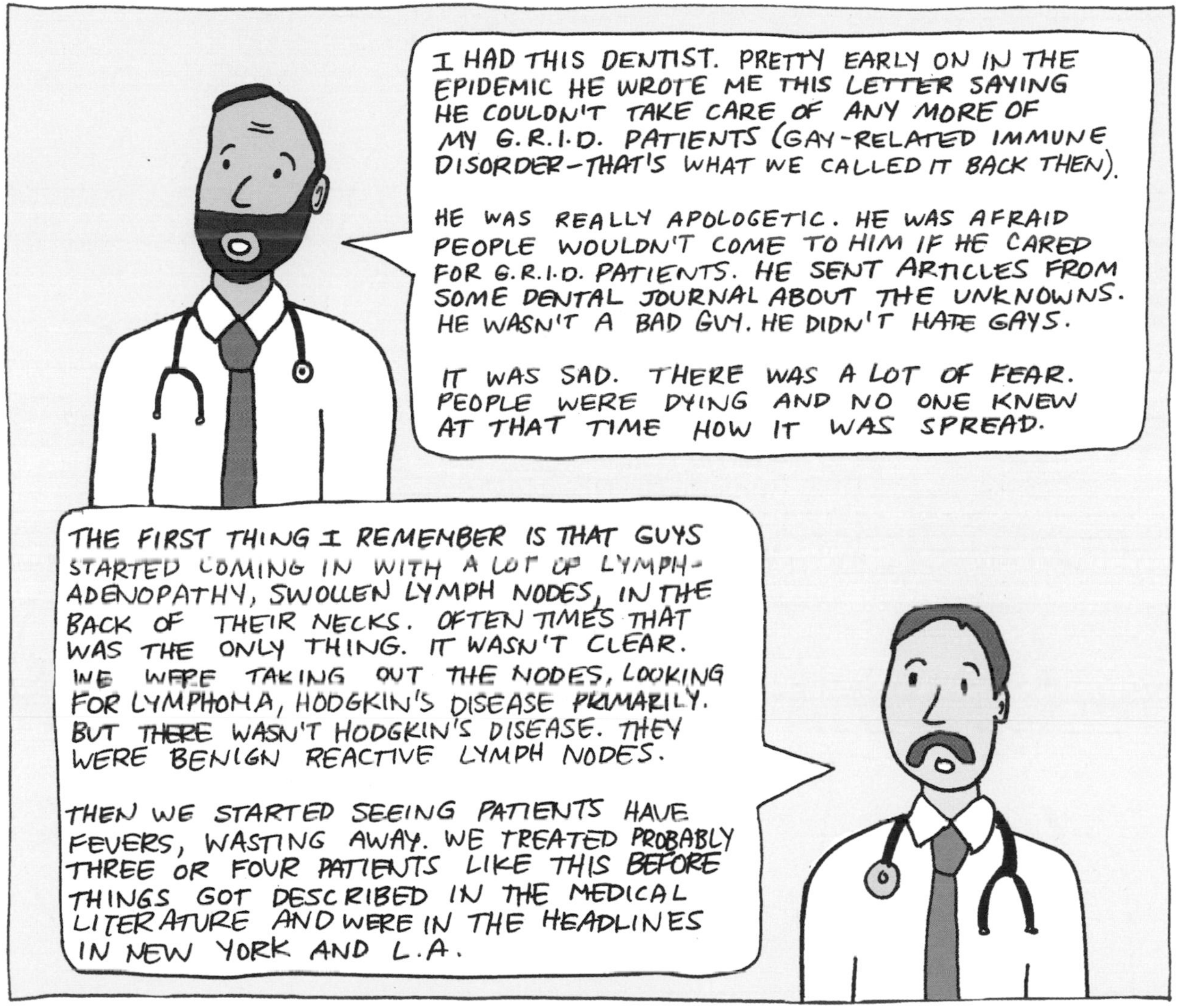
I HAD THIS DENTIST. PRETTY EARLY ON IN THE EPIDEMIC HE WROTE ME THIS LETTER SAYING HE COULDN'T TAKE CARE OF ANY MORE OF MY G.R.I.D. PATIENTS (GAY-RELATED IMMUNE DISORDER—THAT'S WHAT WE CALLED IT BACK THEN).
HE WAS REALLY APOLOGETIC. HE WAS AFRAID PEOPLE WOULDN'T COME TO HIM IF HE CARED FOR G.R.I.D. PATIENTS. HE SENT ARTICLES FROM SOME DENTAL JOURNAL ABOUT THE UNKNOWNS. HE WASN'T A BAD GUY. HE DIDN'T HATE GAYS.
IT WAS SAD. THERE WAS A LOT OF FEAR. PEOPLE WERE DYING AND NO ONE KNEW AT THAT TIME HOW IT WAS SPREAD.
THE FIRST THING I REMEMBER IS THAT GUYS STARTED COMING IN WITH A LOT OF LYMPH-ADENOPATHY, SWOLLEN LYMPH NODES, IN THE BACK OF THEIR NECKS. OFTEN TIMES THAT WAS THE ONLY THING. IT WASN'T CLEAR. WE WERE TAKING OUT THE NODES, LOOKING FOR LYMPHOMA, HODGKIN'S DISEASE PRIMARILY. BUT THERE WASN'T HODGKIN'S DISEASE. THEY WERE BENIGN REACTIVE LYMPH NODES.
THEN WE STARTED SEEING PATIENTS HAVE FEVERS, WASTING AWAY. WE TREATED PROBABLY THREE OR FOUR PATIENTS LIKE THIS BEFORE THINGS GOT DESCRIBED IN THE MEDICAL LITERATURE AND WERE IN THE HEADLINES IN NEW YORK AND L.A.

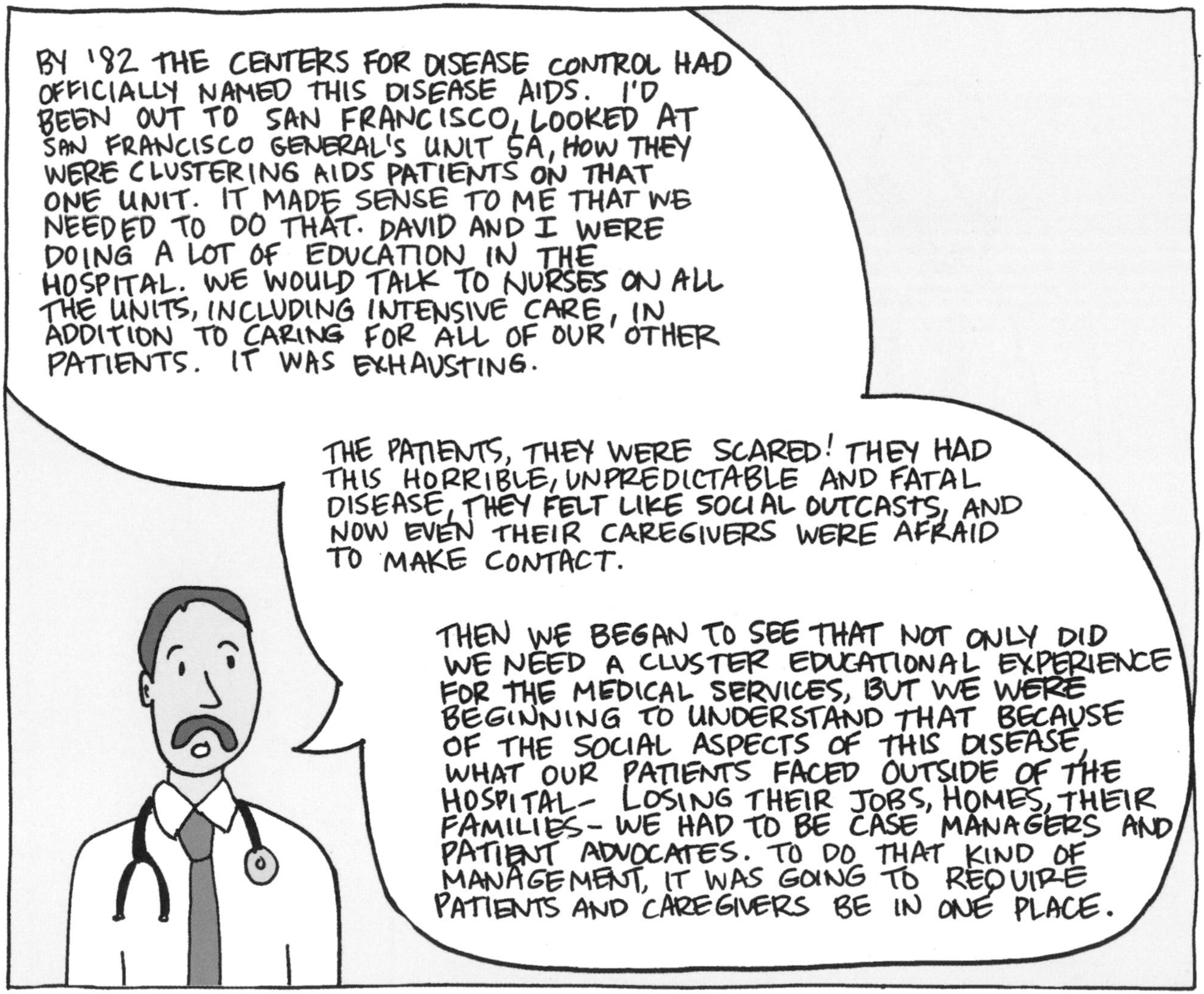

BY '82 THE CENTERS FOR DISEASE CONTROL HAD OFFICIALLY NAMED THIS DISEASE AIDS. I'D BEEN OUT TO SAN FRANCISCO, LOOKED AT SAN FRANCISCO GENERAL'S UNIT 5A, HOW THEY WERE CLUSTERING AIDS PATIENTS ON THAT ONE UNIT. IT MADE SENSE TO ME THAT WE NEEDED TO DO THAT. DAVID AND I WERE DOING A LOT OF EDUCATION IN THE HOSPITAL. WE WOULD TALK TO NURSES ON ALL THE UNITS, INCLUDING INTENSIVE CARE, IN ADDITION TO CARING FOR ALL OF OUR OTHER PATIENTS. IT WAS EXHAUSTING.

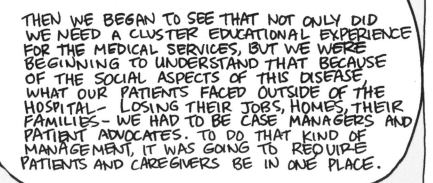

THE PATIENTS, THEY WERE SCARED! THEY HAD THIS HORRIBLE, UNPREDICTABLE AND FATAL DISEASE, THEY FELT LIKE SOCIAL OUTCASTS, AND NOW EVEN THEIR CAREGIVERS WERE AFRAID TO MAKE CONTACT.

THEN WE BEGAN TO SEE THAT NOT ONLY DID WE NEED A CLUSTER EDUCATIONAL EXPERIENCE FOR THE MEDICAL SERVICES, BUT WE WERE BEGINNING TO UNDERSTAND THAT BECAUSE OF THE SOCIAL ASPECTS OF THIS DISEASE, WHAT OUR PATIENTS FACED OUTSIDE OF THE HOSPITAL— LOSING THEIR JOBS, HOMES, THEIR FAMILIES— WE HAD TO BE CASE MANAGERS AND PATIENT ADVOCATES. TO DO THAT KIND OF MANAGEMENT, IT WAS GOING TO REQUIRE PATIENTS AND CAREGIVERS BE IN ONE PLACE.

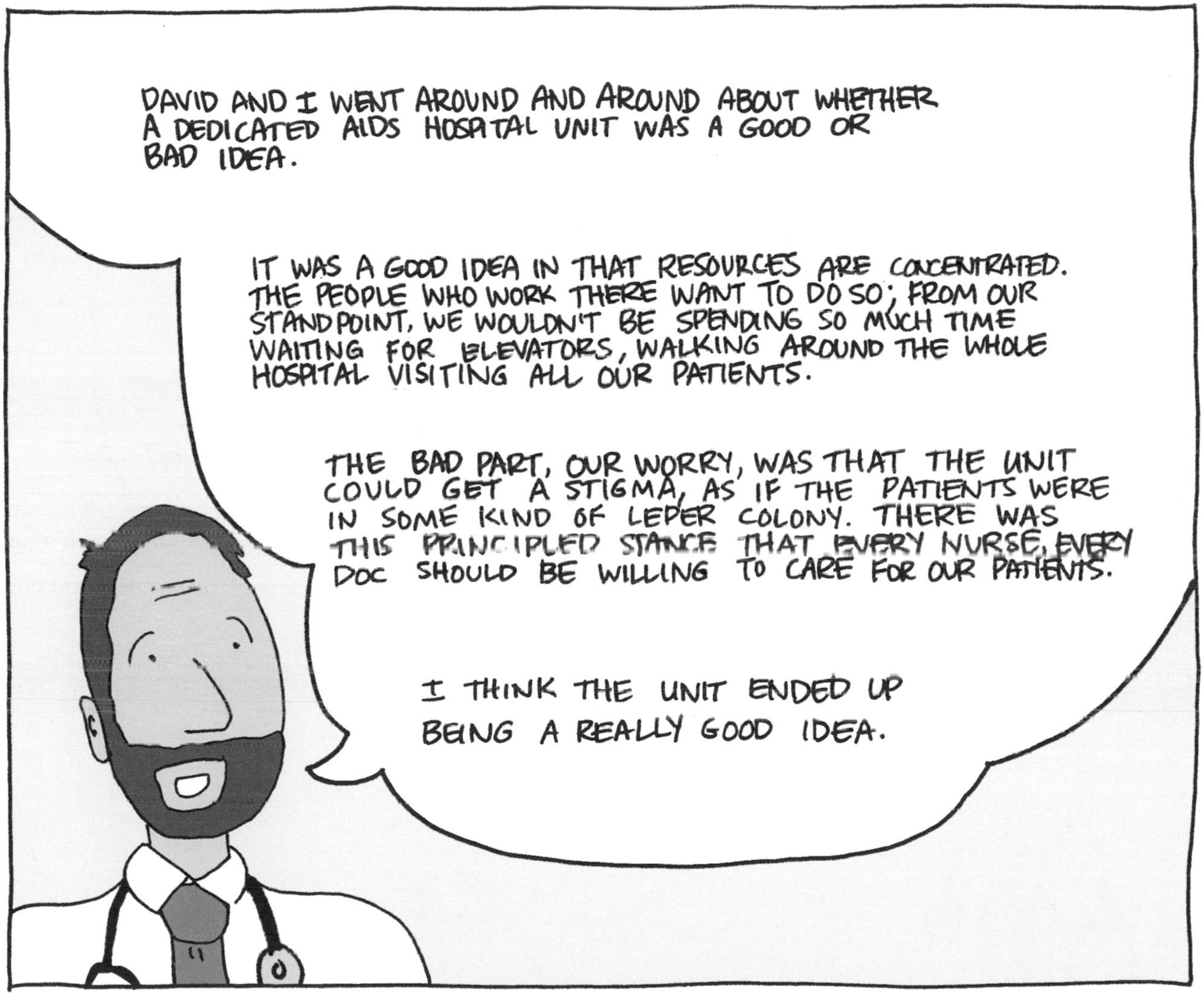
DAVID AND I WENT AROUND AND AROUND ABOUT WHETHER A DEDICATED AIDS HOSPITAL UNIT WAS A GOOD OR BAD IDEA.
IT WAS A GOOD IDEA IN THAT RESOURCES ARE CONCENTRATED. THE PEOPLE WHO WORK THERE WANT TO DO SO; FROM OUR STANDPOINT, WE WOULDN'T BE SPENDING SO MUCH TIME WAITING FOR ELEVATORS, WALKING AROUND THE WHOLE HOSPITAL VISITING ALL OUR PATIENTS.
THE BAD PART, OUR WORRY, WAS THAT THE UNIT COULD GET A STIGMA, AS IF THE PATIENTS WERE IN SOME KIND OF LEPER COLONY. THERE WAS THIS PRINCIPLED STANCE THAT EVERY NURSE, EVERY DOC SHOULD BE WILLING TO CARE FOR OUR PATIENTS.
I THINK THE UNIT ENDED UP BEING A REALLY GOOD IDEA.

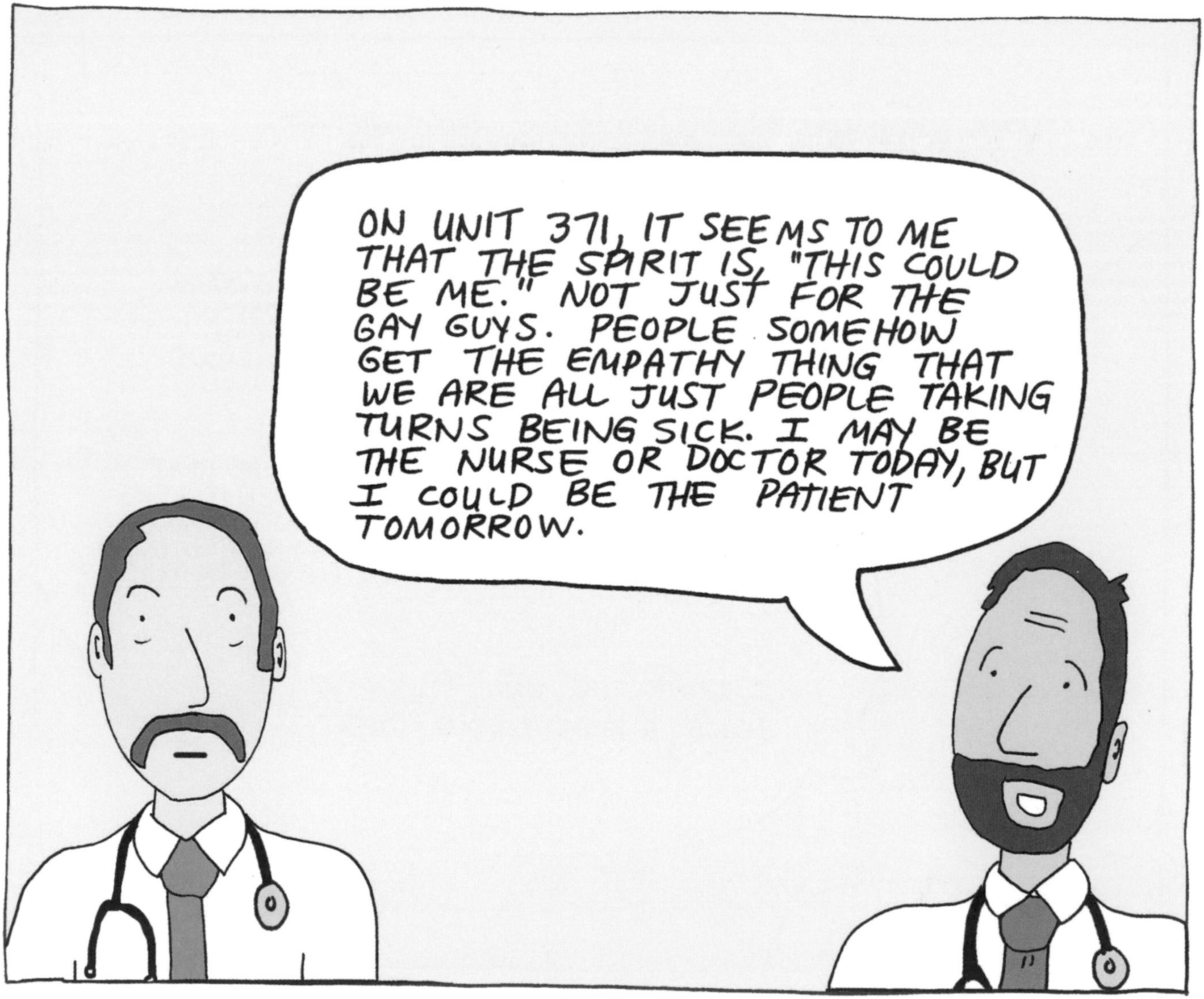
ON UNIT 371, IT SEEMS TO ME THAT THE SPIRIT IS, "THIS COULD BE ME." NOT JUST FOR THE GAY GUYS. PEOPLE SOMEHOW GET THE EMPATHY THING THAT WE ARE ALL JUST PEOPLE TAKING TURNS BEING SICK. I MAY BE THE NURSE OR DOCTOR TODAY, BUT I COULD BE THE PATIENT TOMORROW.

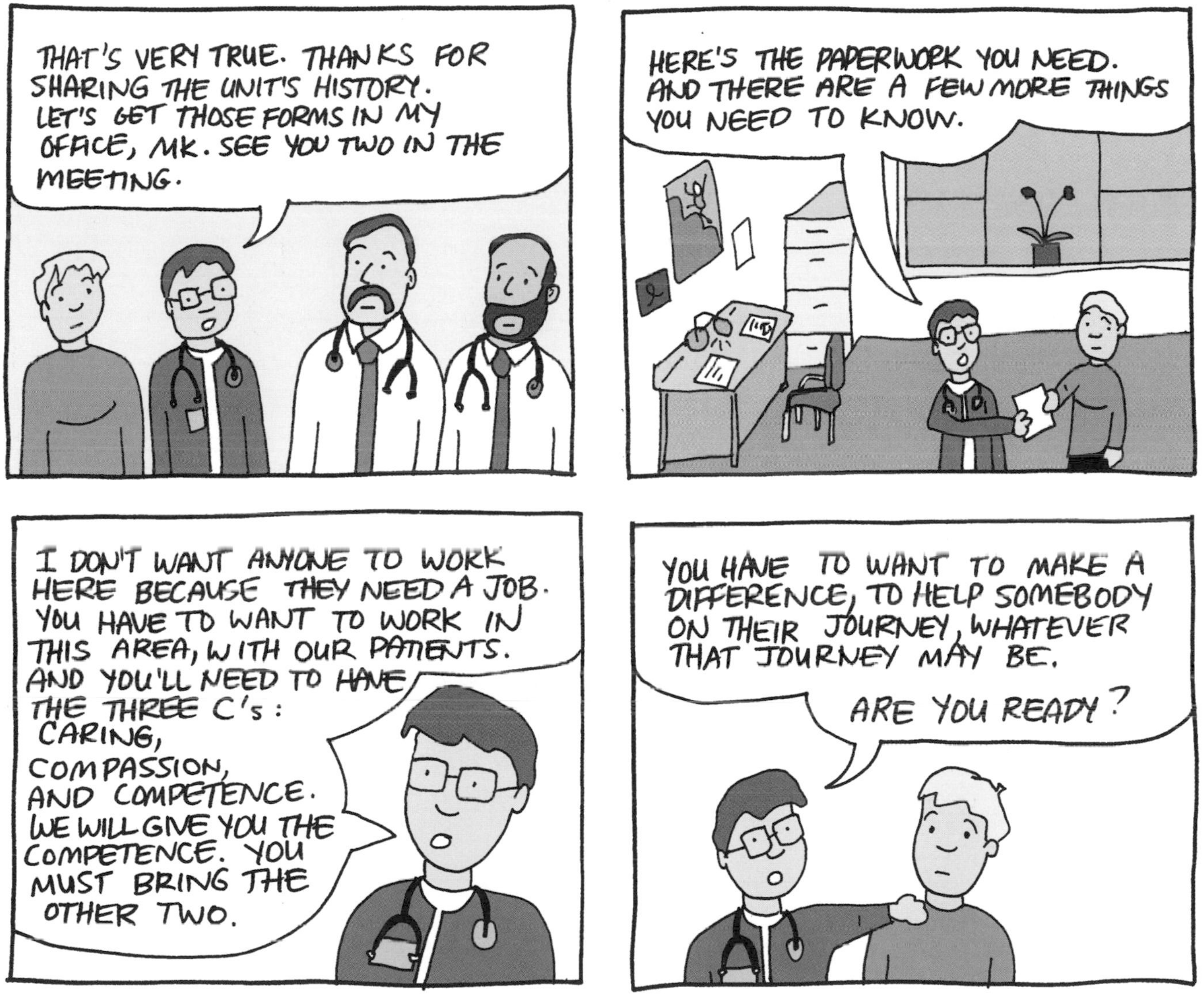
THAT'S VERY TRUE. THANKS FOR SHARING THE UNIT'S HISTORY. LET'S GET THOSE FORMS IN MY OFFICE, MK. SEE YOU TWO IN THE MEETING.
HERE'S THE PAPERWORK YOU NEED. AND THERE ARE A FEW MORE THINGS YOU NEED TO KNOW.
I DON'T WANT ANYONE TO WORK HERE BECAUSE THEY NEED A JOB. YOU HAVE TO WANT TO WORK IN THIS AREA, WITH OUR PATIENTS. AND YOU'LL NEED TO HAVE THE THREE C's: CARING, COMPASSION, AND COMPETENCE. WE WILL GIVE YOU THE COMPETENCE. YOU MUST BRING THE OTHER TWO.
YOU HAVE TO WANT TO MAKE A DIFFERENCE, TO HELP SOMEBODY ON THEIR JOURNEY, WHATEVER THAT JOURNEY MAY BE.
ARE YOU READY?

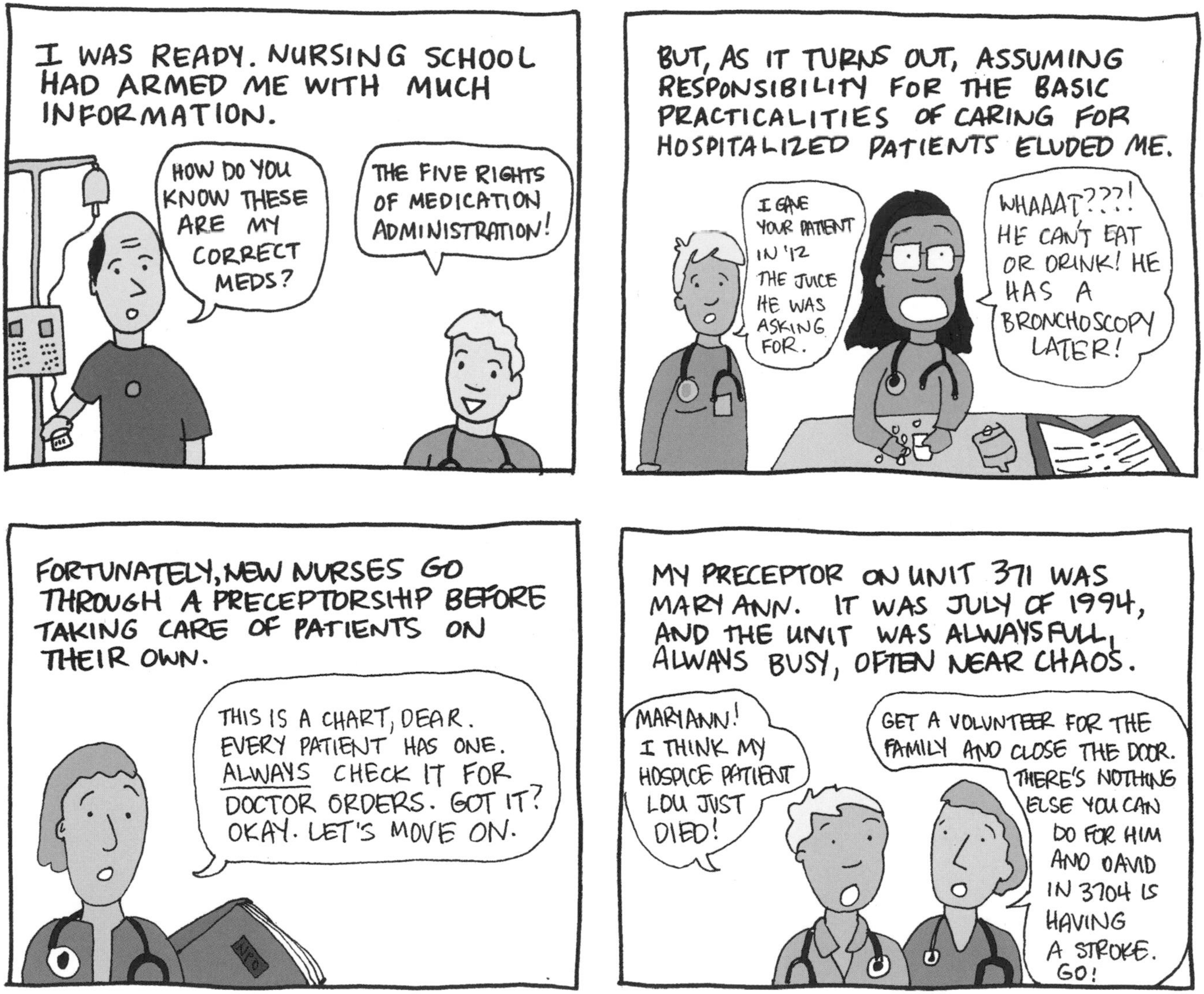
I WAS READY. NURSING SCHOOL HAD ARMED ME WITH MUCH INFORMATION.
HOW DO YOU KNOW THESE ARE MY CORRECT MEDS?
THE FIVE RIGHTS OF MEDICATION ADMINISTRATION!
BUT, AS IT TURNS OUT, ASSUMING RESPONSIBILITY FOR THE BASIC PRACTICALITIES OF CARING FOR HOSPITALIZED PATIENTS ELUDED ME.
I GAVE YOUR PATIENT IN '12 THE JUICE HE WAS ASKING FOR.
WHAAAT???! HE CAN'T EAT OR DRINK! HE HAS A BRONCHOSCOPY LATER!
FORTUNATELY, NEW NURSES GO THROUGH A PRECEPTORSHIP BEFORE TAKING CARE OF PATIENTS ON THEIR OWN.
THIS IS A CHART, DEAR. EVERY PATIENT HAS ONE. ALWAYS CHECK IT FOR DOCTOR ORDERS. GOT IT? OKAY. LET'S MOVE ON.
MY PRECEPTOR ON UNIT 371 WAS MARY ANN. IT WAS JULY OF 1994, AND THE UNIT WAS ALWAYS FULL, ALWAYS BUSY, OFTEN NEAR CHAOS.
MARY ANN! I THINK MY HOSPICE PATIENT LOU JUST DIED!
GET A VOLUNTEER FOR THE FAMILY AND CLOSE THE DOOR. THERE'S NOTHING ELSE YOU CAN DO FOR HIM AND DAVID IN 3704 IS HAVING A STROKE. GO!

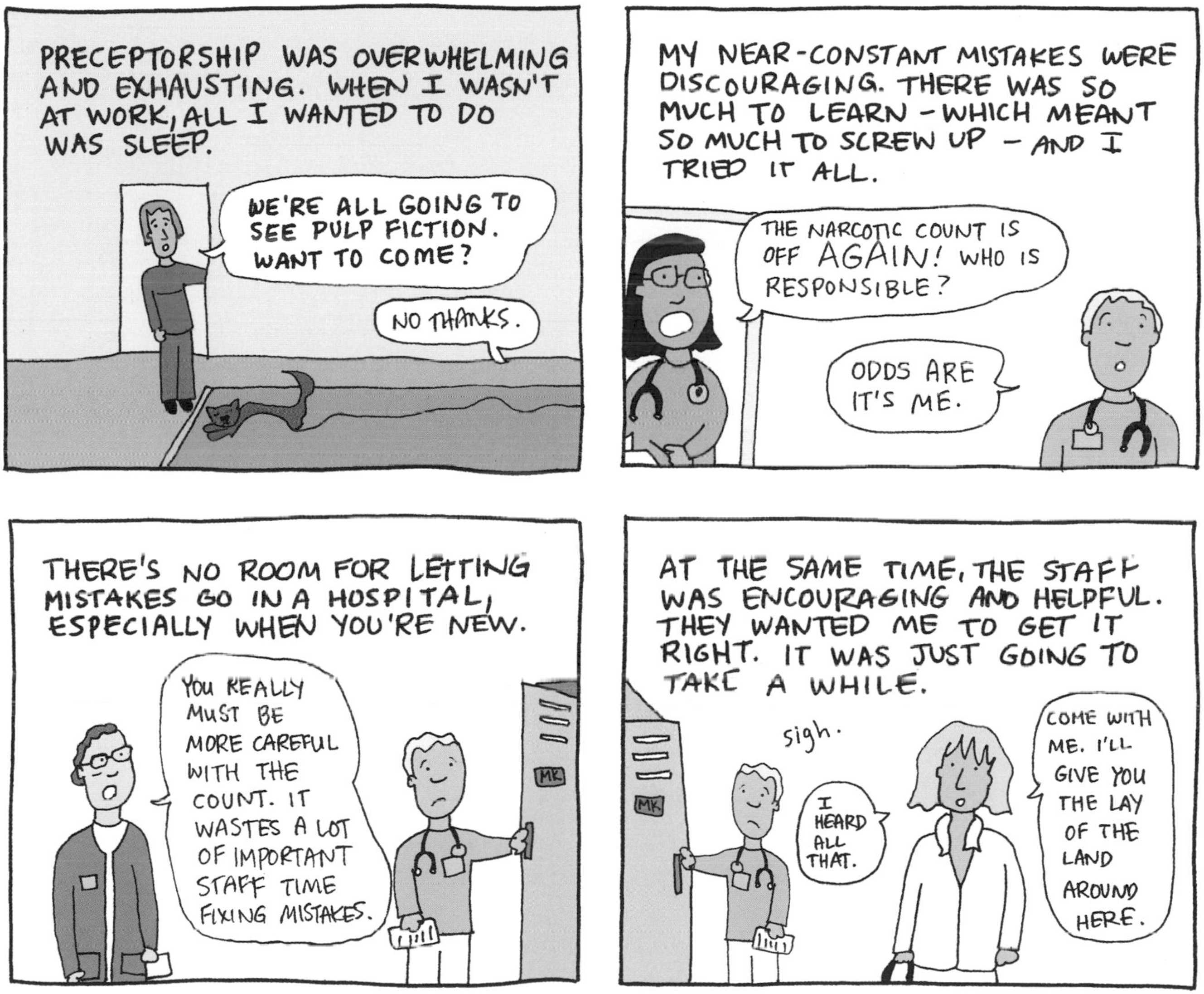
PRECEPTORSHIP WAS OVERWHELMING AND EXHAUSTING. WHEN I WASN'T AT WORK, ALL I WANTED TO DO WAS SLEEP.
WE'RE ALL GOING TO SEE PULP FICTION. WANT TO COME?
NO THANKS.
MY NEAR-CONSTANT MISTAKES WERE DISCOURAGING. THERE WAS SO MUCH TO LEARN - WHICH MEANT SO MUCH TO SCREW UP - AND I TRIED IT ALL.
THE NARCOTIC COUNT IS OFF AGAIN! WHO IS RESPONSIBLE?
ODDS ARE IT'S ME.
THERE'S NO ROOM FOR LETTING MISTAKES GO IN A HOSPITAL, ESPECIALLY WHEN YOU'RE NEW.
YOU REALLY MUST BE MORE CAREFUL WITH THE COUNT. IT WASTES A LOT OF IMPORTANT STAFF TIME FIXING MISTAKES.
MK
AT THE SAME TIME, THE STAFF WAS ENCOURAGING AND HELPFUL. THEY WANTED ME TO GET IT RIGHT. IT WAS JUST GOING TO TAKE A WHILE.
sigh.
MK
I HEARD ALL THAT.
COME WITH ME. I'LL GIVE YOU THE LAY OF THE LAND AROUND HERE.

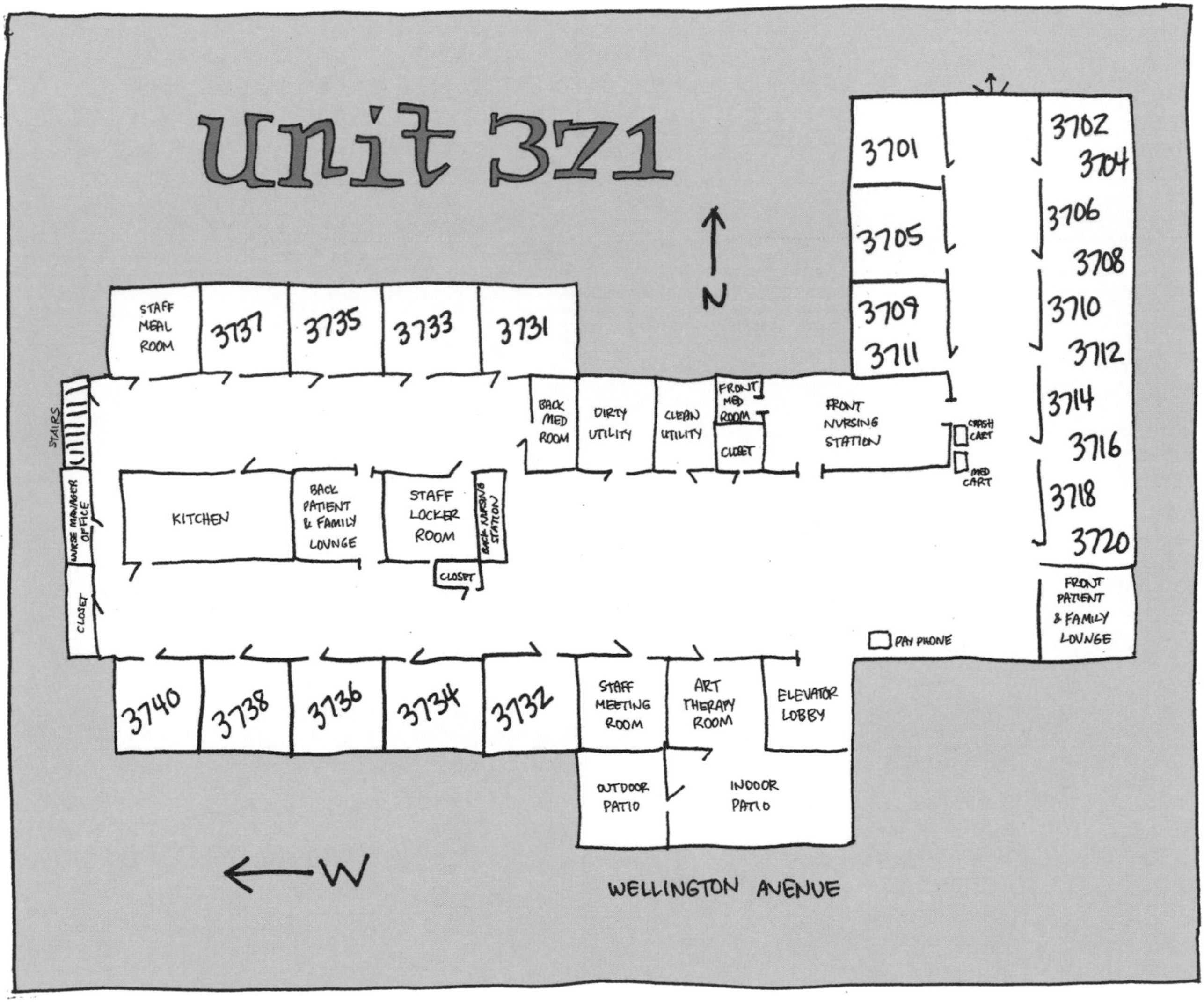
Unit 371
N
W
STAFF MEAL ROOM
3737
3735
3733
3731
3701
3702
3704
3705
3706
3708
3709
3711
3710
3712
3714
3716
3718
3720
STAIRS
NURSE MANAGER OFFICE
CLOSET
BACK MED ROOM
DIRTY UTILITY
CLEAN UTILITY
FRONT MED ROOM
CLOSET
FRONT NURSING STATION
CRASH CART
MED CART
KITCHEN
BACK PATIENT & FAMILY LOUNGE
STAFF LOCKER ROOM
BACK NURSING STATION
CLOSET
FRONT PATIENT & FAMILY LOUNGE
PAY PHONE
3740
3738
3736
3734
3732
STAFF MEETING ROOM
ART THERAPY ROOM
ELEVATOR LOBBY
OUTDOOR PATIO
INDOOR PATIO
WELLINGTON AVENUE

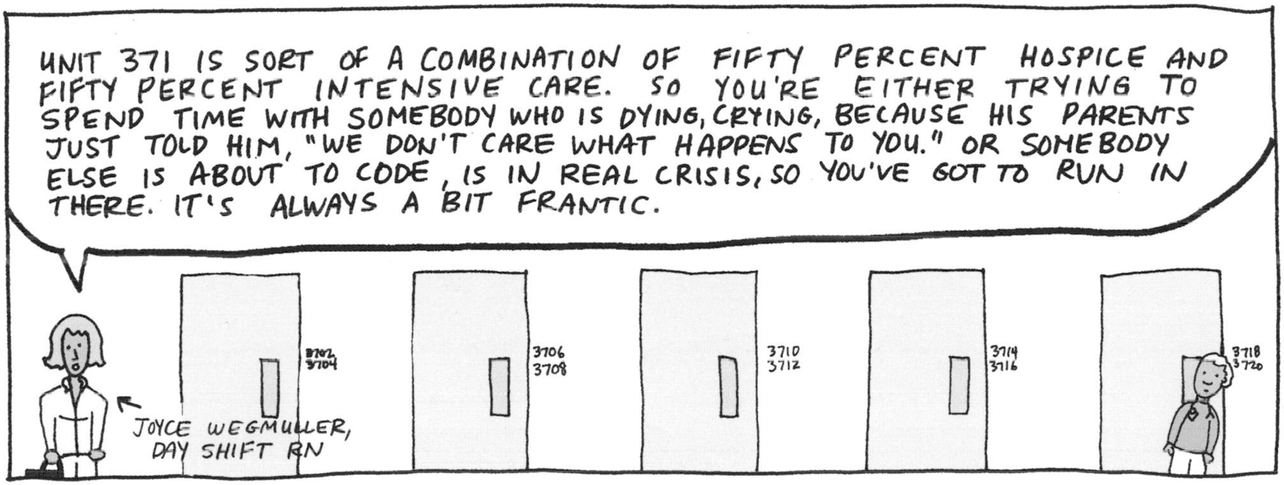
UNIT 371 IS SORT OF A COMBINATION OF FIFTY PERCENT HOSPICE AND FIFTY PERCENT INTENSIVE CARE. SO YOU'RE EITHER TRYING TO SPEND TIME WITH SOMEBODY WHO IS DYING, CRYING, BECAUSE HIS PARENTS JUST TOLD HIM, "WE DON'T CARE WHAT HAPPENS TO YOU." OR SOMEBODY ELSE IS ABOUT TO CODE, IS IN REAL CRISIS, SO YOU'VE GOT TO RUN IN THERE. IT'S ALWAYS A BIT FRANTIC.
JOYCE WEGMULLER, DAY SHIFT RN
3702 3704
3706 3708
3710 3712
3714 3716
3718 3720

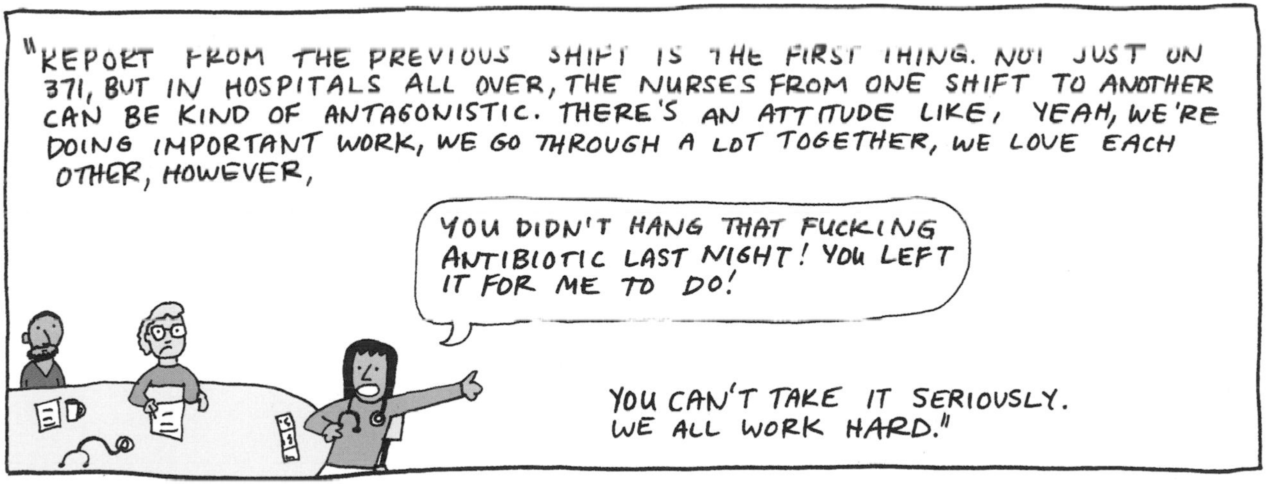
"REPORT FROM THE PREVIOUS SHIFT IS THE FIRST THING. NOT JUST ON 371, BUT IN HOSPITALS ALL OVER, THE NURSES FROM ONE SHIFT TO ANOTHER CAN BE KIND OF ANTAGONISTIC. THERE'S AN ATTITUDE LIKE, YEAH, WE'RE DOING IMPORTANT WORK, WE GO THROUGH A LOT TOGETHER, WE LOVE EACH OTHER, HOWEVER,
YOU DIDN'T HANG THAT FUCKING ANTIBIOTIC LAST NIGHT! YOU LEFT IT FOR ME TO DO!
YOU CAN'T TAKE IT SERIOUSLY. WE ALL WORK HARD."

"THE MEDICATIONS ARE A NIGHTMARE. EVERY YEAR THERE ARE MORE MEDS COMING ALONG. ONLY ONE TREATS THE VIRUS ITSELF, AZT. THE OTHERS ARE FOR INFECTIONS, OR TO TREAT SIDE EFFECTS OF THE MEDS THEMSELVES.

IMAGINE TWENTY PILLS WITH BREAKFAST! AND THE INTRAVENOUS MEDS? CRAZY! — WE HAVE TO FIGURE OUT HOW TO GET ALL THIS INFUSED, WORKING AROUND BRONCHO-SCOPIES, CAT SCANS, MRI EXAMS, ETC..."

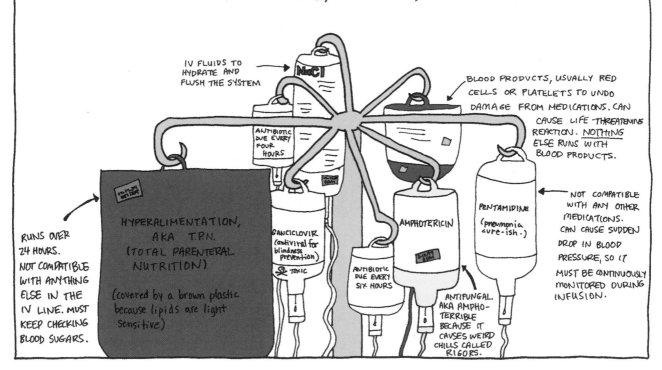

IV FLUIDS TO HYDRATE AND FLUSH THE SYSTEM

NaCl

BLOOD PRODUCTS, USUALLY RED CELLS OR PLATELETS TO UNDO DAMAGE FROM MEDICATIONS. CAN CAUSE LIFE-THREATENING REACTION. NOTHING ELSE RUNS WITH BLOOD PRODUCTS.

ANTIBIOTIC DUE EVERY FOUR HOURS

RUNS OVER 24 HOURS. NOT COMPATIBLE WITH ANYTHING ELSE IN THE IV LINE. MUST KEEP CHECKING BLOOD SUGARS.

HYPERALIMENTATION, AKA T.P.N. (TOTAL PARENTERAL NUTRITION)

(covered by a brown plastic because lipids are light sensitive)

GANCICLOVIR (antiviral for blindness prevention)

TOXIC

ANTIBIOTIC DUE EVERY SIX HOURS

AMPHOTERICIN

STEADY RATE

ANTIFUNGAL. AKA AMPHO-TERRIBLE BECAUSE IT CAUSES WEIRD CHILLS CALLED RIGORS.

PENTAMIDINE (pneumonia cure-ish.)

NOT COMPATIBLE WITH ANY OTHER MEDICATIONS. CAN CAUSE SUDDEN DROP IN BLOOD PRESSURE, SO IT MUST BE CONTINUOUSLY MONITORED DURING INFUSION.

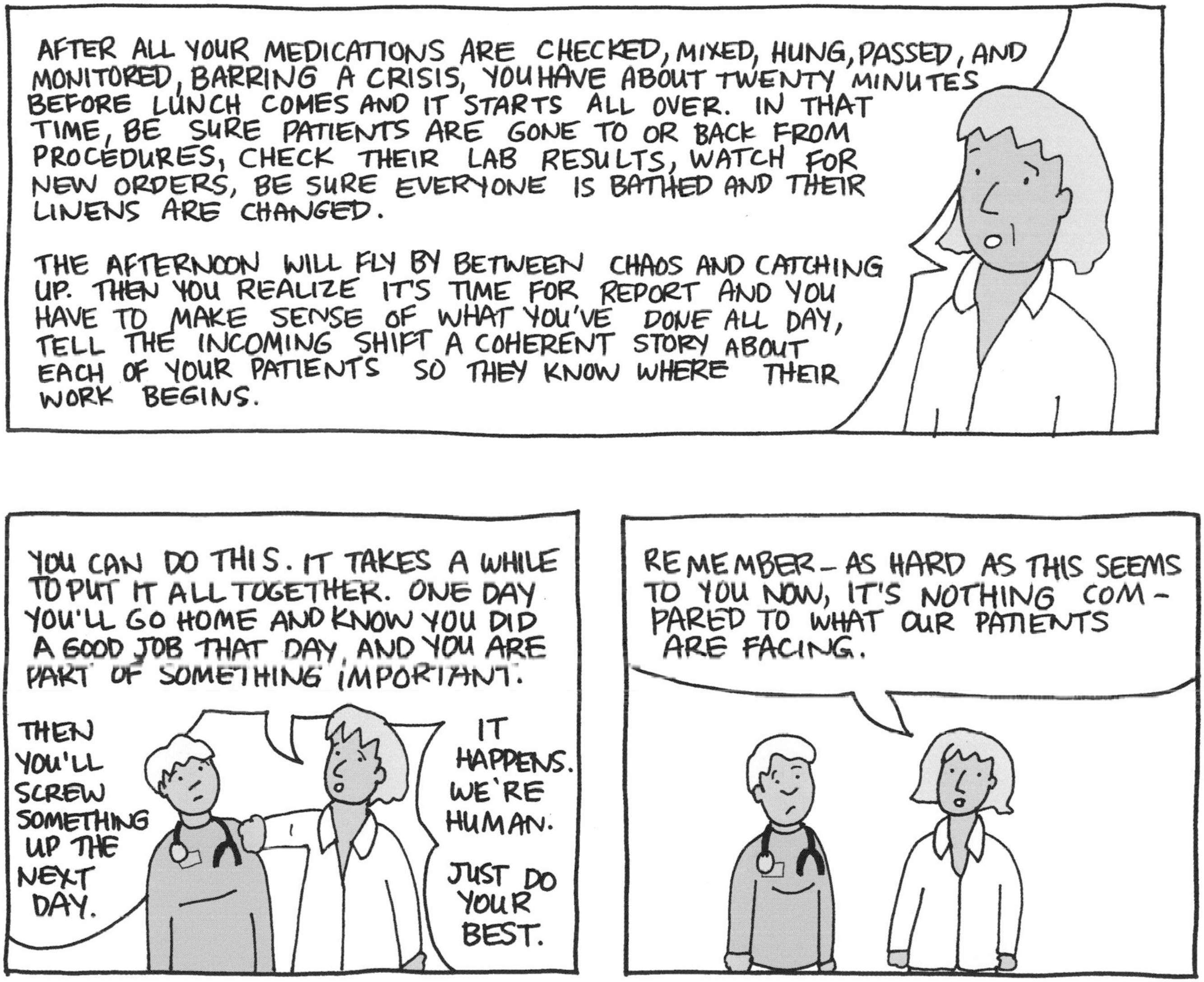
AFTER ALL YOUR MEDICATIONS ARE CHECKED, MIXED, HUNG, PASSED, AND MONITORED, BARRING A CRISIS, YOU HAVE ABOUT TWENTY MINUTES BEFORE LUNCH COMES AND IT STARTS ALL OVER. IN THAT TIME, BE SURE PATIENTS ARE GONE TO OR BACK FROM PROCEDURES, CHECK THEIR LAB RESULTS, WATCH FOR NEW ORDERS, BE SURE EVERYONE IS BATHED AND THEIR LINENS ARE CHANGED.
THE AFTERNOON WILL FLY BY BETWEEN CHAOS AND CATCHING UP. THEN YOU REALIZE IT'S TIME FOR REPORT AND YOU HAVE TO MAKE SENSE OF WHAT YOU'VE DONE ALL DAY, TELL THE INCOMING SHIFT A COHERENT STORY ABOUT EACH OF YOUR PATIENTS SO THEY KNOW WHERE THEIR WORK BEGINS.
YOU CAN DO THIS. IT TAKES A WHILE TO PUT IT ALL TOGETHER. ONE DAY YOU'LL GO HOME AND KNOW YOU DID A GOOD JOB THAT DAY, AND YOU ARE PART OF SOMETHING IMPORTANT.
THEN YOU'LL SCREW SOMETHING UP THE NEXT DAY.
IT HAPPENS. WE'RE HUMAN.
JUST DO YOUR BEST.
REMEMBER — AS HARD AS THIS SEEMS TO YOU NOW, IT'S NOTHING COMPARED TO WHAT OUR PATIENTS ARE FACING.

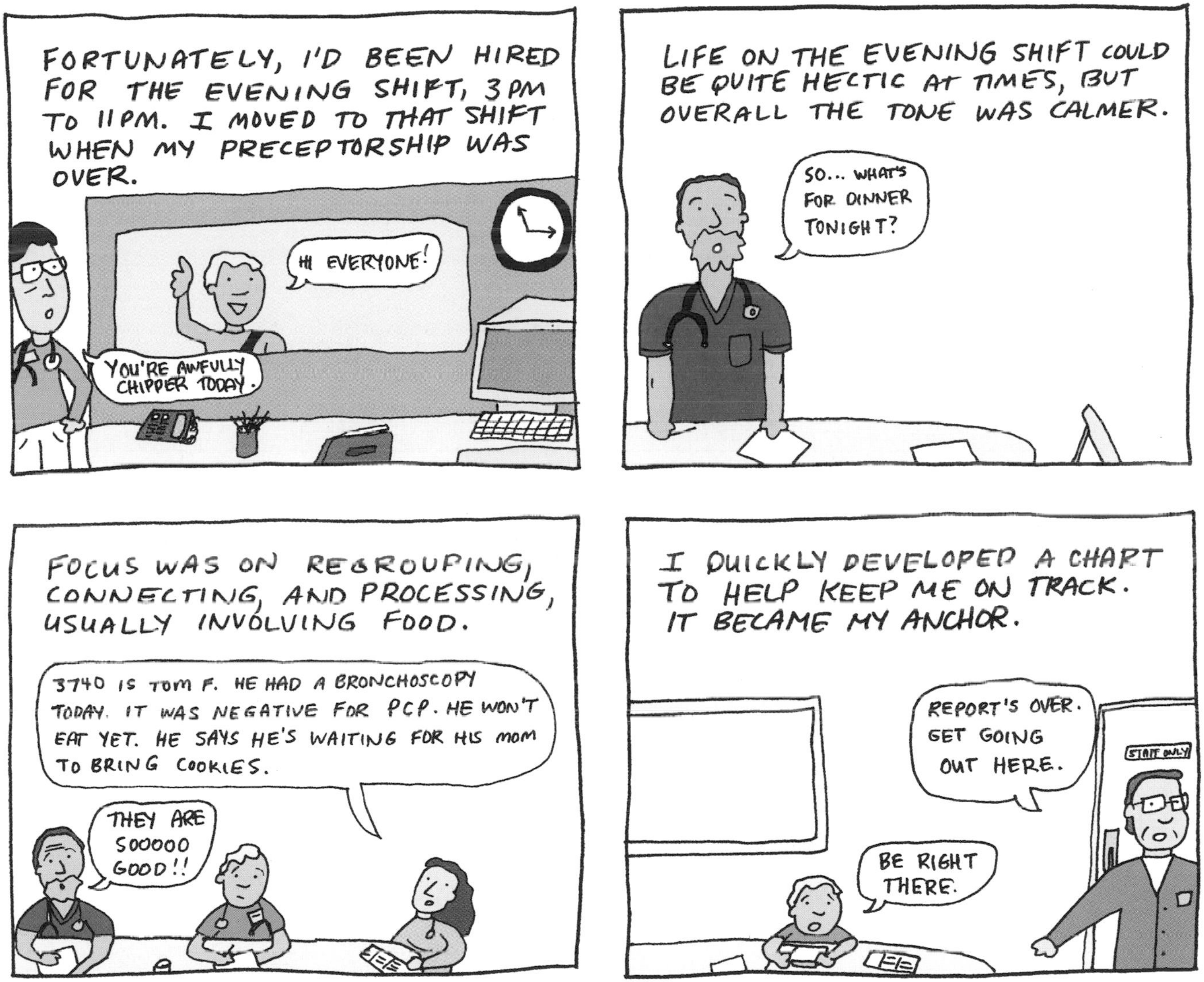
FORTUNATELY, I'D BEEN HIRED FOR THE EVENING SHIFT, 3PM TO 11PM. I MOVED TO THAT SHIFT WHEN MY PRECEPTORSHIP WAS OVER.
HI EVERYONE!
YOU'RE AWFULLY CHIPPER TODAY.
LIFE ON THE EVENING SHIFT COULD BE QUITE HECTIC AT TIMES, BUT OVERALL THE TONE WAS CALMER.
SO... WHAT'S FOR DINNER TONIGHT?
FOCUS WAS ON REGROUPING, CONNECTING, AND PROCESSING, USUALLY INVOLVING FOOD.
3740 IS TOM F. HE HAD A BRONCHOSCOPY TODAY. IT WAS NEGATIVE FOR PCP. HE WON'T EAT YET. HE SAYS HE'S WAITING FOR HIS MOM TO BRING COOKIES.
THEY ARE SOOOOO GOOD!!
I QUICKLY DEVELOPED A CHART TO HELP KEEP ME ON TRACK. IT BECAME MY ANCHOR.
REPORT'S OVER. GET GOING OUT HERE.
STAFF ONLY
BE RIGHT THERE.

	5pm	6pm	7pm	8pm	9pm	10pm
3701 MICHAEL STEVENS seizures	IV ANTIBIOTIC	DISCHARGE ———————————————				
3702 DONNA HULTZ pneumonia	PILLS IV ANTIBIOTIC	FAMILY CONFERENCE			PILLS PREP FOR BRONCHOSCOPY IN AM	
3704 TED BLAKE CMV retinitis	PILLS	FOLLOW UP ON LABS			PILLS	
3706 RANDY HARPER end stage	TURN		TURN FATHER MAY VISIT		TURN	
3708 ANDY TIMMINS KS legs, diarrhea	PILLS			PILLS	IV NUTRITION	

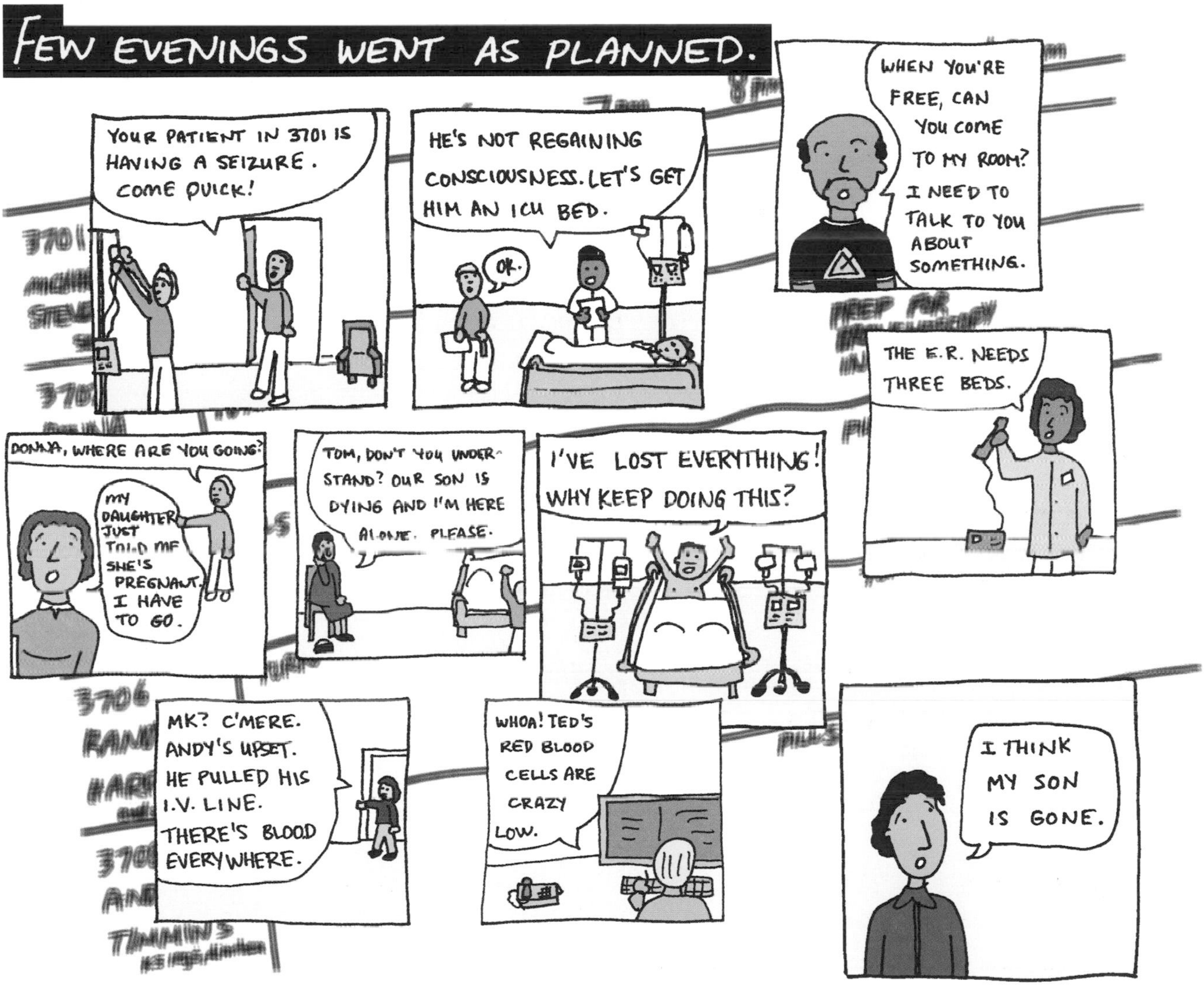
FEW EVENINGS WENT AS PLANNED.
YOUR PATIENT IN 3701 IS HAVING A SEIZURE. COME QUICK!
HE'S NOT REGAINING CONSCIOUSNESS. LET'S GET HIM AN ICU BED.
OK.
WHEN YOU'RE FREE, CAN YOU COME TO MY ROOM? I NEED TO TALK TO YOU ABOUT SOMETHING.
THE E.R. NEEDS THREE BEDS.
DONNA, WHERE ARE YOU GOING?
MY DAUGHTER JUST TOLD ME SHE'S PREGNANT. I HAVE TO GO.
TOM, DON'T YOU UNDERSTAND? OUR SON IS DYING AND I'M HERE ALONE. PLEASE.
I'VE LOST EVERYTHING! WHY KEEP DOING THIS?
MK? C'MERE. ANDY'S UPSET. HE PULLED HIS I.V. LINE. THERE'S BLOOD EVERYWHERE.
WHOA! TED'S RED BLOOD CELLS ARE CRAZY LOW.
I THINK MY SON IS GONE.

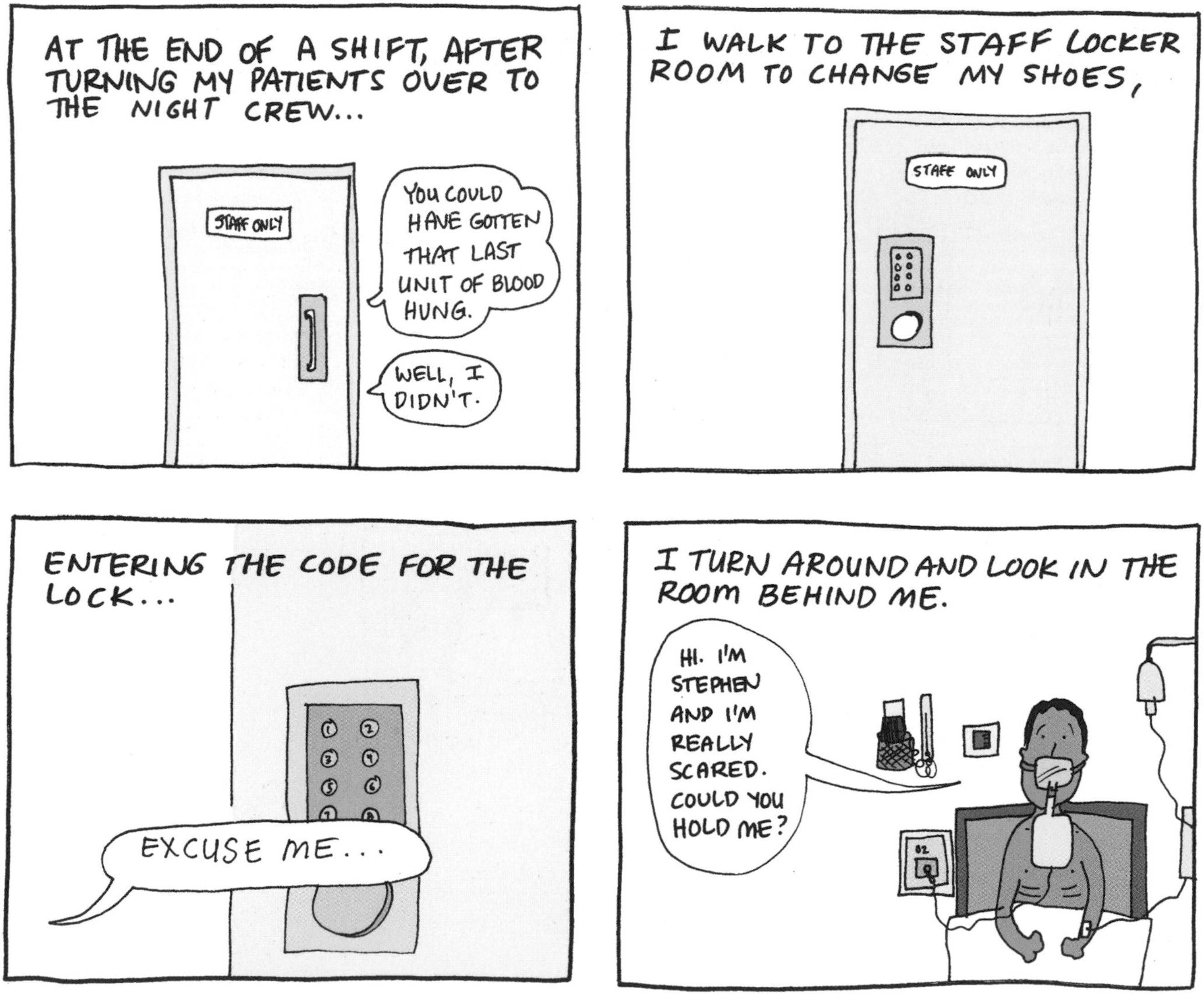
AT THE END OF A SHIFT, AFTER TURNING MY PATIENTS OVER TO THE NIGHT CREW...
STAFF ONLY
YOU COULD HAVE GOTTEN THAT LAST UNIT OF BLOOD HUNG.
WELL, I DIDN'T.
I WALK TO THE STAFF LOCKER ROOM TO CHANGE MY SHOES,
STAFF ONLY
ENTERING THE CODE FOR THE LOCK...
EXCUSE ME...
I TURN AROUND AND LOOK IN THE ROOM BEHIND ME.
HI. I'M STEPHEN AND I'M REALLY SCARED. COULD YOU HOLD ME?

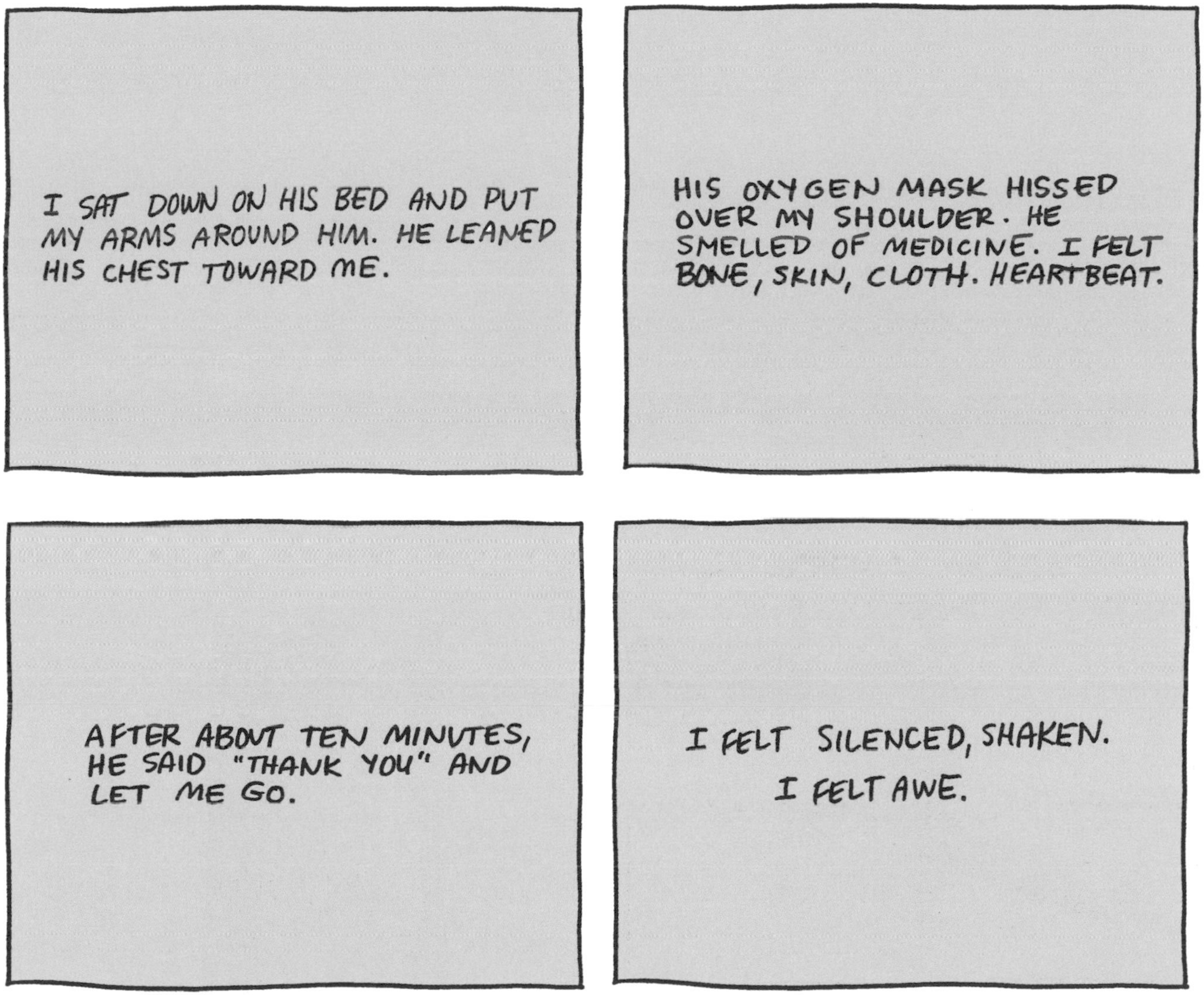
I SAT DOWN ON HIS BED AND PUT MY ARMS AROUND HIM. HE LEANED HIS CHEST TOWARD ME.
HIS OXYGEN MASK HISSED OVER MY SHOULDER. HE SMELLED OF MEDICINE. I FELT BONE, SKIN, CLOTH. HEARTBEAT.
AFTER ABOUT TEN MINUTES, HE SAID "THANK YOU" AND LET ME GO.
I FELT SILENCED, SHAKEN.
I FELT AWE.

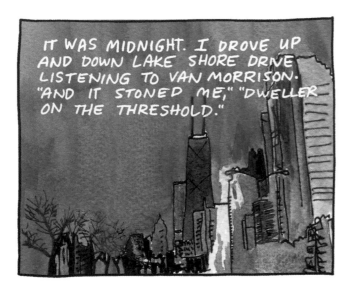

IT WAS MIDNIGHT. I DROVE UP AND DOWN LAKE SHORE DRIVE LISTENING TO VAN MORRISON. "AND IT STONED ME," "DWELLER ON THE THRESHOLD."

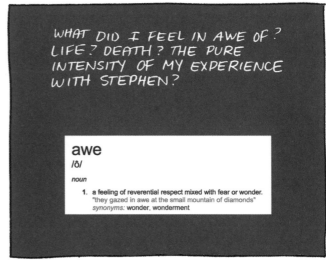

WHAT DID I FEEL IN AWE OF? LIFE? DEATH? THE PURE INTENSITY OF MY EXPERIENCE WITH STEPHEN?

awe
/ô/

noun

1. a feeling of reverential respect mixed with fear or wonder.
   "they gazed in awe at the small mountain of diamonds"
   synonyms: **wonder, wonderment**

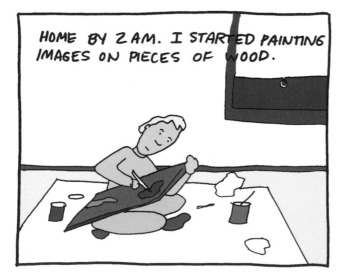

HOME BY 2 AM. I STARTED PAINTING IMAGES ON PIECES OF WOOD.

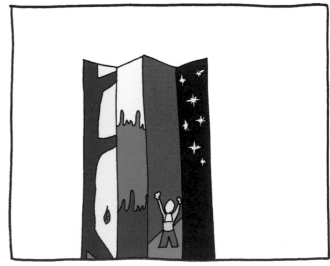

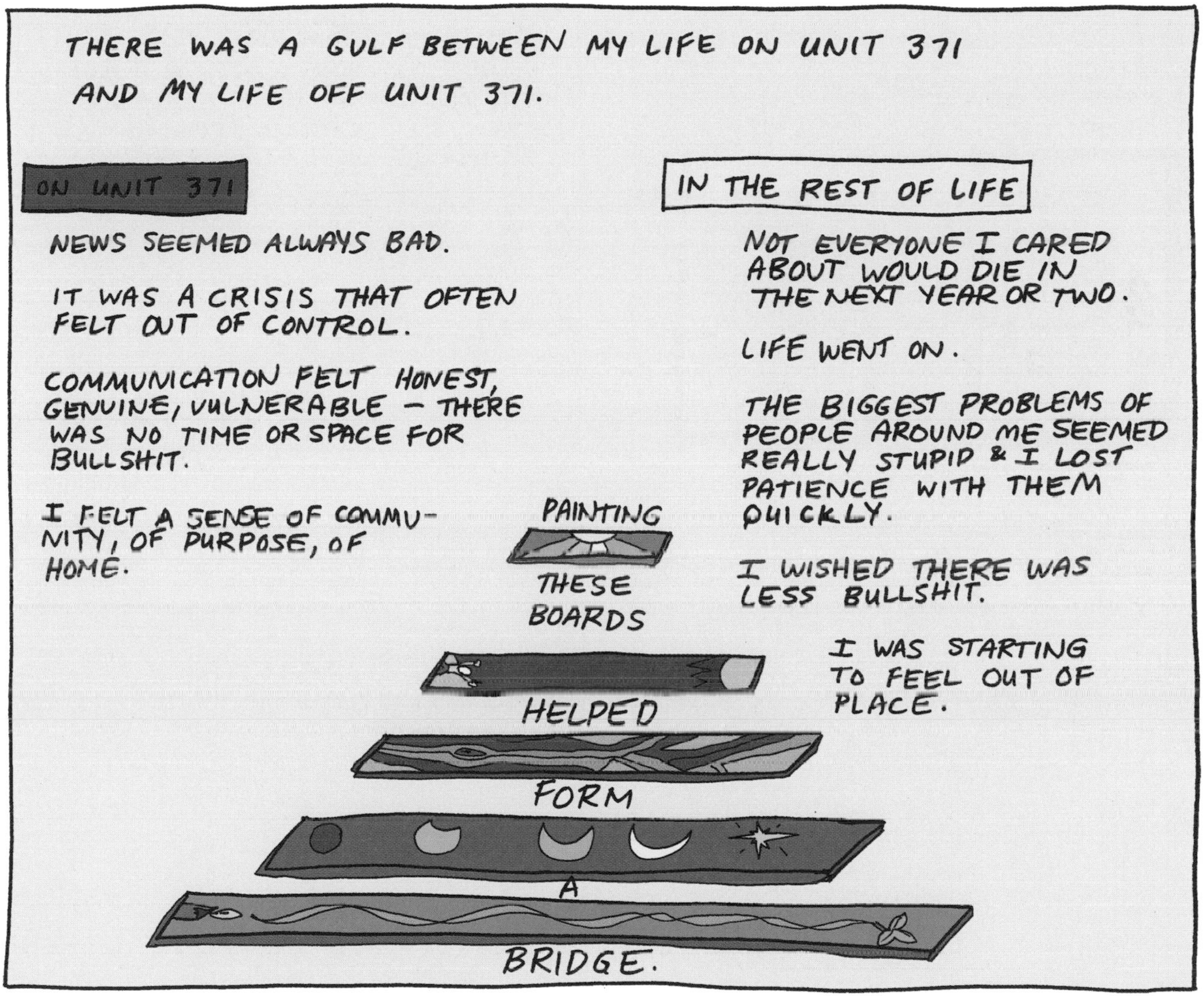

THERE WAS A GULF BETWEEN MY LIFE ON UNIT 371
AND MY LIFE OFF UNIT 371.

ON UNIT 371

NEWS SEEMED ALWAYS BAD.

IT WAS A CRISIS THAT OFTEN FELT OUT OF CONTROL.

COMMUNICATION FELT HONEST, GENUINE, VULNERABLE — THERE WAS NO TIME OR SPACE FOR BULLSHIT.

I FELT A SENSE OF COMMUNITY, OF PURPOSE, OF HOME.

IN THE REST OF LIFE

NOT EVERYONE I CARED ABOUT WOULD DIE IN THE NEXT YEAR OR TWO.

LIFE WENT ON.

THE BIGGEST PROBLEMS OF PEOPLE AROUND ME SEEMED REALLY STUPID & I LOST PATIENCE WITH THEM QUICKLY.

I WISHED THERE WAS LESS BULLSHIT.

I WAS STARTING TO FEEL OUT OF PLACE.

PAINTING

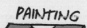

THESE BOARDS

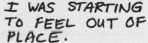

HELPED

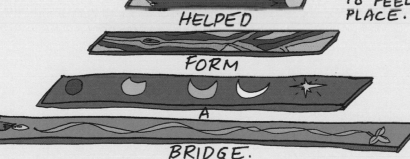

FORM

A

BRIDGE.

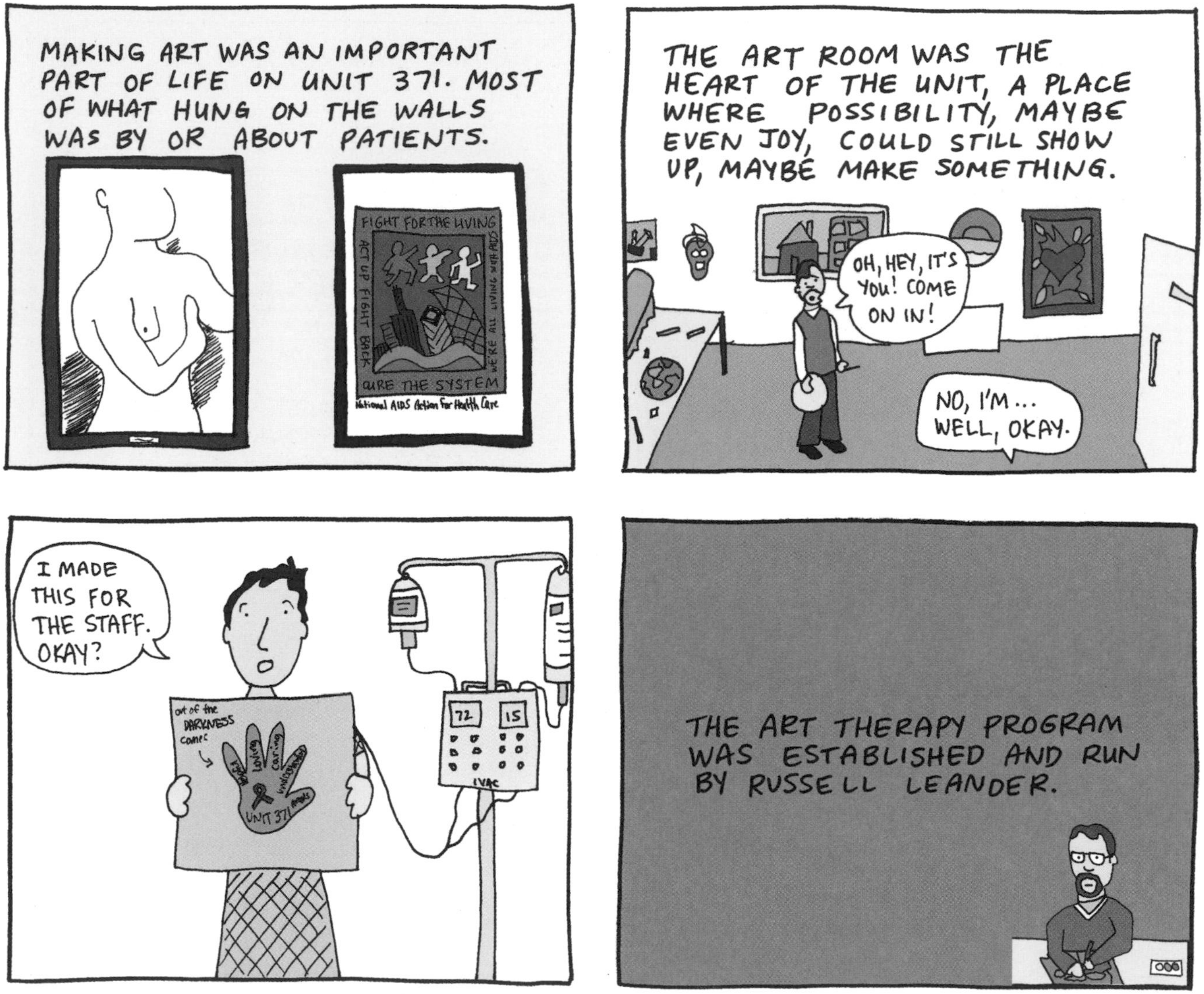
MAKING ART WAS AN IMPORTANT PART OF LIFE ON UNIT 371. MOST OF WHAT HUNG ON THE WALLS WAS BY OR ABOUT PATIENTS.
FIGHT FOR THE LIVING
ACT UP FIGHT BACK
WE'RE ALL LIVING WITH AIDS
CURE THE SYSTEM
National AIDS Action for Health Care
THE ART ROOM WAS THE HEART OF THE UNIT, A PLACE WHERE POSSIBILITY, MAYBE EVEN JOY, COULD STILL SHOW UP, MAYBE MAKE SOMETHING.
OH, HEY, IT'S YOU! COME ON IN!
NO, I'M... WELL, OKAY.
I MADE THIS FOR THE STAFF. OKAY?
out of the DARKNESS comes
UNIT 371
72
15
IVAC
THE ART THERAPY PROGRAM WAS ESTABLISHED AND RUN BY RUSSELL LEANDER.

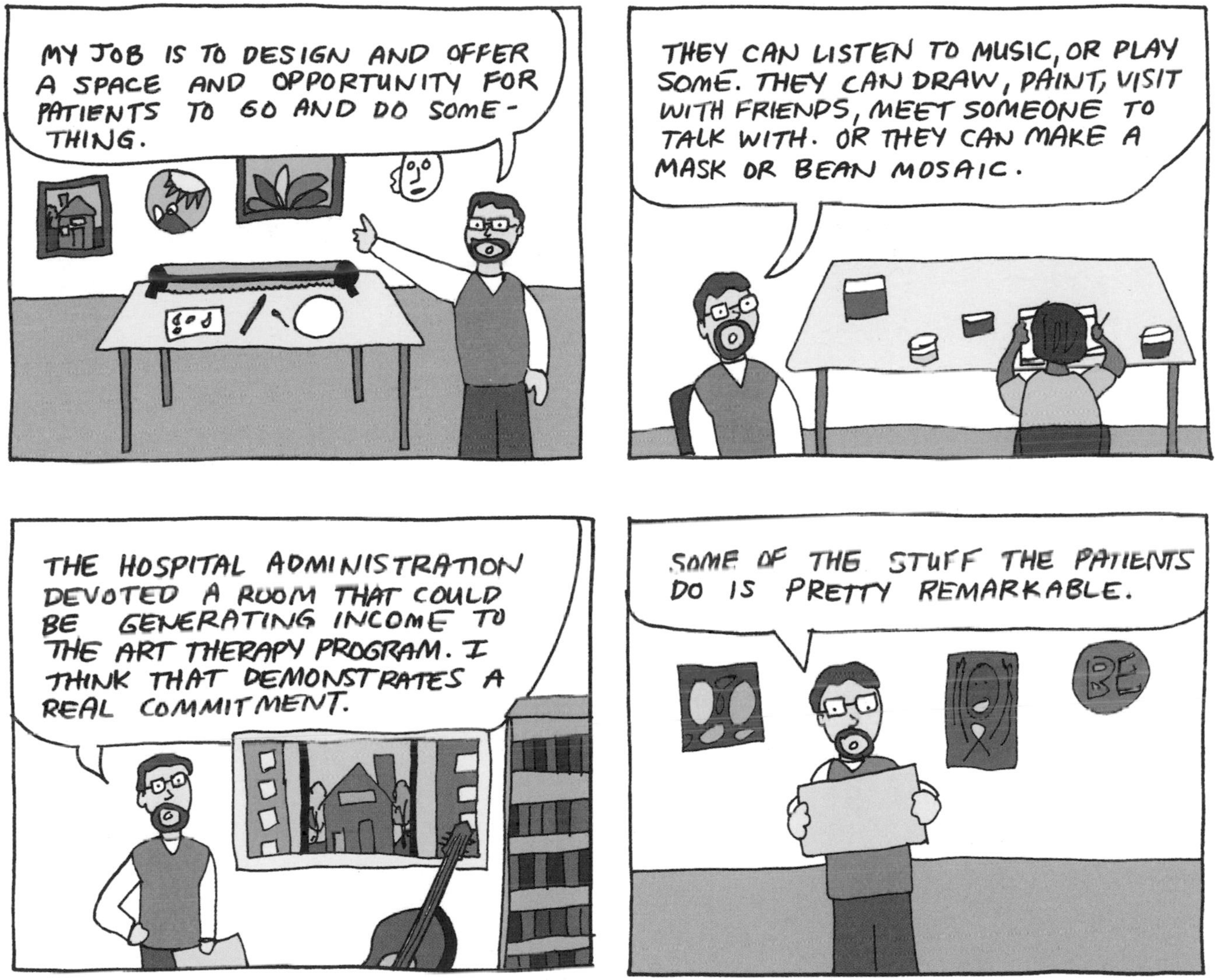
MY JOB IS TO DESIGN AND OFFER A SPACE AND OPPORTUNITY FOR PATIENTS TO GO AND DO SOME-THING.
THEY CAN LISTEN TO MUSIC, OR PLAY SOME. THEY CAN DRAW, PAINT, VISIT WITH FRIENDS, MEET SOMEONE TO TALK WITH. OR THEY CAN MAKE A MASK OR BEAN MOSAIC.
THE HOSPITAL ADMINISTRATION DEVOTED A ROOM THAT COULD BE GENERATING INCOME TO THE ART THERAPY PROGRAM. I THINK THAT DEMONSTRATES A REAL COMMITMENT.
SOME OF THE STUFF THE PATIENTS DO IS PRETTY REMARKABLE.
BE

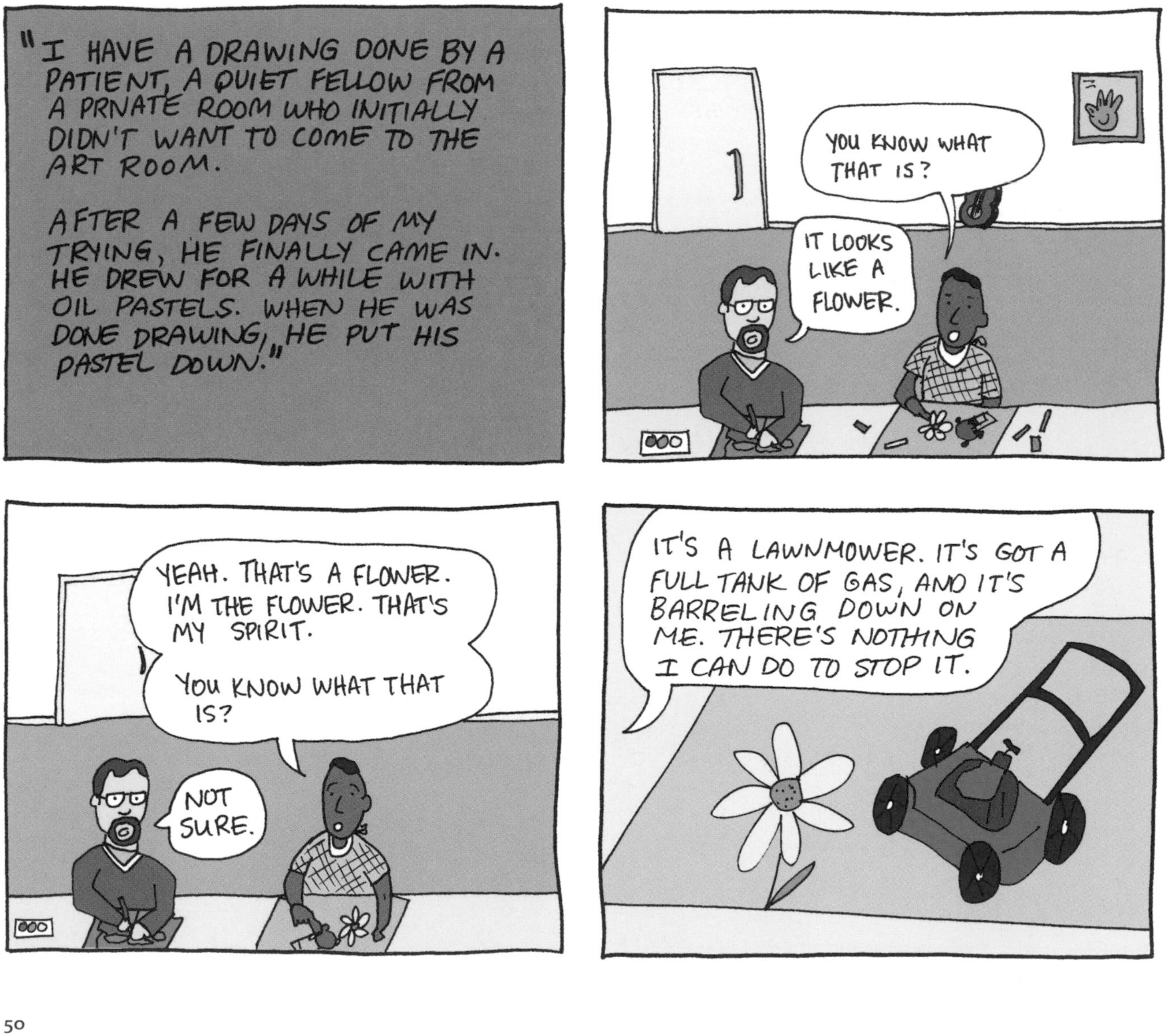
"I HAVE A DRAWING DONE BY A PATIENT, A QUIET FELLOW FROM A PRIVATE ROOM WHO INITIALLY DIDN'T WANT TO COME TO THE ART ROOM.
AFTER A FEW DAYS OF MY TRYING, HE FINALLY CAME IN. HE DREW FOR A WHILE WITH OIL PASTELS. WHEN HE WAS DONE DRAWING, HE PUT HIS PASTEL DOWN."
YOU KNOW WHAT THAT IS?
IT LOOKS LIKE A FLOWER.
YEAH. THAT'S A FLOWER. I'M THE FLOWER. THAT'S MY SPIRIT.
YOU KNOW WHAT THAT IS?
NOT SURE.
IT'S A LAWNMOWER. IT'S GOT A FULL TANK OF GAS, AND IT'S BARRELING DOWN ON ME. THERE'S NOTHING I CAN DO TO STOP IT.

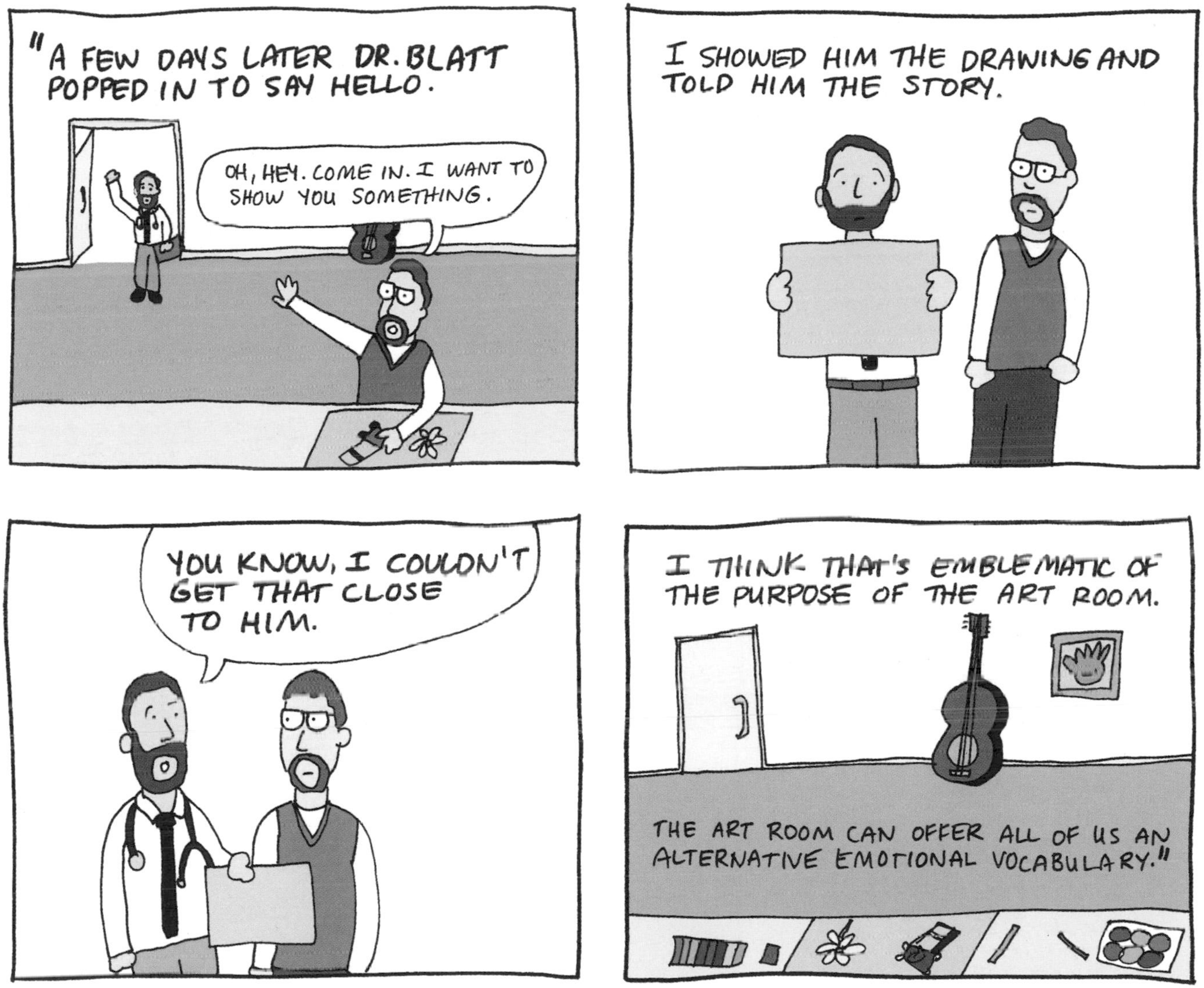
"A FEW DAYS LATER DR. BLATT POPPED IN TO SAY HELLO.
OH, HEY. COME IN. I WANT TO SHOW YOU SOMETHING.
I SHOWED HIM THE DRAWING AND TOLD HIM THE STORY.
YOU KNOW, I COULDN'T GET THAT CLOSE TO HIM.
I THINK THAT'S EMBLEMATIC OF THE PURPOSE OF THE ART ROOM.
THE ART ROOM CAN OFFER ALL OF US AN ALTERNATIVE EMOTIONAL VOCABULARY."

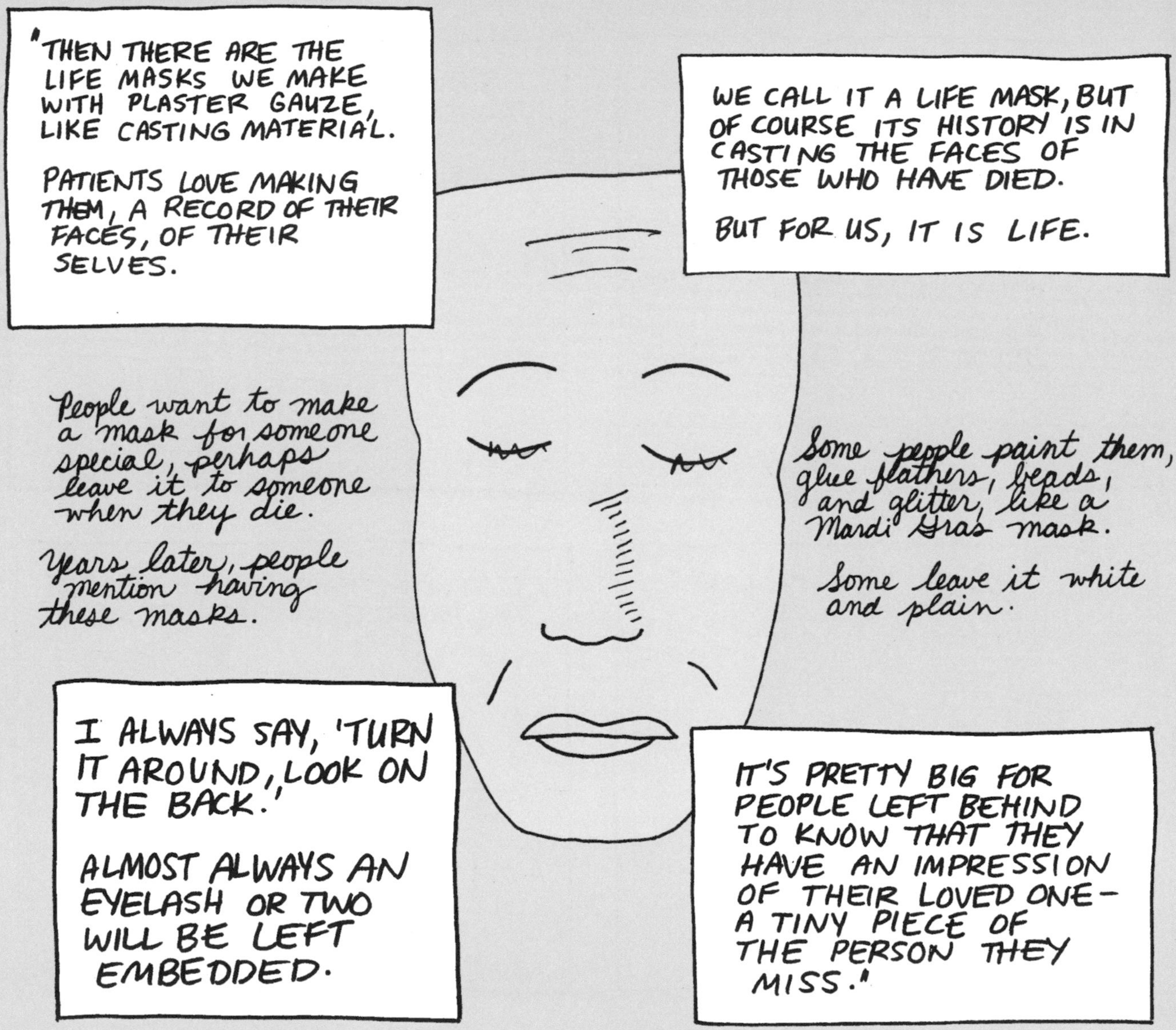
"THEN THERE ARE THE LIFE MASKS WE MAKE WITH PLASTER GAUZE, LIKE CASTING MATERIAL.
PATIENTS LOVE MAKING THEM, A RECORD OF THEIR FACES, OF THEIR SELVES.
WE CALL IT A LIFE MASK, BUT OF COURSE ITS HISTORY IS IN CASTING THE FACES OF THOSE WHO HAVE DIED.
BUT FOR US, IT IS LIFE.
People want to make a mask for someone special, perhaps leave it to someone when they die.
Years later, people mention having these masks.
Some people paint them, glue feathers, beads, and glitter, like a Mardi Gras mask.
Some leave it white and plain.
I ALWAYS SAY, 'TURN IT AROUND, LOOK ON THE BACK.'
ALMOST ALWAYS AN EYELASH OR TWO WILL BE LEFT EMBEDDED.
IT'S PRETTY BIG FOR PEOPLE LEFT BEHIND TO KNOW THAT THEY HAVE AN IMPRESSION OF THEIR LOVED ONE— A TINY PIECE OF THE PERSON THEY MISS."

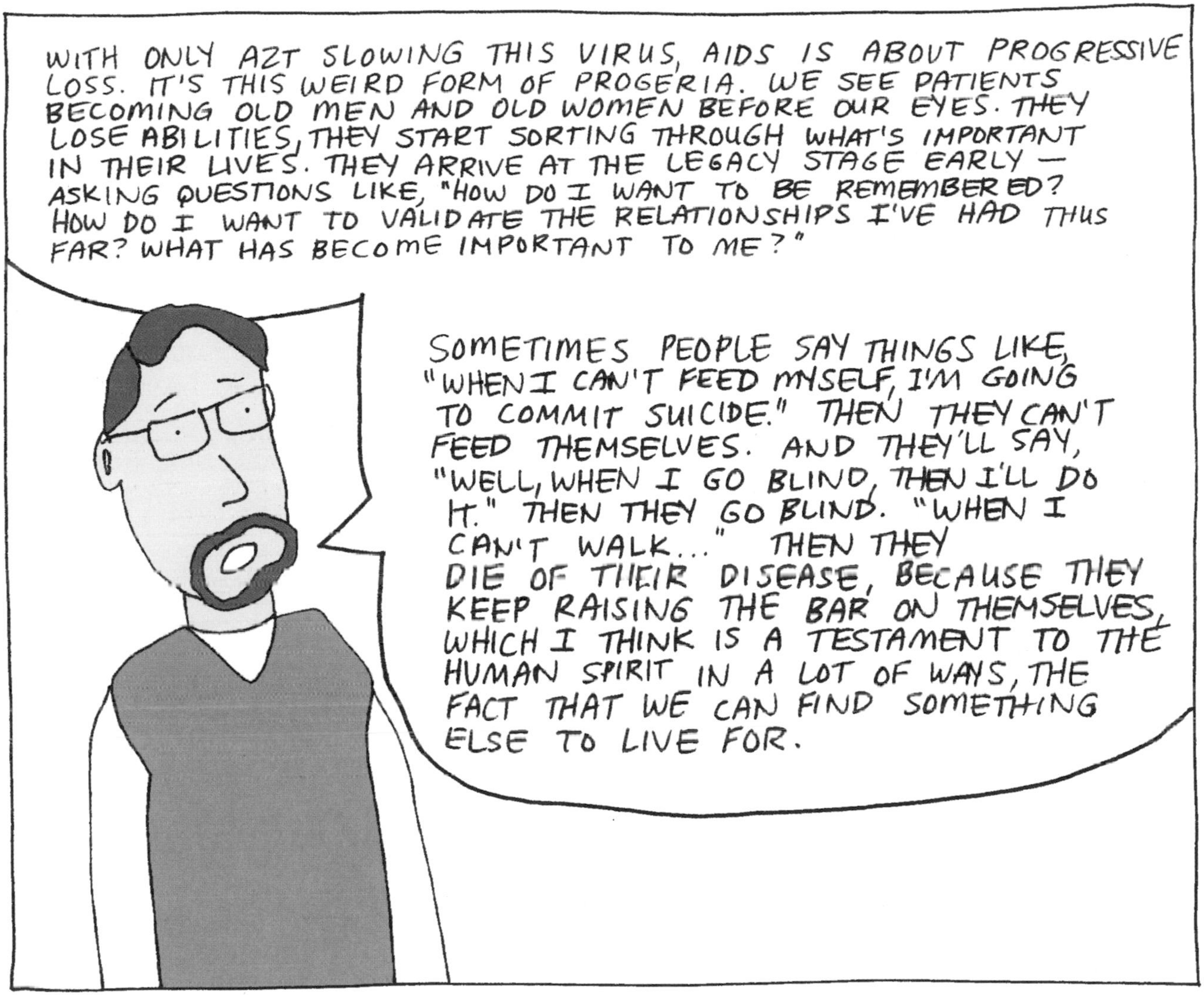
WITH ONLY AZT SLOWING THIS VIRUS, AIDS IS ABOUT PROGRESSIVE LOSS. IT'S THIS WEIRD FORM OF PROGERIA. WE SEE PATIENTS BECOMING OLD MEN AND OLD WOMEN BEFORE OUR EYES. THEY LOSE ABILITIES, THEY START SORTING THROUGH WHAT'S IMPORTANT IN THEIR LIVES. THEY ARRIVE AT THE LEGACY STAGE EARLY — ASKING QUESTIONS LIKE, "HOW DO I WANT TO BE REMEMBERED? HOW DO I WANT TO VALIDATE THE RELATIONSHIPS I'VE HAD THUS FAR? WHAT HAS BECOME IMPORTANT TO ME?"
SOMETIMES PEOPLE SAY THINGS LIKE, "WHEN I CAN'T FEED MYSELF, I'M GOING TO COMMIT SUICIDE." THEN THEY CAN'T FEED THEMSELVES. AND THEY'LL SAY, "WELL, WHEN I GO BLIND, THEN I'LL DO IT." THEN THEY GO BLIND. "WHEN I CAN'T WALK..." THEN THEY DIE OF THEIR DISEASE, BECAUSE THEY KEEP RAISING THE BAR ON THEMSELVES, WHICH I THINK IS A TESTAMENT TO THE HUMAN SPIRIT IN A LOT OF WAYS, THE FACT THAT WE CAN FIND SOMETHING ELSE TO LIVE FOR.

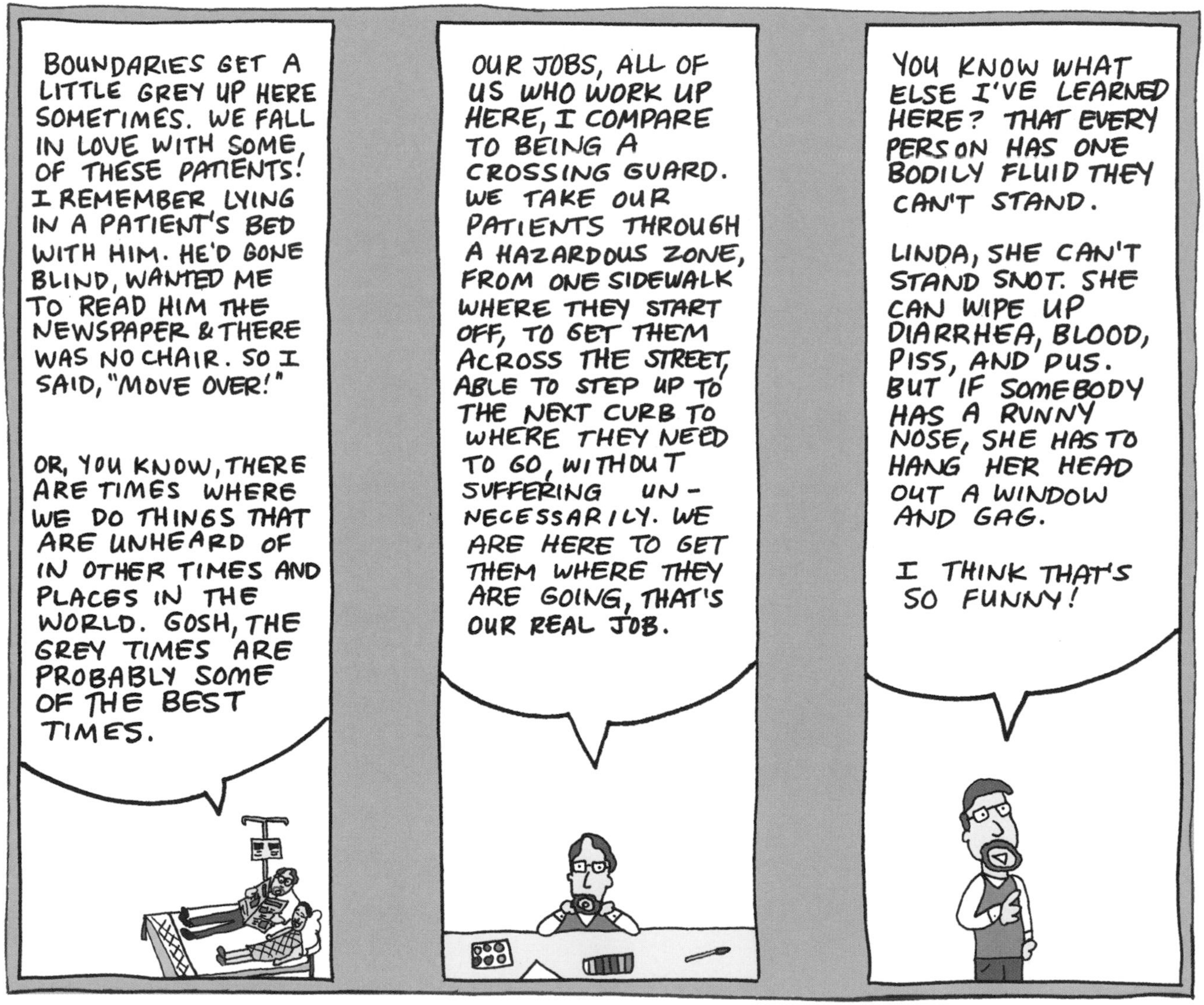
BOUNDARIES GET A LITTLE GREY UP HERE SOMETIMES. WE FALL IN LOVE WITH SOME OF THESE PATIENTS! I REMEMBER LYING IN A PATIENT'S BED WITH HIM. HE'D GONE BLIND, WANTED ME TO READ HIM THE NEWSPAPER & THERE WAS NO CHAIR. SO I SAID, "MOVE OVER!"
OR, YOU KNOW, THERE ARE TIMES WHERE WE DO THINGS THAT ARE UNHEARD OF IN OTHER TIMES AND PLACES IN THE WORLD. GOSH, THE GREY TIMES ARE PROBABLY SOME OF THE BEST TIMES.
OUR JOBS, ALL OF US WHO WORK UP HERE, I COMPARE TO BEING A CROSSING GUARD. WE TAKE OUR PATIENTS THROUGH A HAZARDOUS ZONE, FROM ONE SIDEWALK WHERE THEY START OFF, TO GET THEM ACROSS THE STREET, ABLE TO STEP UP TO THE NEXT CURB TO WHERE THEY NEED TO GO, WITHOUT SUFFERING UN-NECESSARILY. WE ARE HERE TO GET THEM WHERE THEY ARE GOING, THAT'S OUR REAL JOB.
YOU KNOW WHAT ELSE I'VE LEARNED HERE? THAT EVERY PERSON HAS ONE BODILY FLUID THEY CAN'T STAND.
LINDA, SHE CAN'T STAND SNOT. SHE CAN WIPE UP DIARRHEA, BLOOD, PISS, AND PUS. BUT IF SOMEBODY HAS A RUNNY NOSE, SHE HAS TO HANG HER HEAD OUT A WINDOW AND GAG.
I THINK THAT'S SO FUNNY!

1995

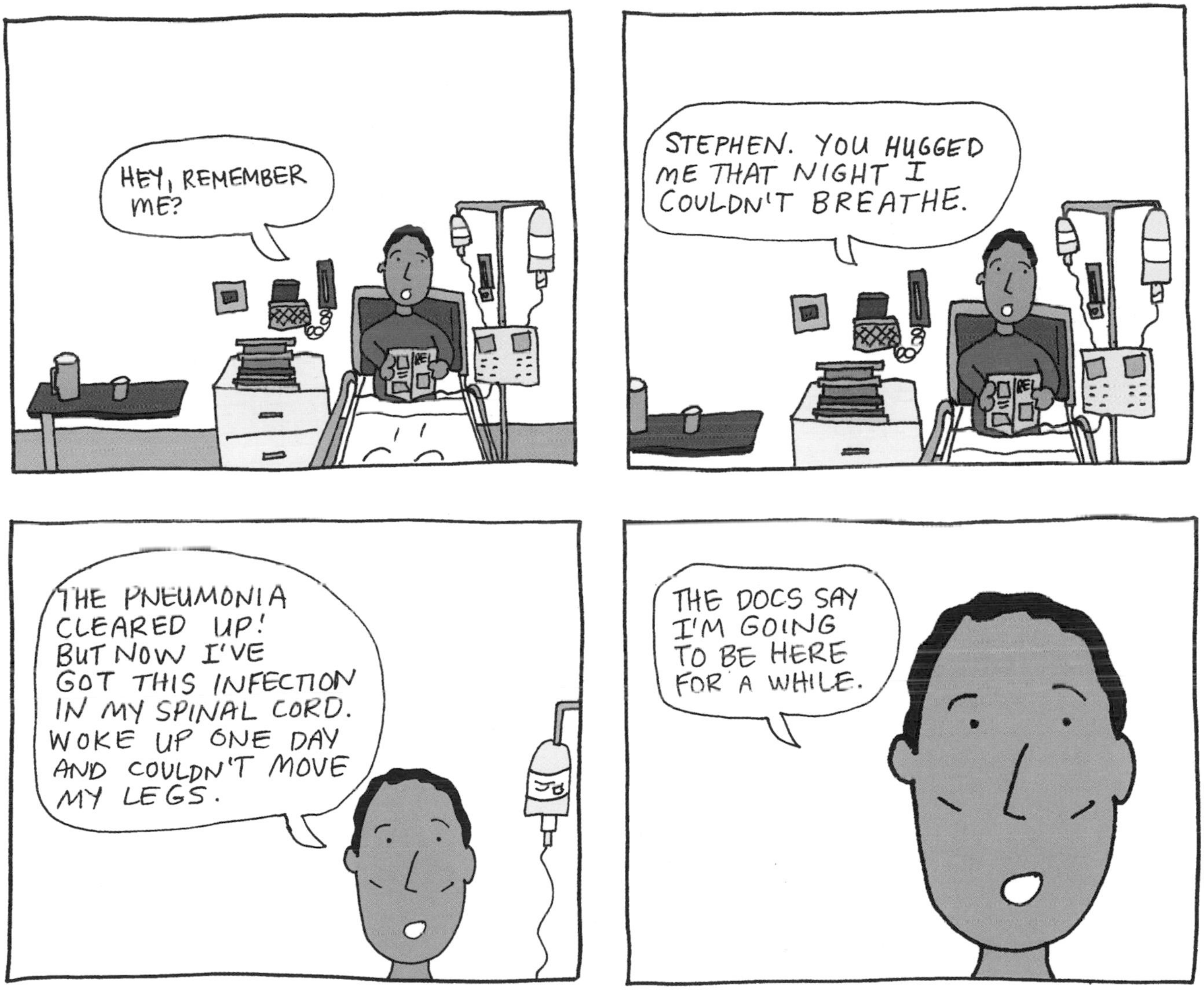
HEY, REMEMBER ME?
STEPHEN. YOU HUGGED ME THAT NIGHT I COULDN'T BREATHE.
THE PNEUMONIA CLEARED UP! BUT NOW I'VE GOT THIS INFECTION IN MY SPINAL CORD. WOKE UP ONE DAY AND COULDN'T MOVE MY LEGS.
THE DOCS SAY I'M GOING TO BE HERE FOR A WHILE.

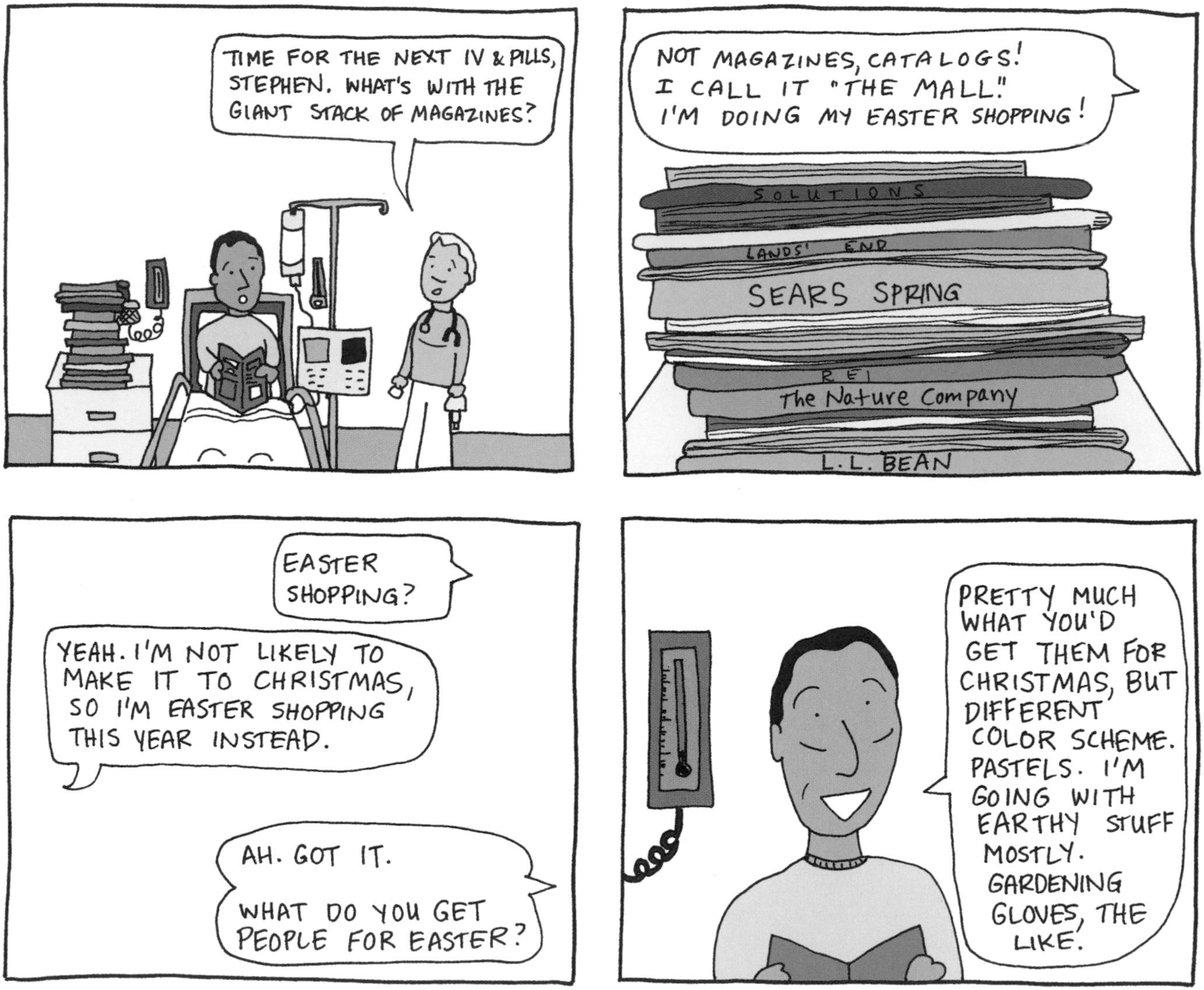
TIME FOR THE NEXT IV & PILLS, STEPHEN. WHAT'S WITH THE GIANT STACK OF MAGAZINES?
NOT MAGAZINES, CATALOGS! I CALL IT "THE MALL." I'M DOING MY EASTER SHOPPING!
SOLUTIONS
LANDS' END
SEARS SPRING
REI
The Nature Company
L.L. BEAN
EASTER SHOPPING?
YEAH. I'M NOT LIKELY TO MAKE IT TO CHRISTMAS, SO I'M EASTER SHOPPING THIS YEAR INSTEAD.
AH. GOT IT.
WHAT DO YOU GET PEOPLE FOR EASTER?
PRETTY MUCH WHAT YOU'D GET THEM FOR CHRISTMAS, BUT DIFFERENT COLOR SCHEME. PASTELS. I'M GOING WITH EARTHY STUFF MOSTLY. GARDENING GLOVES, THE LIKE.

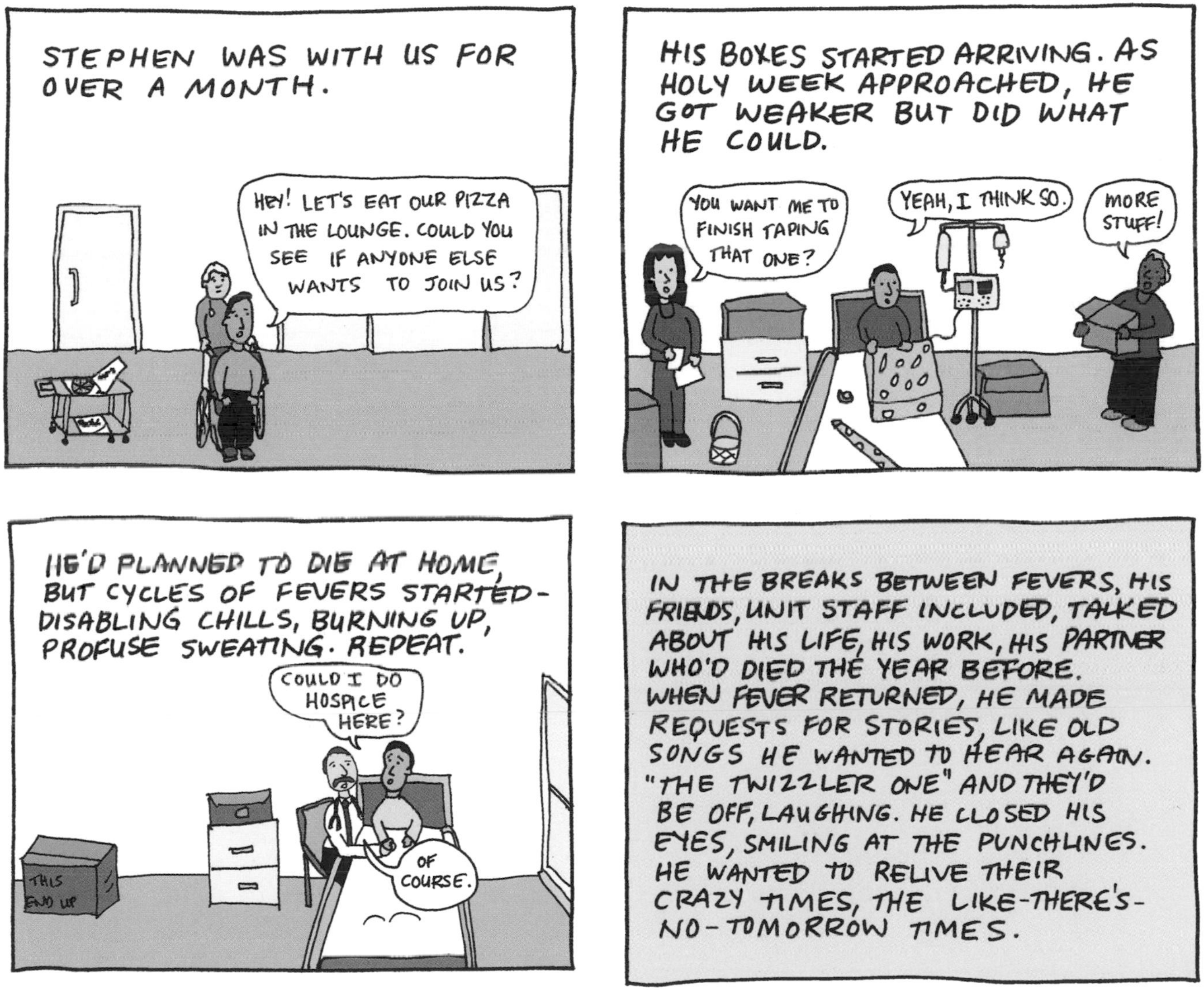
STEPHEN WAS WITH US FOR OVER A MONTH.
HEY! LET'S EAT OUR PIZZA IN THE LOUNGE. COULD YOU SEE IF ANYONE ELSE WANTS TO JOIN US?
HIS BOXES STARTED ARRIVING. AS HOLY WEEK APPROACHED, HE GOT WEAKER BUT DID WHAT HE COULD.
YOU WANT ME TO FINISH TAPING THAT ONE?
YEAH, I THINK SO.
MORE STUFF!
HE'D PLANNED TO DIE AT HOME, BUT CYCLES OF FEVERS STARTED - DISABLING CHILLS, BURNING UP, PROFUSE SWEATING. REPEAT.
COULD I DO HOSPICE HERE?
OF COURSE.
THIS END UP
IN THE BREAKS BETWEEN FEVERS, HIS FRIENDS, UNIT STAFF INCLUDED, TALKED ABOUT HIS LIFE, HIS WORK, HIS PARTNER WHO'D DIED THE YEAR BEFORE. WHEN FEVER RETURNED, HE MADE REQUESTS FOR STORIES, LIKE OLD SONGS HE WANTED TO HEAR AGAIN. "THE TWIZZLER ONE" AND THEY'D BE OFF, LAUGHING. HE CLOSED HIS EYES, SMILING AT THE PUNCHLINES. HE WANTED TO RELIVE THEIR CRAZY TIMES, THE LIKE-THERE'S-NO-TOMORROW TIMES.

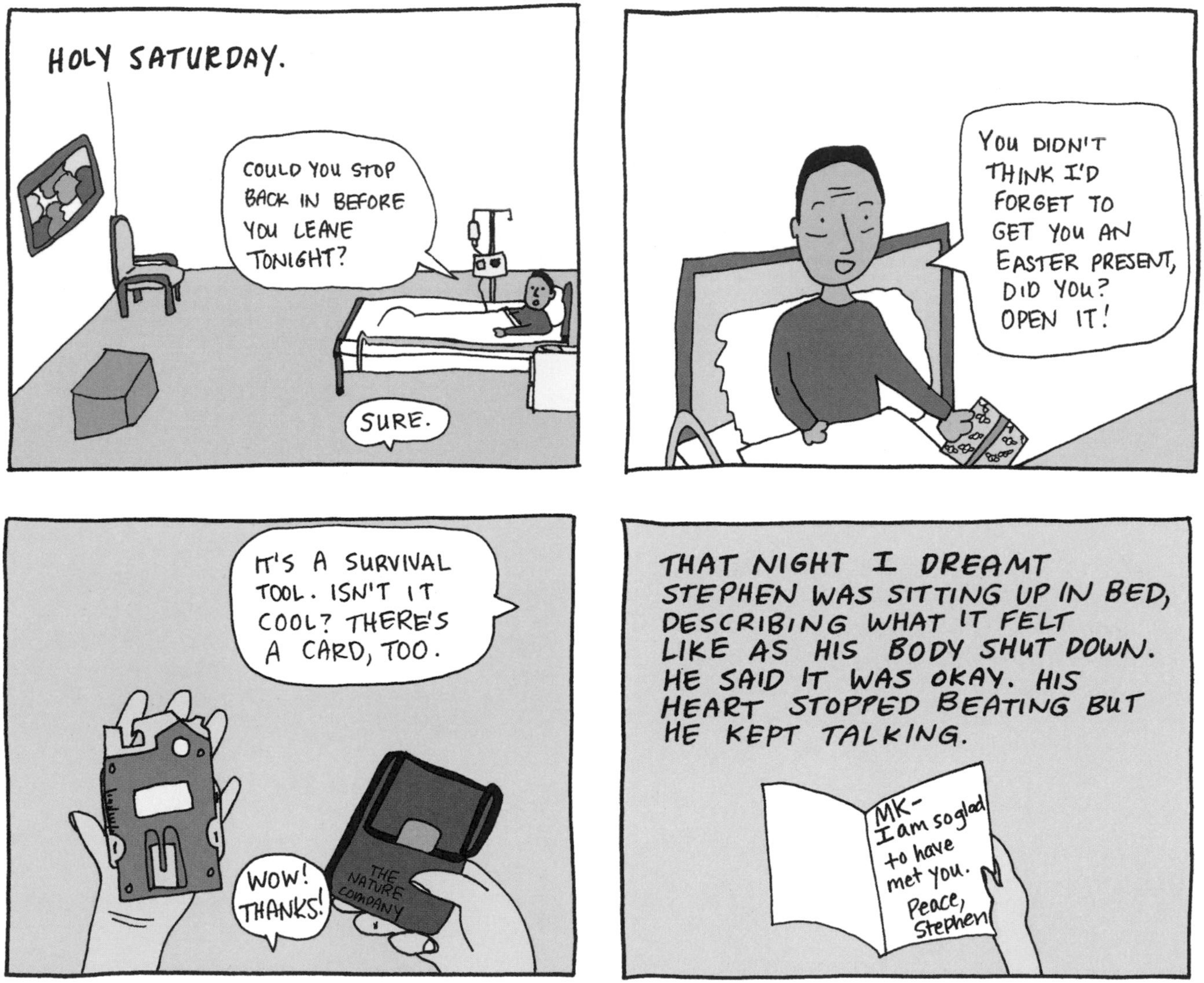
HOLY SATURDAY.
COULD YOU STOP BACK IN BEFORE YOU LEAVE TONIGHT?
SURE.
YOU DIDN'T THINK I'D FORGET TO GET YOU AN EASTER PRESENT, DID YOU? OPEN IT!
IT'S A SURVIVAL TOOL. ISN'T IT COOL? THERE'S A CARD, TOO.
WOW! THANKS!
THE NATURE COMPANY
THAT NIGHT I DREAMT STEPHEN WAS SITTING UP IN BED, DESCRIBING WHAT IT FELT LIKE AS HIS BODY SHUT DOWN. HE SAID IT WAS OKAY. HIS HEART STOPPED BEATING BUT HE KEPT TALKING.
MK- I am so glad to have met you. Peace, Stephen

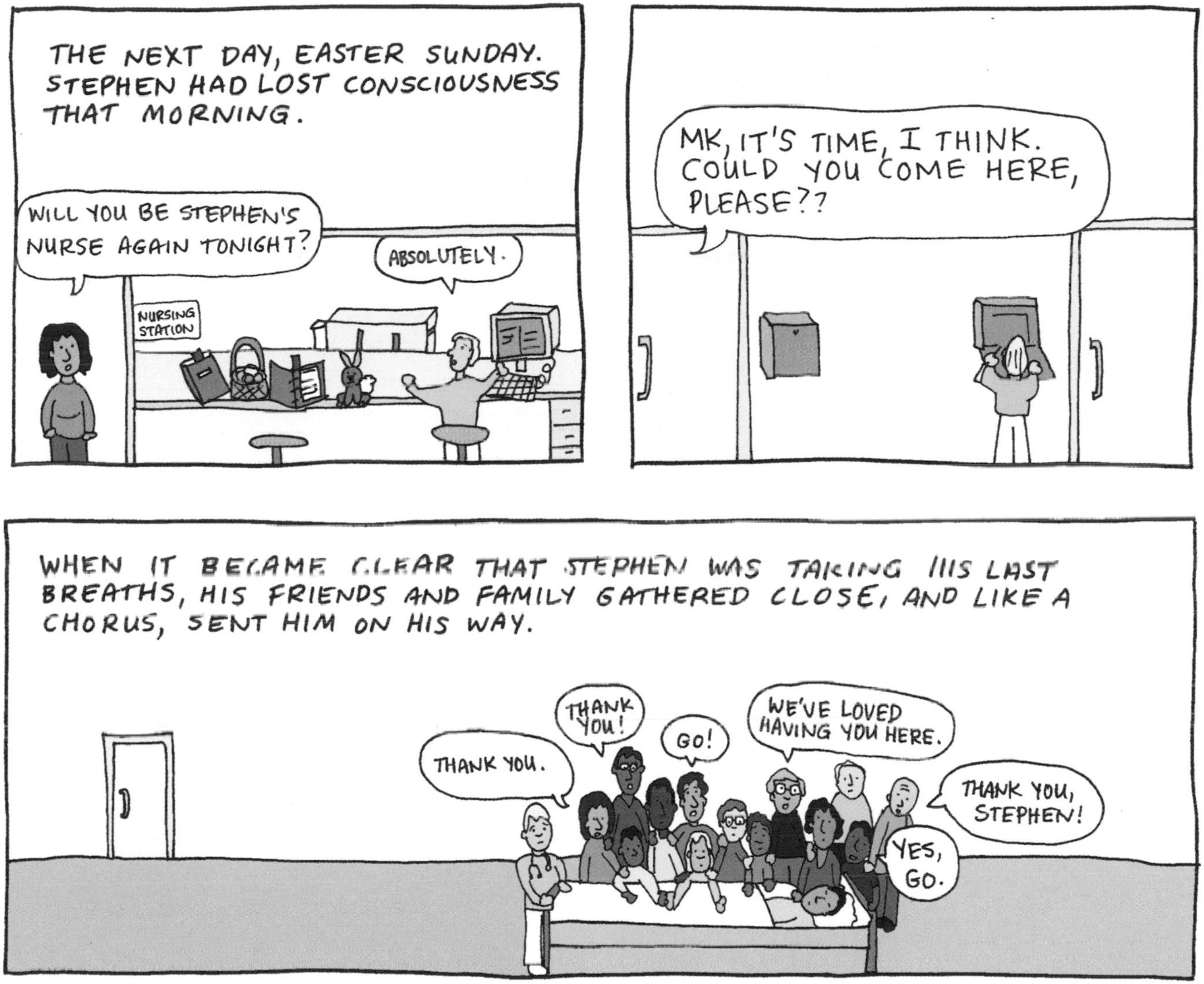
THE NEXT DAY, EASTER SUNDAY. STEPHEN HAD LOST CONSCIOUSNESS THAT MORNING.
WILL YOU BE STEPHEN'S NURSE AGAIN TONIGHT?
ABSOLUTELY.
NURSING STATION
MK, IT'S TIME, I THINK. COULD YOU COME HERE, PLEASE??
WHEN IT BECAME CLEAR THAT STEPHEN WAS TAKING HIS LAST BREATHS, HIS FRIENDS AND FAMILY GATHERED CLOSE, AND LIKE A CHORUS, SENT HIM ON HIS WAY.
THANK YOU.
THANK YOU!
GO!
WE'VE LOVED HAVING YOU HERE.
THANK YOU, STEPHEN!
YES, GO.

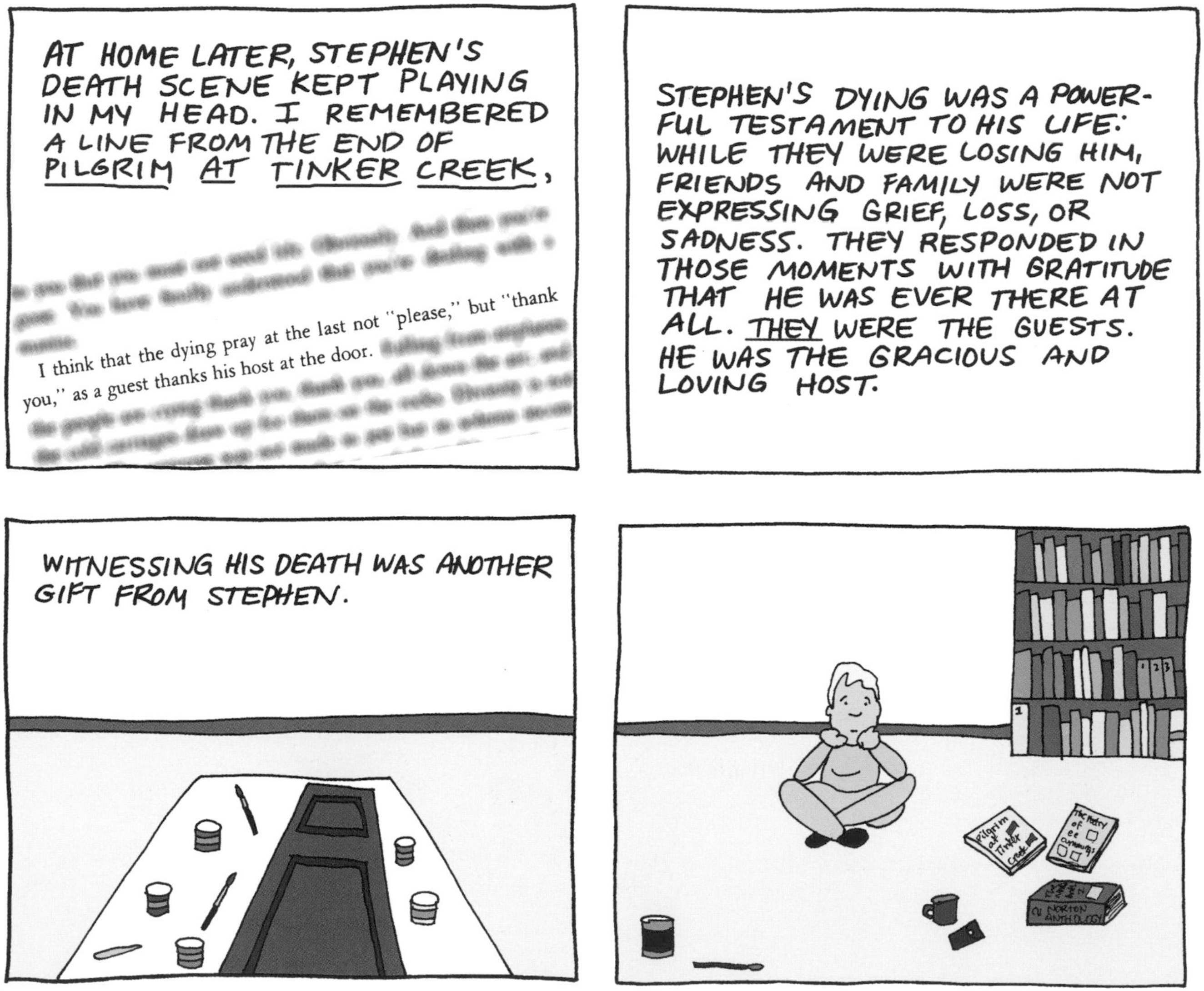
AT HOME LATER, STEPHEN'S DEATH SCENE KEPT PLAYING IN MY HEAD. I REMEMBERED A LINE FROM THE END OF PILGRIM AT TINKER CREEK,
I think that the dying pray at the last not "please," but "thank you," as a guest thanks his host at the door.
STEPHEN'S DYING WAS A POWERFUL TESTAMENT TO HIS LIFE: WHILE THEY WERE LOSING HIM, FRIENDS AND FAMILY WERE NOT EXPRESSING GRIEF, LOSS, OR SADNESS. THEY RESPONDED IN THOSE MOMENTS WITH GRATITUDE THAT HE WAS EVER THERE AT ALL. THEY WERE THE GUESTS. HE WAS THE GRACIOUS AND LOVING HOST.
WITNESSING HIS DEATH WAS ANOTHER GIFT FROM STEPHEN.
Pilgrim at Tinker Creek
NORTON ANTHOLOGY

NORTON ANTHOLOGY

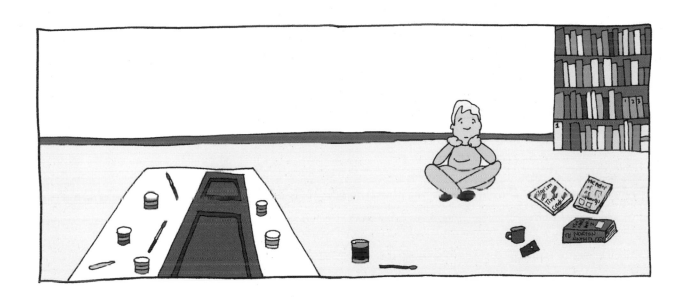

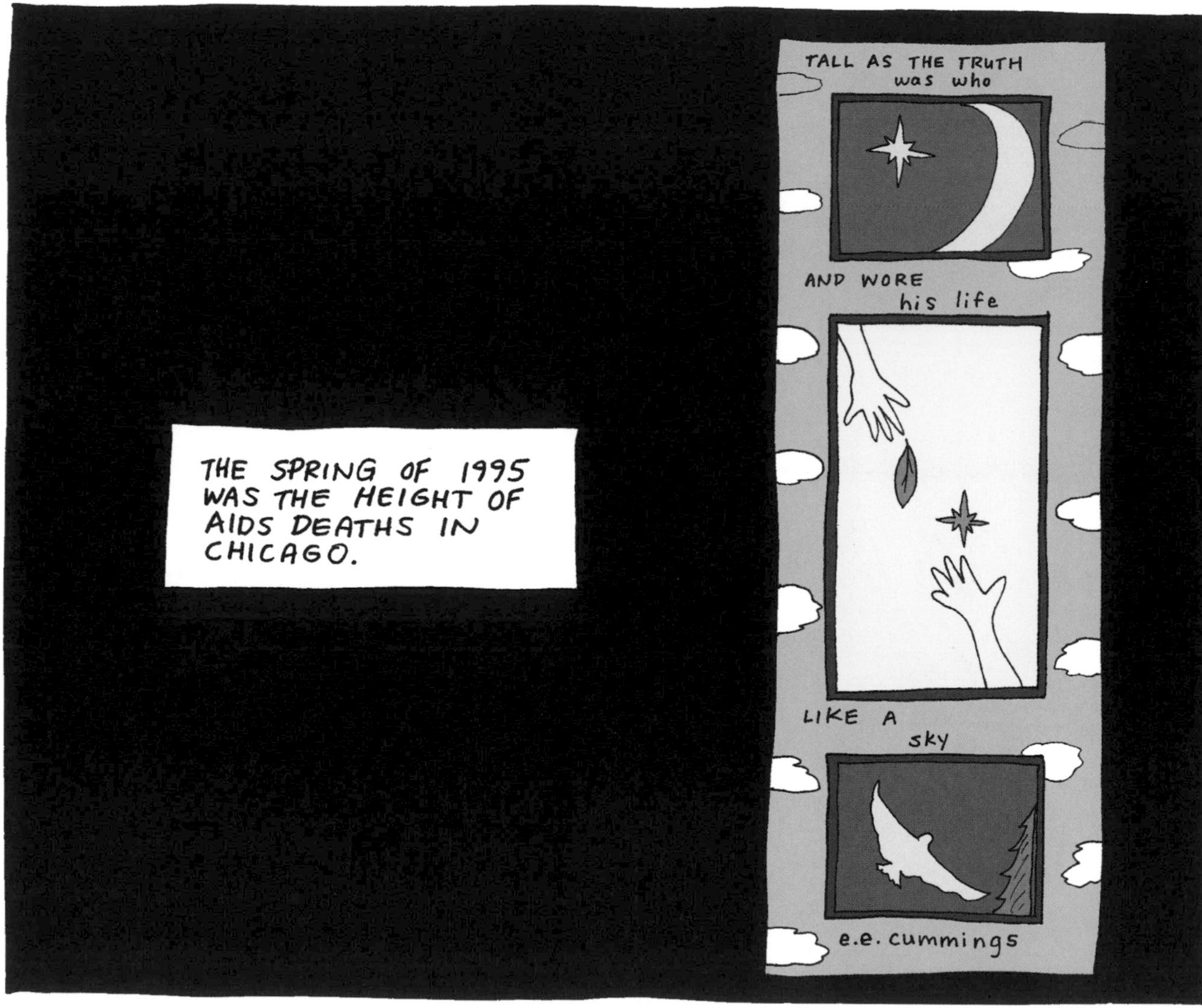
THE SPRING OF 1995 WAS THE HEIGHT OF AIDS DEATHS IN CHICAGO.
TALL AS THE TRUTH
was who
AND WORE
his life
LIKE A
sky
e.e. cummings

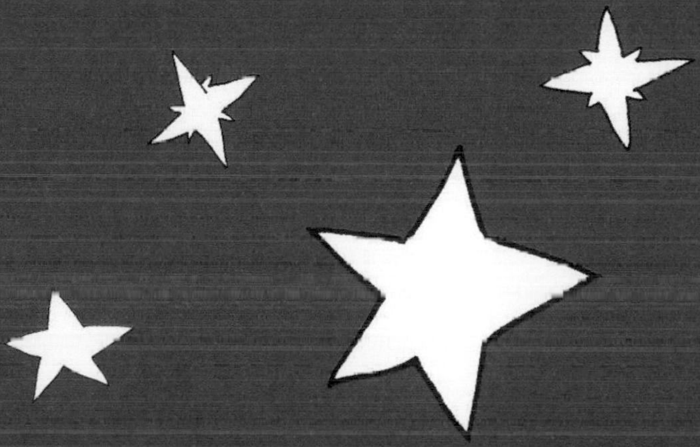

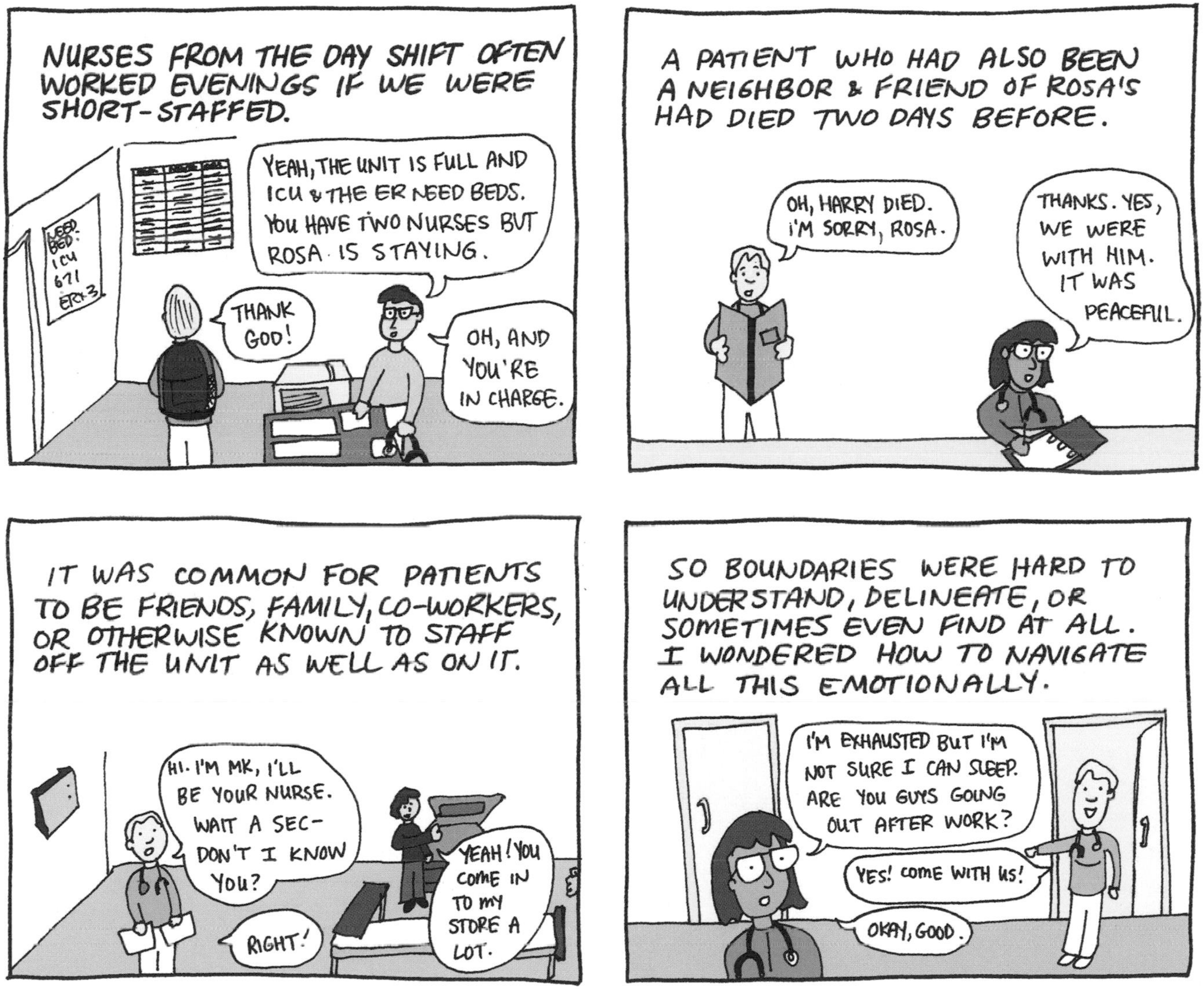
NURSES FROM THE DAY SHIFT OFTEN WORKED EVENINGS IF WE WERE SHORT-STAFFED.
YEAH, THE UNIT IS FULL AND ICU & THE ER NEED BEDS. YOU HAVE TWO NURSES BUT ROSA IS STAYING.
THANK GOD!
OH, AND YOU'RE IN CHARGE.
A PATIENT WHO HAD ALSO BEEN A NEIGHBOR & FRIEND OF ROSA'S HAD DIED TWO DAYS BEFORE.
OH, HARRY DIED. I'M SORRY, ROSA.
THANKS. YES, WE WERE WITH HIM. IT WAS PEACEFUL.
IT WAS COMMON FOR PATIENTS TO BE FRIENDS, FAMILY, CO-WORKERS, OR OTHERWISE KNOWN TO STAFF OFF THE UNIT AS WELL AS ON IT.
HI. I'M MK, I'LL BE YOUR NURSE. WAIT A SEC- DON'T I KNOW YOU?
RIGHT!
YEAH! YOU COME IN TO MY STORE A LOT.
SO BOUNDARIES WERE HARD TO UNDERSTAND, DELINEATE, OR SOMETIMES EVEN FIND AT ALL. I WONDERED HOW TO NAVIGATE ALL THIS EMOTIONALLY.
I'M EXHAUSTED BUT I'M NOT SURE I CAN SLEEP. ARE YOU GUYS GOING OUT AFTER WORK?
YES! COME WITH US!
OKAY, GOOD.

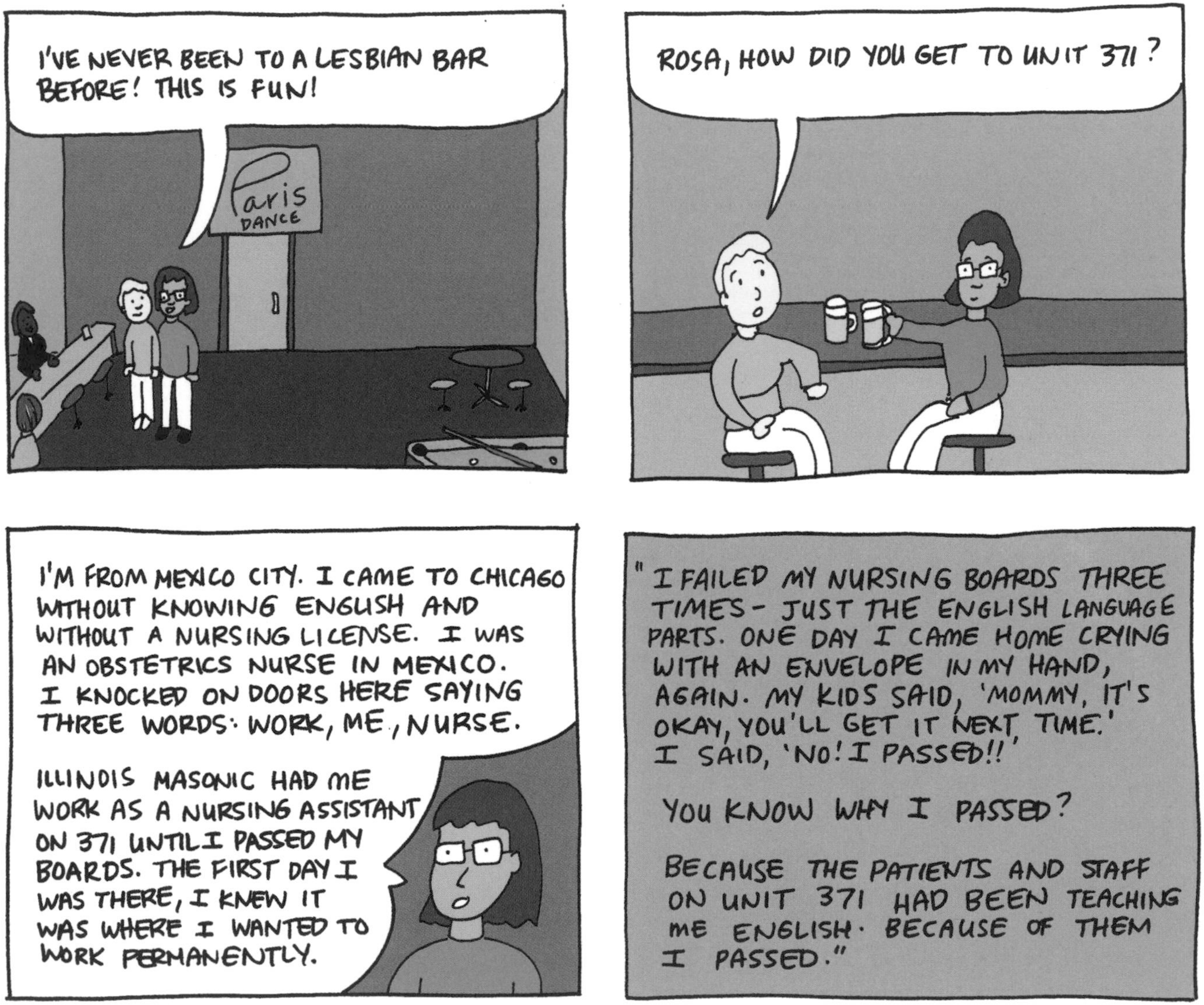
I'VE NEVER BEEN TO A LESBIAN BAR BEFORE! THIS IS FUN!
Paris DANCE
ROSA, HOW DID YOU GET TO UNIT 371?
I'M FROM MEXICO CITY. I CAME TO CHICAGO WITHOUT KNOWING ENGLISH AND WITHOUT A NURSING LICENSE. I WAS AN OBSTETRICS NURSE IN MEXICO. I KNOCKED ON DOORS HERE SAYING THREE WORDS: WORK, ME, NURSE.
ILLINOIS MASONIC HAD ME WORK AS A NURSING ASSISTANT ON 371 UNTIL I PASSED MY BOARDS. THE FIRST DAY I WAS THERE, I KNEW IT WAS WHERE I WANTED TO WORK PERMANENTLY.
"I FAILED MY NURSING BOARDS THREE TIMES - JUST THE ENGLISH LANGUAGE PARTS. ONE DAY I CAME HOME CRYING WITH AN ENVELOPE IN MY HAND, AGAIN. MY KIDS SAID, 'MOMMY, IT'S OKAY, YOU'LL GET IT NEXT TIME.' I SAID, 'NO! I PASSED!!'
YOU KNOW WHY I PASSED?
BECAUSE THE PATIENTS AND STAFF ON UNIT 371 HAD BEEN TEACHING ME ENGLISH. BECAUSE OF THEM I PASSED."

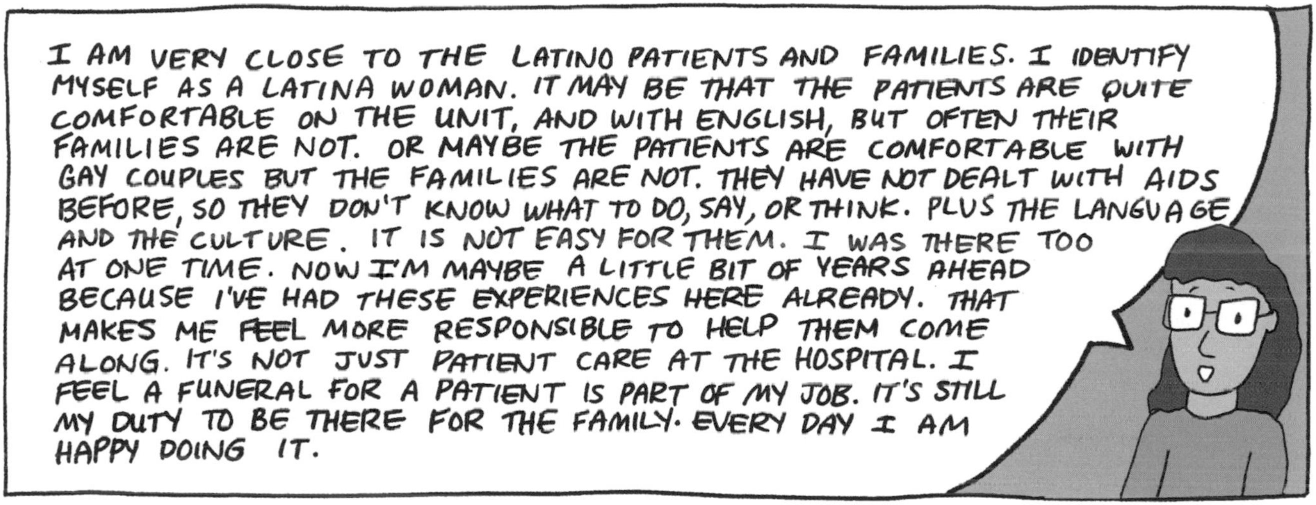
I AM VERY CLOSE TO THE LATINO PATIENTS AND FAMILIES. I IDENTIFY MYSELF AS A LATINA WOMAN. IT MAY BE THAT THE PATIENTS ARE QUITE COMFORTABLE ON THE UNIT, AND WITH ENGLISH, BUT OFTEN THEIR FAMILIES ARE NOT. OR MAYBE THE PATIENTS ARE COMFORTABLE WITH GAY COUPLES BUT THE FAMILIES ARE NOT. THEY HAVE NOT DEALT WITH AIDS BEFORE, SO THEY DON'T KNOW WHAT TO DO, SAY, OR THINK. PLUS THE LANGUAGE AND THE CULTURE. IT IS NOT EASY FOR THEM. I WAS THERE TOO AT ONE TIME. NOW I'M MAYBE A LITTLE BIT OF YEARS AHEAD BECAUSE I'VE HAD THESE EXPERIENCES HERE ALREADY. THAT MAKES ME FEEL MORE RESPONSIBLE TO HELP THEM COME ALONG. IT'S NOT JUST PATIENT CARE AT THE HOSPITAL. I FEEL A FUNERAL FOR A PATIENT IS PART OF MY JOB. IT'S STILL MY DUTY TO BE THERE FOR THE FAMILY. EVERY DAY I AM HAPPY DOING IT.

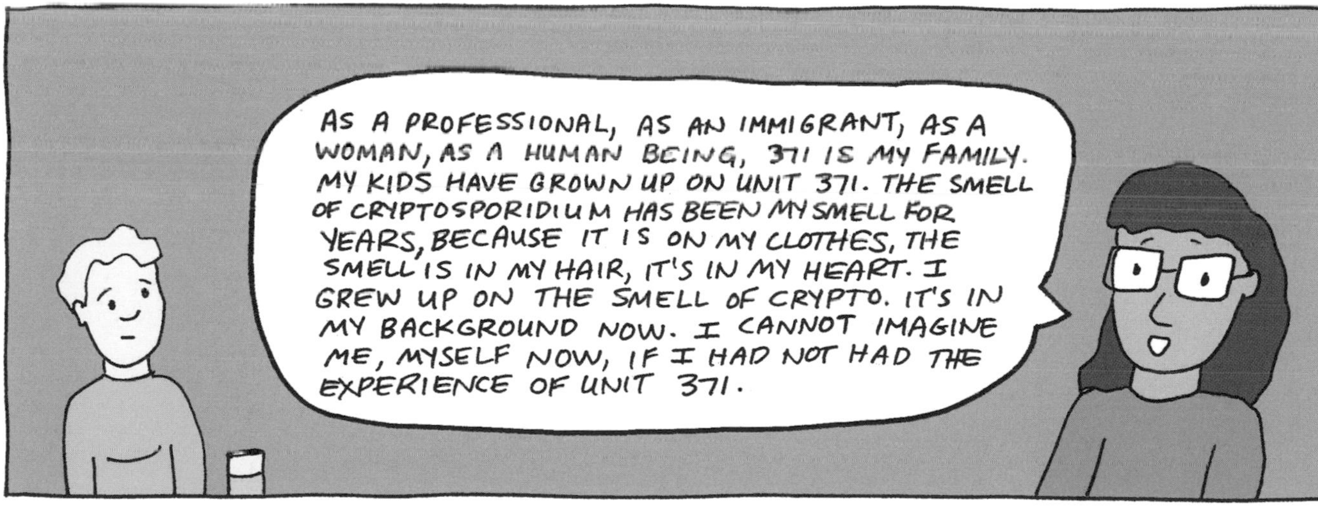
AS A PROFESSIONAL, AS AN IMMIGRANT, AS A WOMAN, AS A HUMAN BEING, 371 IS MY FAMILY. MY KIDS HAVE GROWN UP ON UNIT 371. THE SMELL OF CRYPTOSPORIDIUM HAS BEEN MY SMELL FOR YEARS, BECAUSE IT IS ON MY CLOTHES, THE SMELL IS IN MY HAIR, IT'S IN MY HEART. I GREW UP ON THE SMELL OF CRYPTO. IT'S IN MY BACKGROUND NOW. I CANNOT IMAGINE ME, MYSELF NOW, IF I HAD NOT HAD THE EXPERIENCE OF UNIT 371.

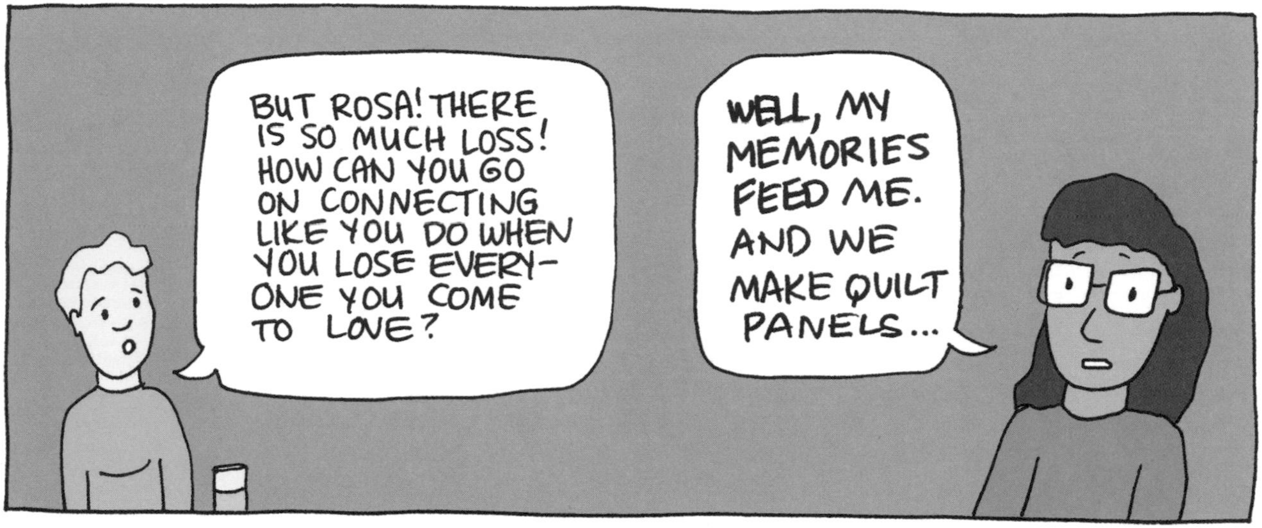
BUT ROSA! THERE IS SO MUCH LOSS! HOW CAN YOU GO ON CONNECTING LIKE YOU DO WHEN YOU LOSE EVERY-ONE YOU COME TO LOVE?
WELL, MY MEMORIES FEED ME. AND WE MAKE QUILT PANELS...

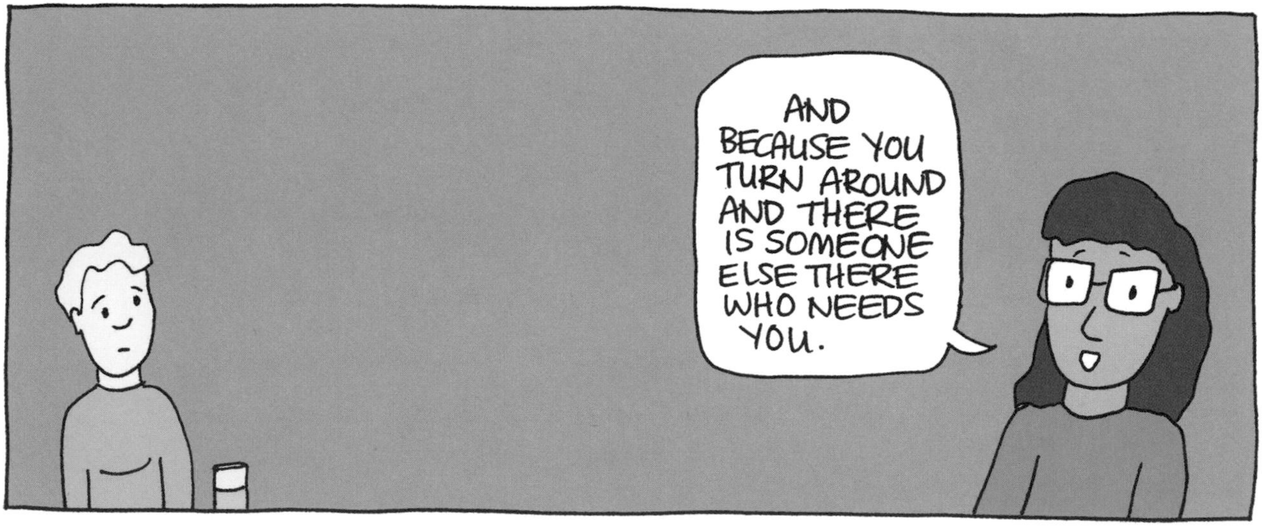
AND BECAUSE YOU TURN AROUND AND THERE IS SOMEONE ELSE THERE WHO NEEDS YOU.

IN A DREAM, I DROVE A ROAD CIRCLING A LARGE BLACK LAKE.

I WAS TO CATCH A TRAIN PULLING INTO A STATION ACROSS THE LAKE.

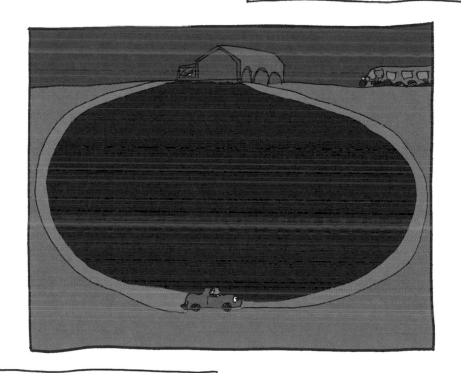

THE ONLY WAY TO MAKE THE TRAIN WAS TO GET OUT OF THE CAR AND SWIM ACROSS THE BLACK LAKE.

SO I DID. IT WAS SILENT, WARM, AND VERY PEACEFUL.

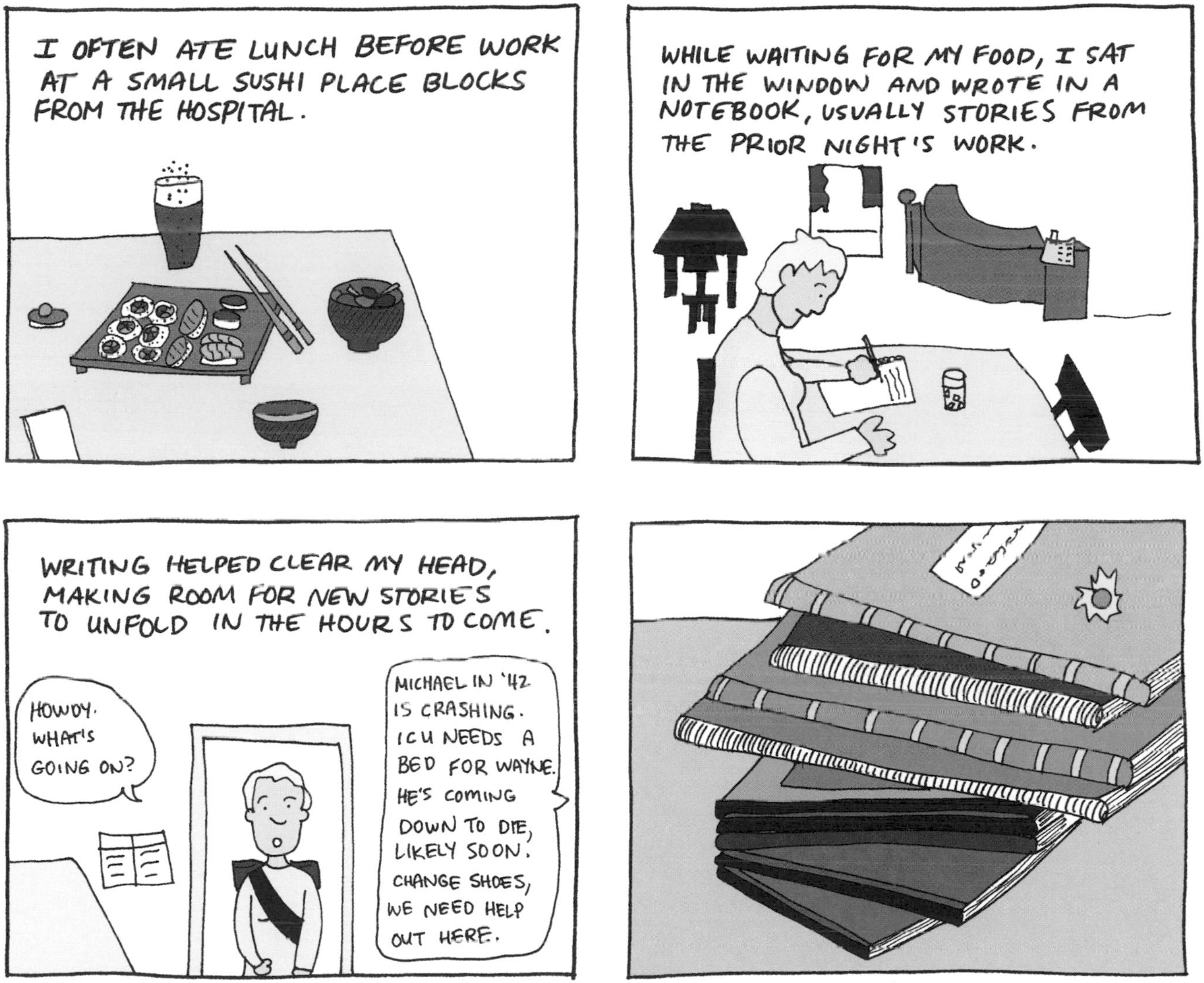
I OFTEN ATE LUNCH BEFORE WORK AT A SMALL SUSHI PLACE BLOCKS FROM THE HOSPITAL.
WHILE WAITING FOR MY FOOD, I SAT IN THE WINDOW AND WROTE IN A NOTEBOOK, USUALLY STORIES FROM THE PRIOR NIGHT'S WORK.
WRITING HELPED CLEAR MY HEAD, MAKING ROOM FOR NEW STORIES TO UNFOLD IN THE HOURS TO COME.
HOWDY. WHAT'S GOING ON?
MICHAEL IN '42 IS CRASHING. ICU NEEDS A BED FOR WAYNE. HE'S COMING DOWN TO DIE, LIKELY SOON. CHANGE SHOES, WE NEED HELP OUT HERE.

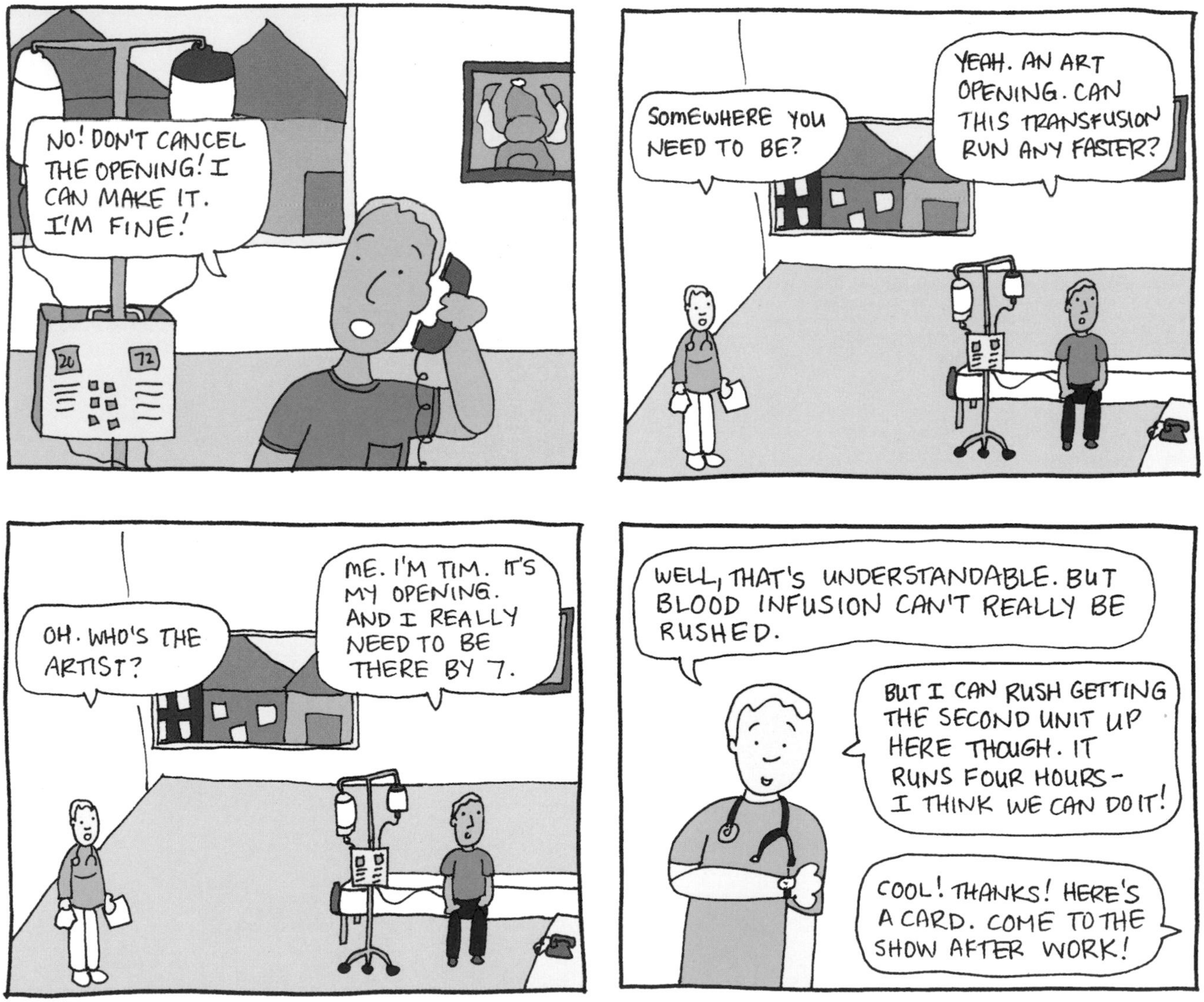
NO! DON'T CANCEL THE OPENING! I CAN MAKE IT. I'M FINE!
20
72
SOMEWHERE YOU NEED TO BE?
YEAH. AN ART OPENING. CAN THIS TRANSFUSION RUN ANY FASTER?
OH. WHO'S THE ARTIST?
ME. I'M TIM. IT'S MY OPENING. AND I REALLY NEED TO BE THERE BY 7.
WELL, THAT'S UNDERSTANDABLE. BUT BLOOD INFUSION CAN'T REALLY BE RUSHED.
BUT I CAN RUSH GETTING THE SECOND UNIT UP HERE THOUGH. IT RUNS FOUR HOURS- I THINK WE CAN DO IT!
COOL! THANKS! HERE'S A CARD. COME TO THE SHOW AFTER WORK!

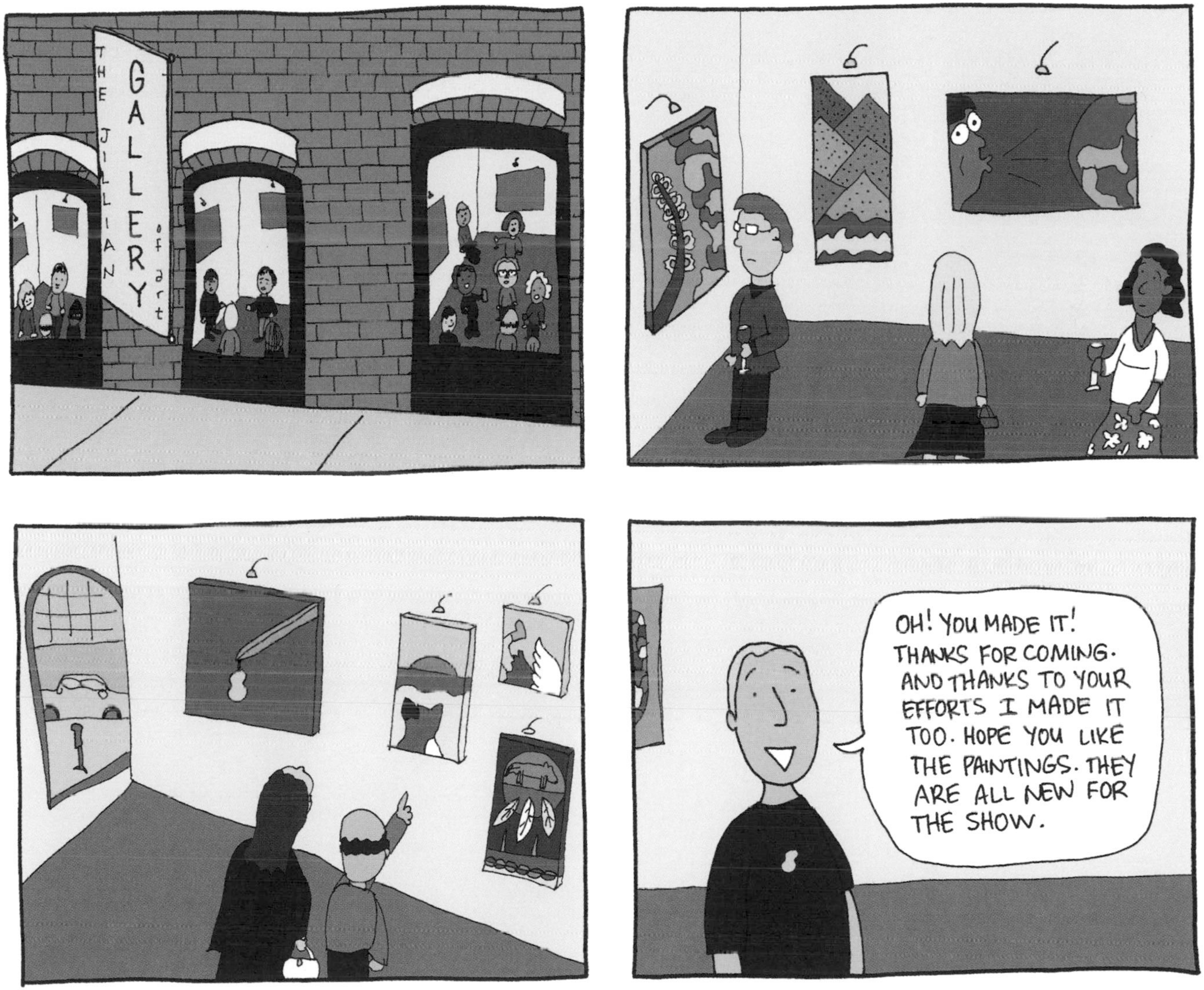
THE JILLIAN GALLERY of art
OH! YOU MADE IT! THANKS FOR COMING. AND THANKS TO YOUR EFFORTS I MADE IT TOO. HOPE YOU LIKE THE PAINTINGS. THEY ARE ALL NEW FOR THE SHOW.

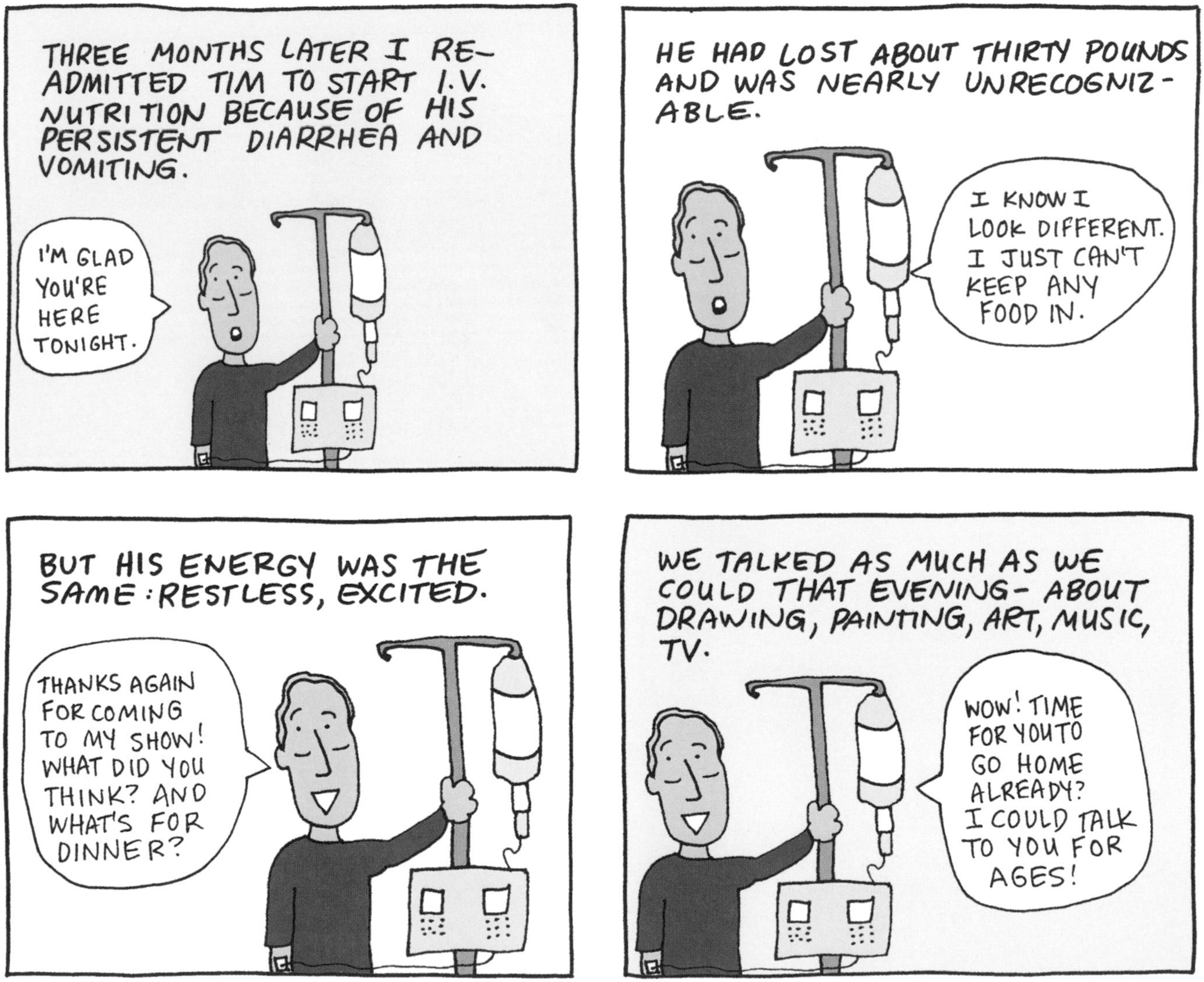
THREE MONTHS LATER I RE-ADMITTED TIM TO START I.V. NUTRITION BECAUSE OF HIS PERSISTENT DIARRHEA AND VOMITING.
I'M GLAD YOU'RE HERE TONIGHT.
HE HAD LOST ABOUT THIRTY POUNDS AND WAS NEARLY UNRECOGNIZ-ABLE.
I KNOW I LOOK DIFFERENT. I JUST CAN'T KEEP ANY FOOD IN.
BUT HIS ENERGY WAS THE SAME: RESTLESS, EXCITED.
THANKS AGAIN FOR COMING TO MY SHOW! WHAT DID YOU THINK? AND WHAT'S FOR DINNER?
WE TALKED AS MUCH AS WE COULD THAT EVENING- ABOUT DRAWING, PAINTING, ART, MUSIC, TV.
WOW! TIME FOR YOU TO GO HOME ALREADY? I COULD TALK TO YOU FOR AGES!

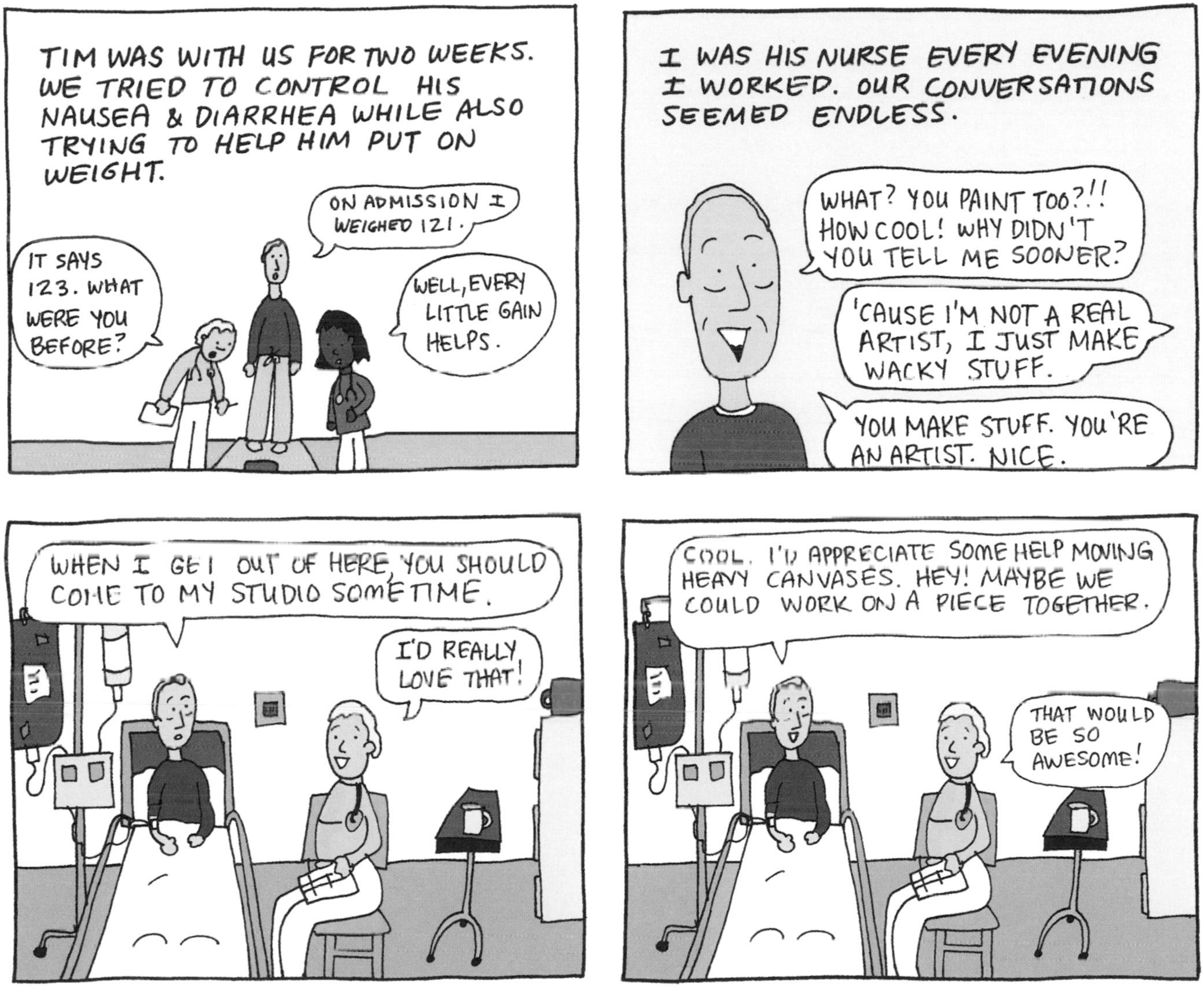
TIM WAS WITH US FOR TWO WEEKS. WE TRIED TO CONTROL HIS NAUSEA & DIARRHEA WHILE ALSO TRYING TO HELP HIM PUT ON WEIGHT.
IT SAYS 123. WHAT WERE YOU BEFORE?
ON ADMISSION I WEIGHED 121.
WELL, EVERY LITTLE GAIN HELPS.
I WAS HIS NURSE EVERY EVENING I WORKED. OUR CONVERSATIONS SEEMED ENDLESS.
WHAT? YOU PAINT TOO?!! HOW COOL! WHY DIDN'T YOU TELL ME SOONER?
'CAUSE I'M NOT A REAL ARTIST, I JUST MAKE WACKY STUFF.
YOU MAKE STUFF. YOU'RE AN ARTIST. NICE.
WHEN I GET OUT OF HERE, YOU SHOULD COME TO MY STUDIO SOMETIME.
I'D REALLY LOVE THAT!
COOL. I'D APPRECIATE SOME HELP MOVING HEAVY CANVASES. HEY! MAYBE WE COULD WORK ON A PIECE TOGETHER.
THAT WOULD BE SO AWESOME!

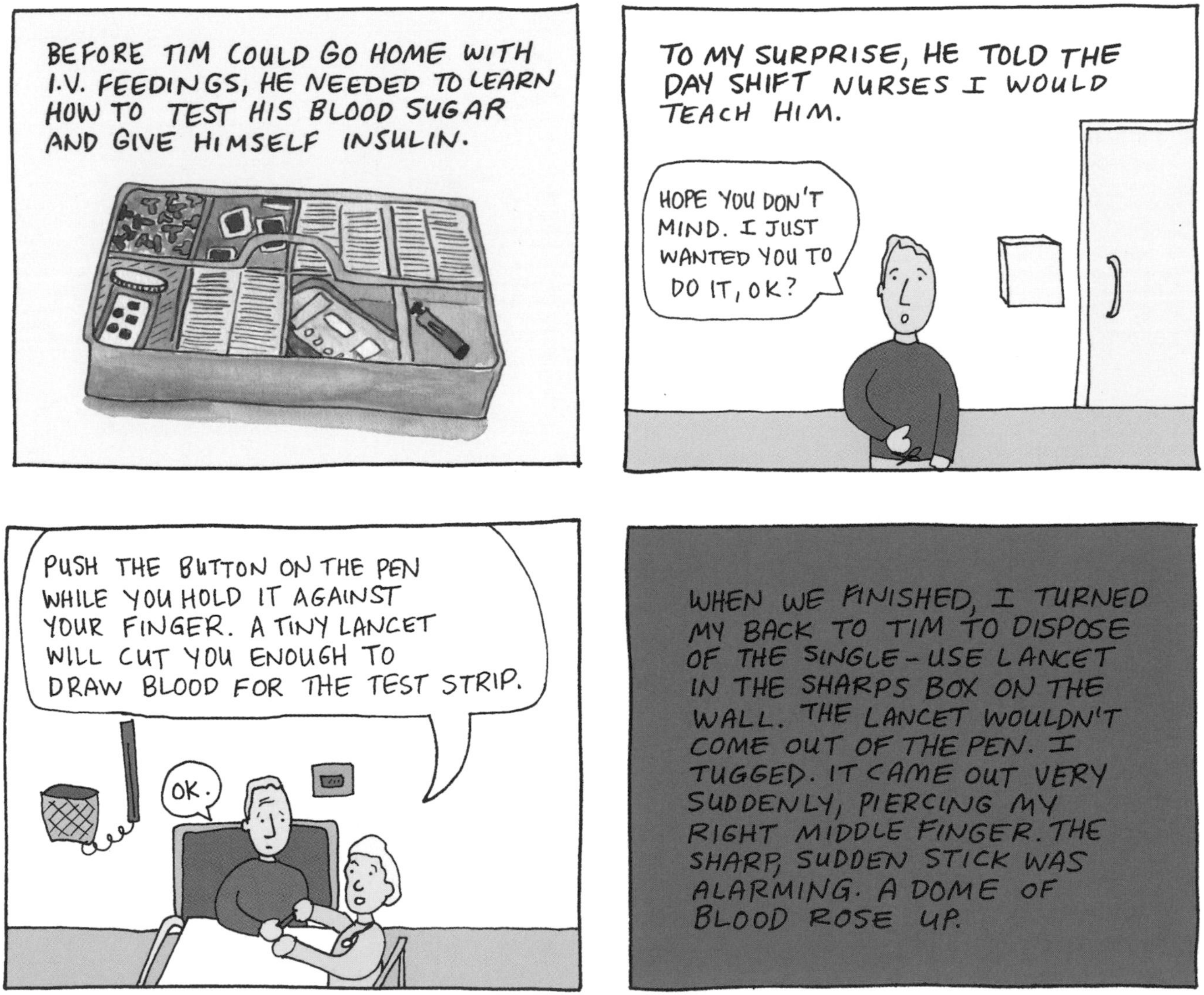
BEFORE TIM COULD GO HOME WITH I.V. FEEDINGS, HE NEEDED TO LEARN HOW TO TEST HIS BLOOD SUGAR AND GIVE HIMSELF INSULIN.
TO MY SURPRISE, HE TOLD THE DAY SHIFT NURSES I WOULD TEACH HIM.
HOPE YOU DON'T MIND. I JUST WANTED YOU TO DO IT, OK?
PUSH THE BUTTON ON THE PEN WHILE YOU HOLD IT AGAINST YOUR FINGER. A TINY LANCET WILL CUT YOU ENOUGH TO DRAW BLOOD FOR THE TEST STRIP.
OK.
WHEN WE FINISHED, I TURNED MY BACK TO TIM TO DISPOSE OF THE SINGLE-USE LANCET IN THE SHARPS BOX ON THE WALL. THE LANCET WOULDN'T COME OUT OF THE PEN. I TUGGED. IT CAME OUT VERY SUDDENLY, PIERCING MY RIGHT MIDDLE FINGER. THE SHARP, SUDDEN STICK WAS ALARMING. A DOME OF BLOOD ROSE UP.

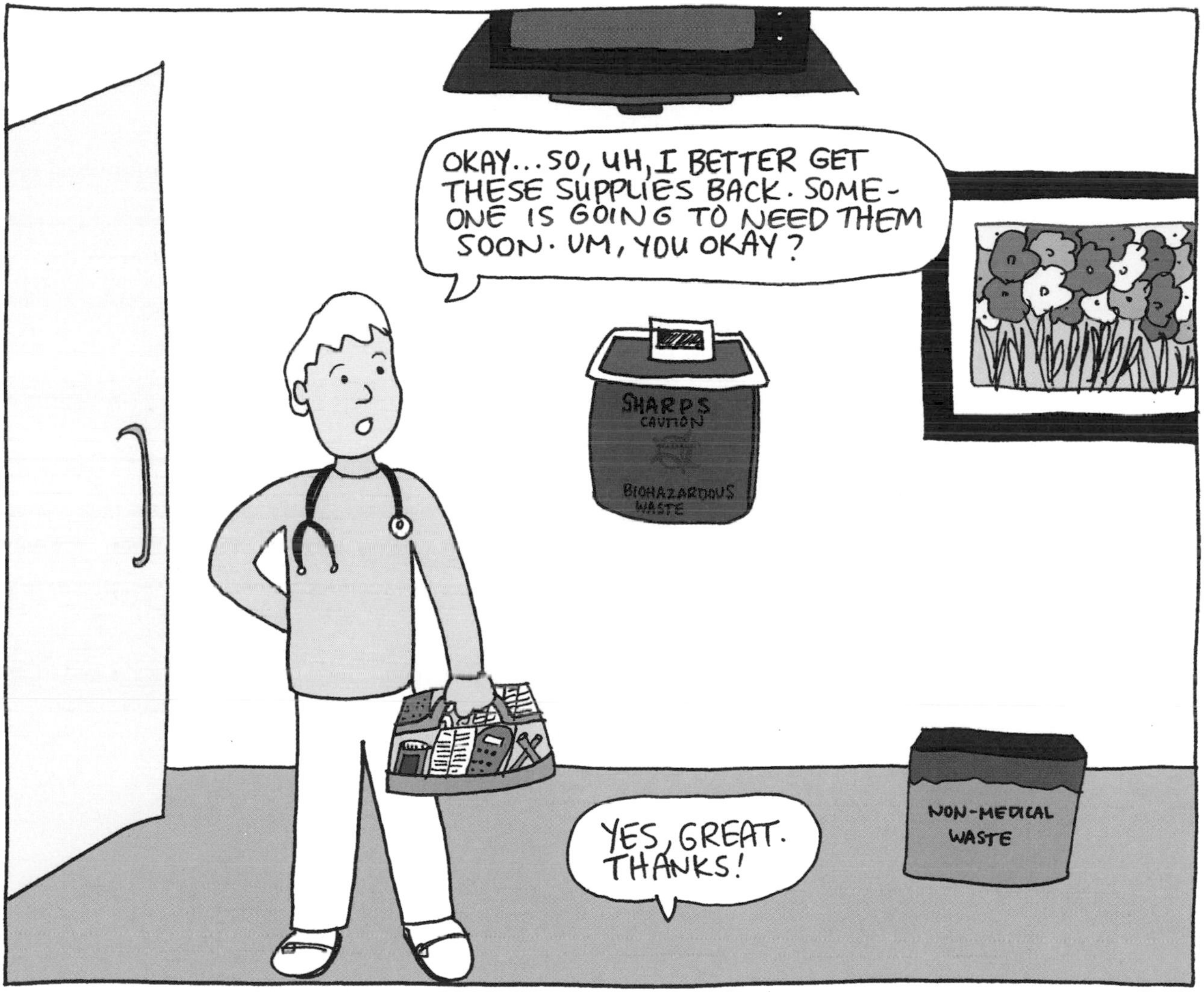
OKAY... SO, UH, I BETTER GET THESE SUPPLIES BACK. SOME-ONE IS GOING TO NEED THEM SOON. UM, YOU OKAY?
SHARPS
CAUTION
BIOHAZARDOUS WASTE
YES, GREAT. THANKS!
NON-MEDICAL WASTE

I RAN
MEDICATION ROOM
STAFF ONLY
AND RINSED
AND SQUEEZED
THEN FROZE.
NOW WHAT?
MEDKARTS

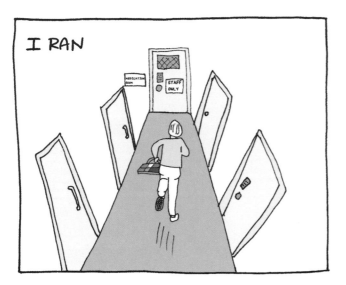

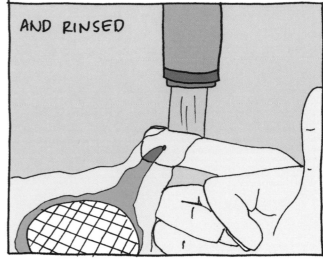

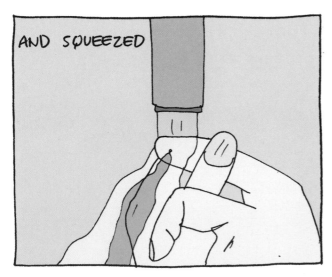

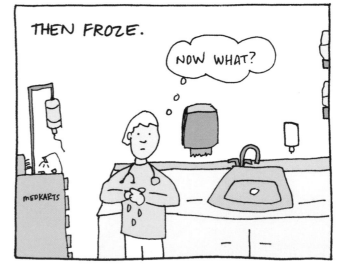

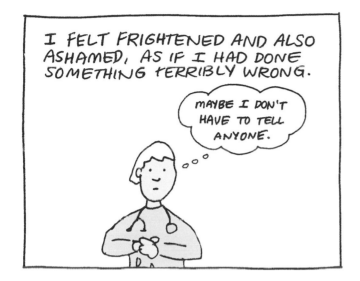

I FELT FRIGHTENED AND ALSO ASHAMED, AS IF I HAD DONE SOMETHING TERRIBLY WRONG.

MAYBE I DON'T HAVE TO TELL ANYONE.

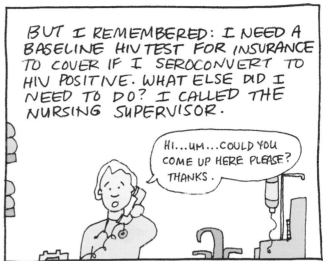

BUT I REMEMBERED: I NEED A BASELINE HIV TEST FOR INSURANCE TO COVER IF I SEROCONVERT TO HIV POSITIVE. WHAT ELSE DID I NEED TO DO? I CALLED THE NURSING SUPERVISOR.

HI...UM...COULD YOU COME UP HERE PLEASE? THANKS.

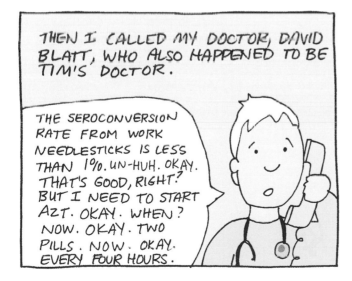

THEN I CALLED MY DOCTOR, DAVID BLATT, WHO ALSO HAPPENED TO BE TIM'S DOCTOR.

THE SEROCONVERSION RATE FROM WORK NEEDLESTICKS IS LESS THAN 1%. UN-HUH. OKAY. THAT'S GOOD, RIGHT? BUT I NEED TO START AZT. OKAY. WHEN? NOW. OKAY. TWO PILLS. NOW. OKAY. EVERY FOUR HOURS.

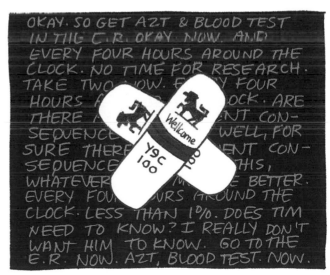

OKAY. SO GET AZT & BLOOD TEST IN THE E.R. OKAY NOW. AND EVERY FOUR HOURS AROUND THE CLOCK. NO TIME FOR RESEARCH. TAKE TWO NOW. EVERY FOUR HOURS AROUND THE CLOCK. ARE THERE ANY DIFFERENT CON- SEQUENCES... WELL, FOR SURE THERE'S DIFFERENT CON- SEQUENCES... TO THIS, WHATEVER MAKES ME BETTER. EVERY FOUR HOURS AROUND THE CLOCK. LESS THAN 1%. DOES TIM NEED TO KNOW? I REALLY DON'T WANT HIM TO KNOW. GO TO THE E.R. NOW. AZT, BLOOD TEST. NOW.

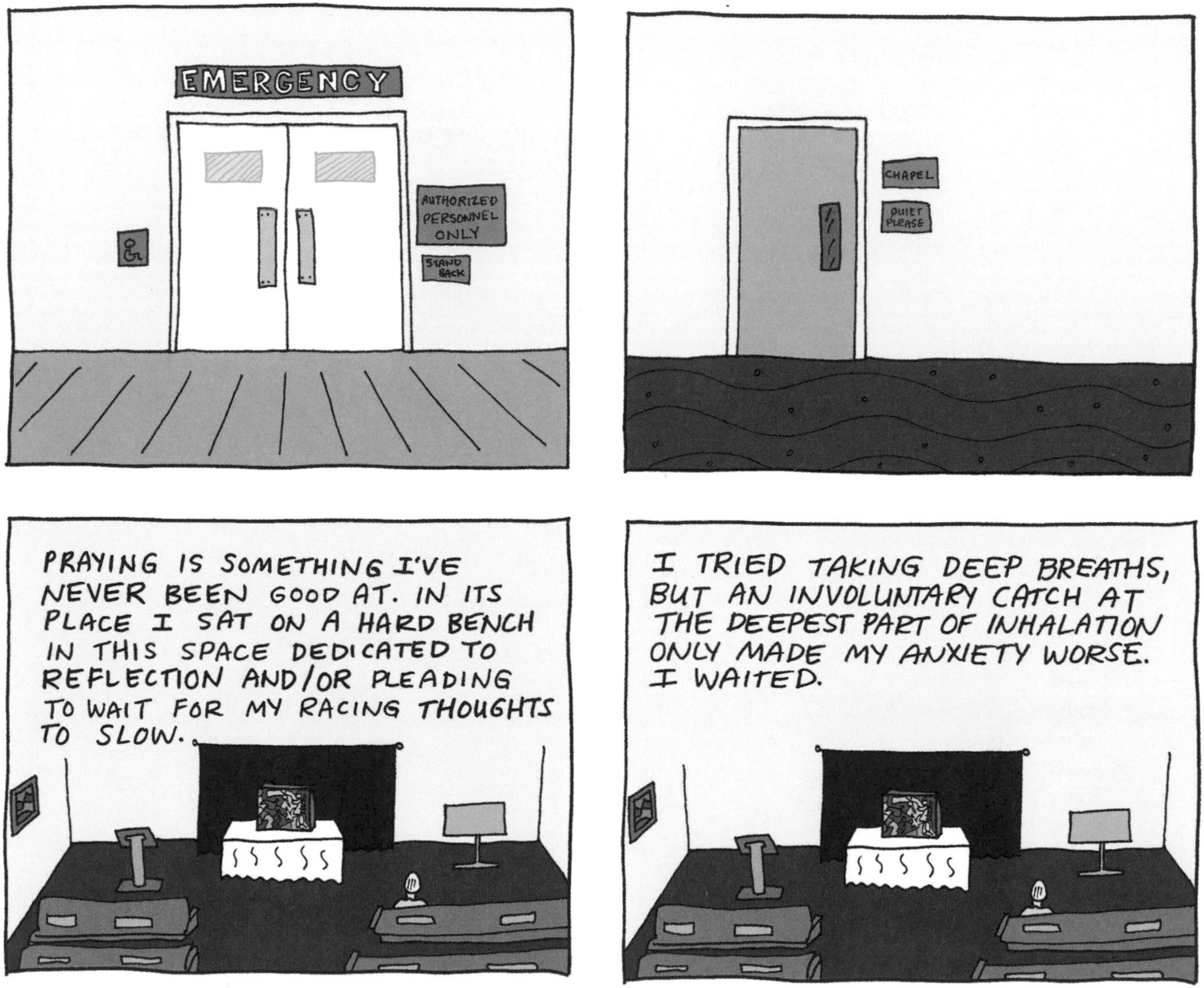
EMERGENCY
AUTHORIZED PERSONNEL ONLY
STAND BACK
CHAPEL
QUIET PLEASE
PRAYING IS SOMETHING I'VE NEVER BEEN GOOD AT. IN ITS PLACE I SAT ON A HARD BENCH IN THIS SPACE DEDICATED TO REFLECTION AND/OR PLEADING TO WAIT FOR MY RACING THOUGHTS TO SLOW.
I TRIED TAKING DEEP BREATHS, BUT AN INVOLUNTARY CATCH AT THE DEEPEST PART OF INHALATION ONLY MADE MY ANXIETY WORSE. I WAITED.

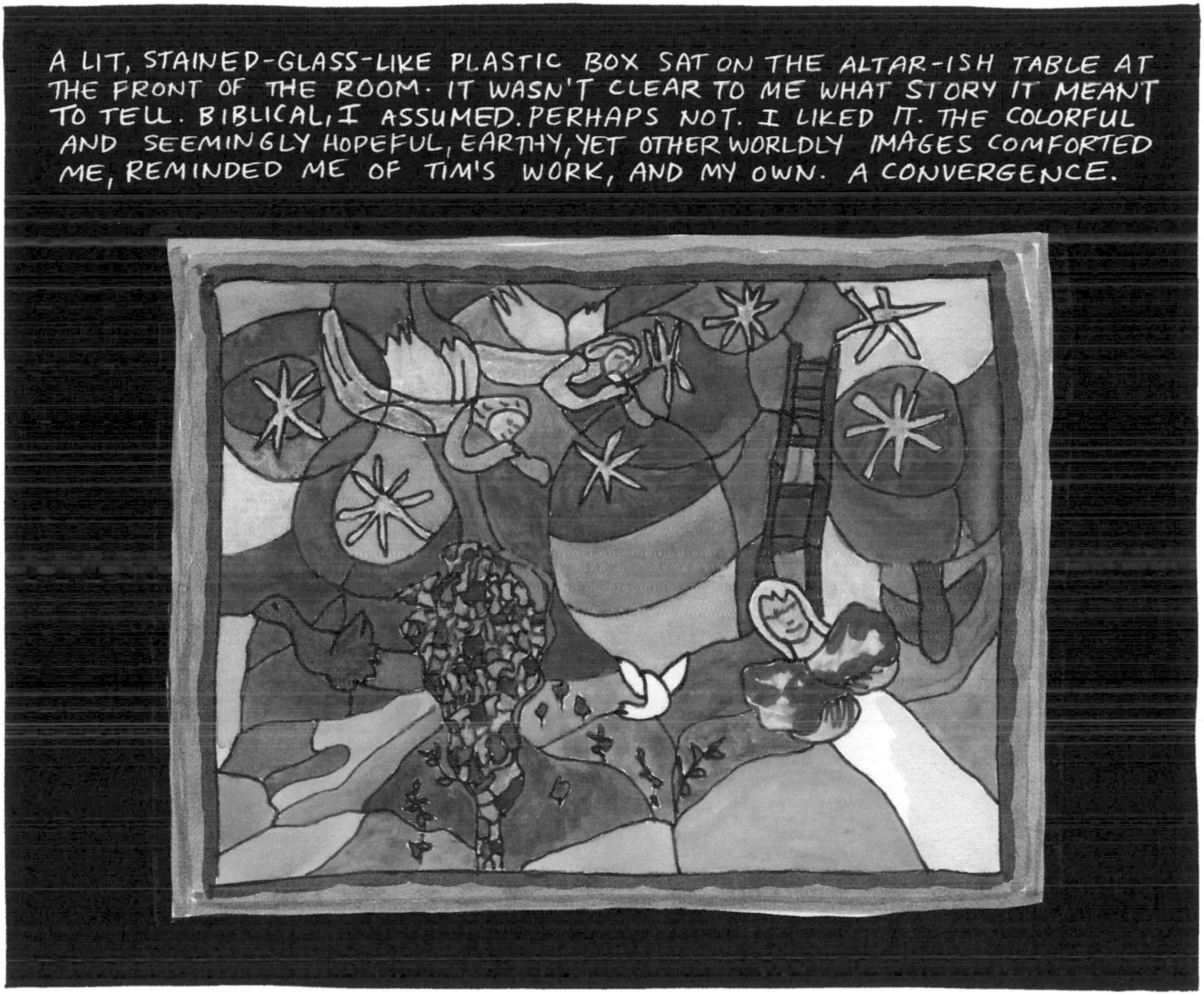
A LIT, STAINED-GLASS-LIKE PLASTIC BOX SAT ON THE ALTAR-ISH TABLE AT THE FRONT OF THE ROOM. IT WASN'T CLEAR TO ME WHAT STORY IT MEANT TO TELL. BIBLICAL, I ASSUMED. PERHAPS NOT. I LIKED IT. THE COLORFUL AND SEEMINGLY HOPEFUL, EARTHY, YET OTHERWORLDLY IMAGES COMFORTED ME, REMINDED ME OF TIM'S WORK, AND MY OWN. A CONVERGENCE.

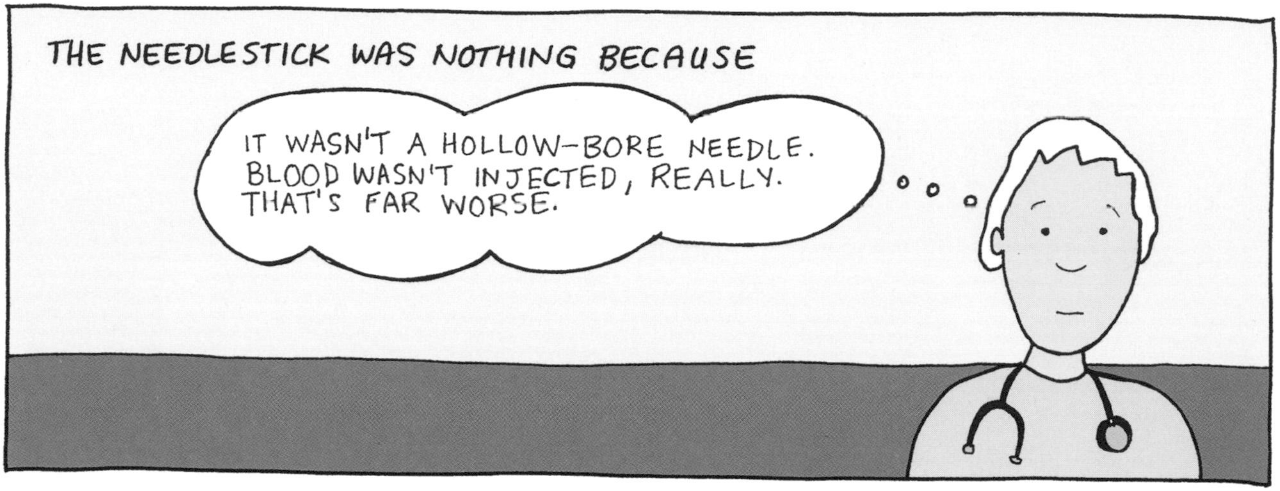
THE NEEDLESTICK WAS NOTHING BECAUSE
IT WASN'T A HOLLOW-BORE NEEDLE. BLOOD WASN'T INJECTED, REALLY. THAT'S FAR WORSE.

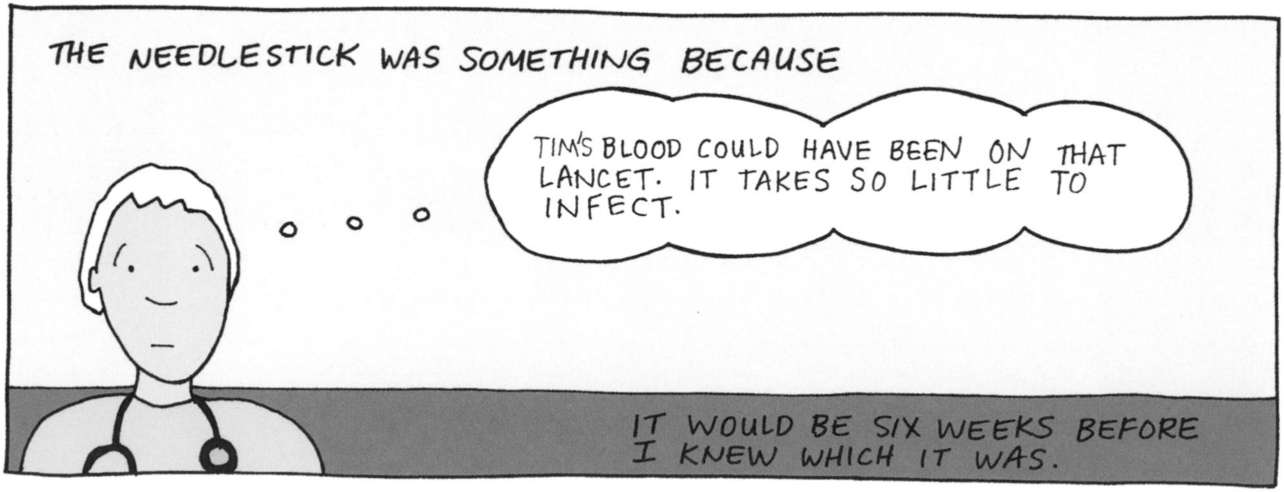
THE NEEDLESTICK WAS SOMETHING BECAUSE
TIM'S BLOOD COULD HAVE BEEN ON THAT LANCET. IT TAKES SO LITTLE TO INFECT.
IT WOULD BE SIX WEEKS BEFORE I KNEW WHICH IT WAS.

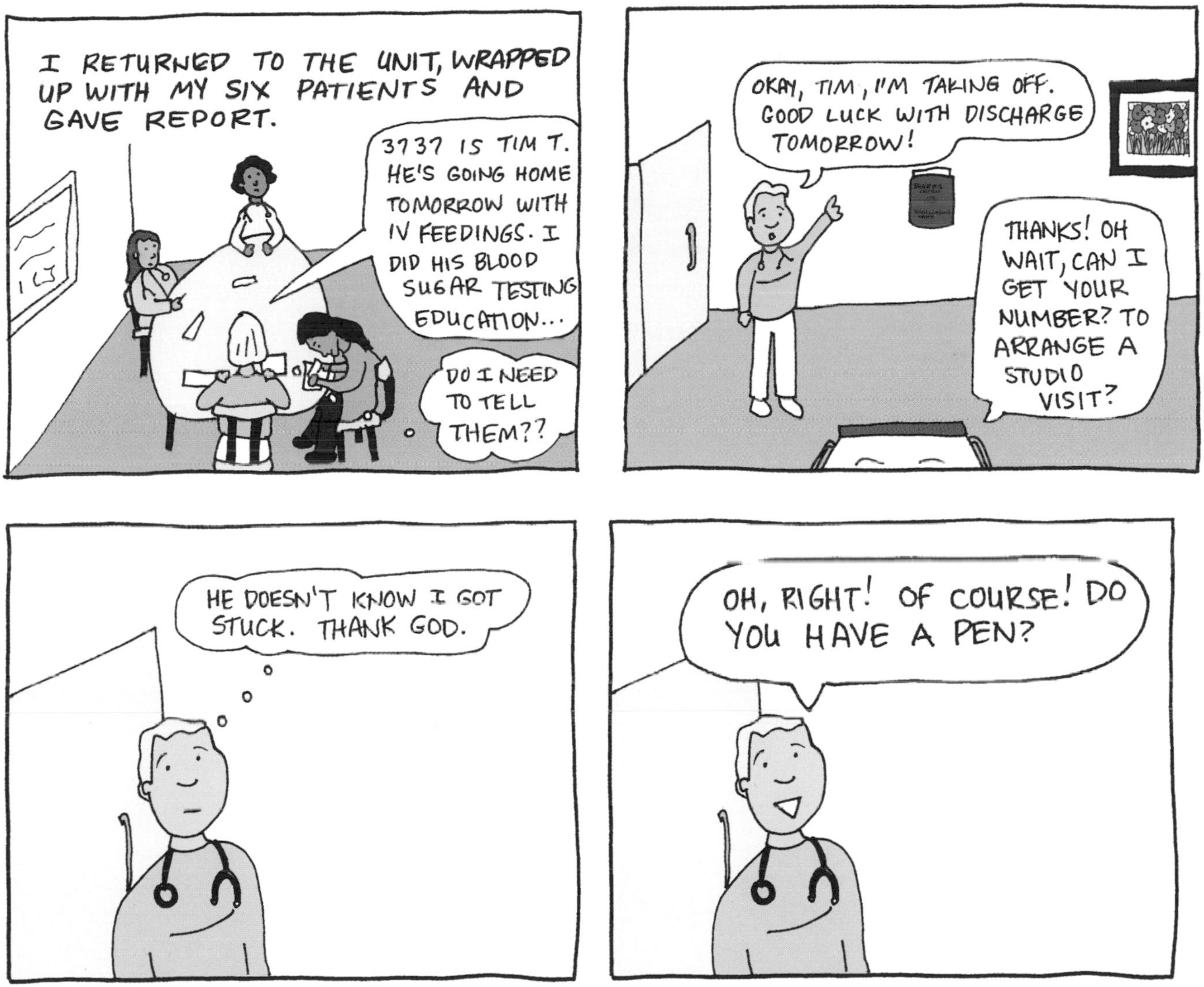
I RETURNED TO THE UNIT, WRAPPED UP WITH MY SIX PATIENTS AND GAVE REPORT.
3737 IS TIM T. HE'S GOING HOME TOMORROW WITH IV FEEDINGS. I DID HIS BLOOD SUGAR TESTING EDUCATION...
DO I NEED TO TELL THEM??
OKAY, TIM, I'M TAKING OFF. GOOD LUCK WITH DISCHARGE TOMORROW!
THANKS! OH WAIT, CAN I GET YOUR NUMBER? TO ARRANGE A STUDIO VISIT?
HE DOESN'T KNOW I GOT STUCK. THANK GOD.
OH, RIGHT! OF COURSE! DO YOU HAVE A PEN?

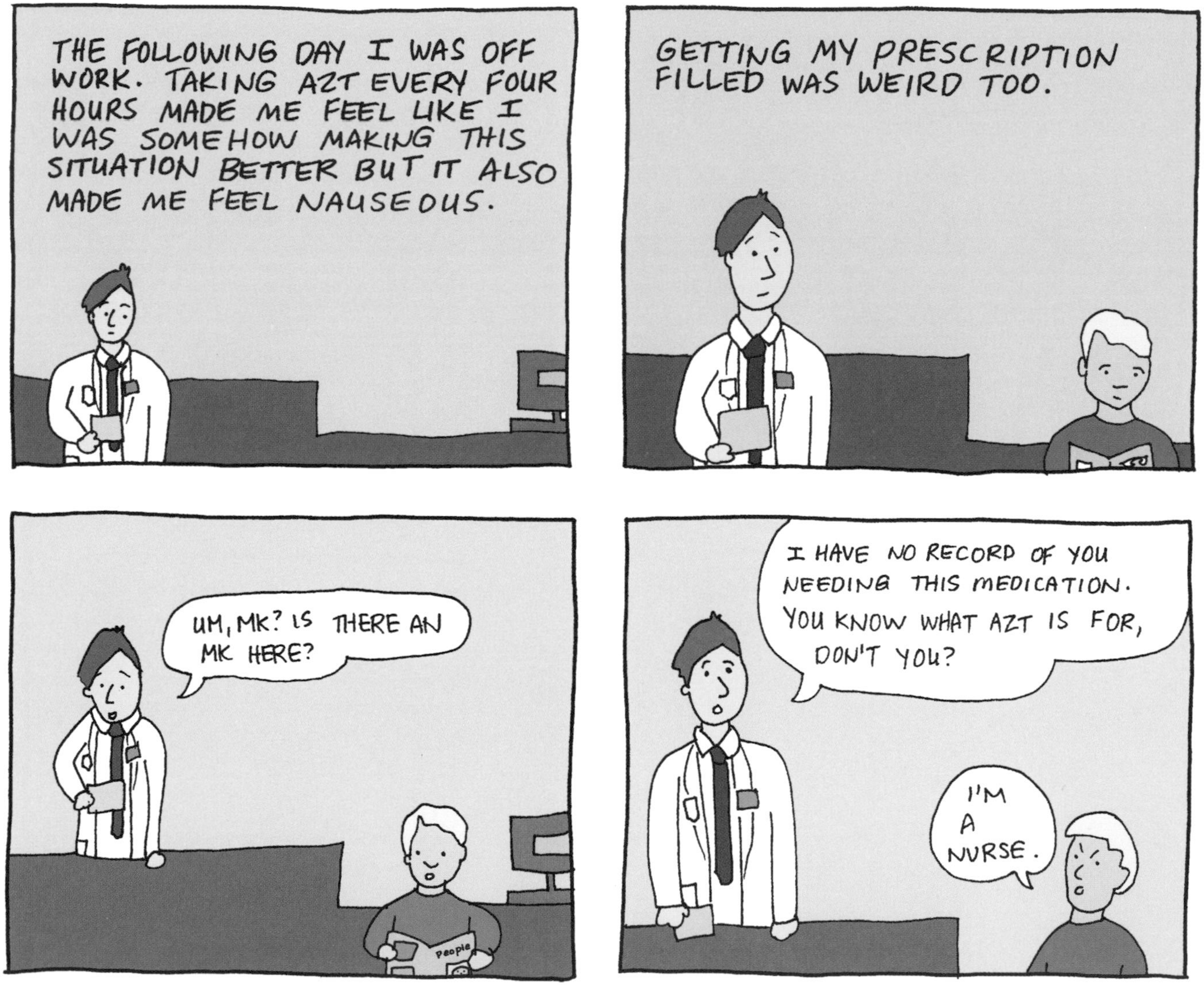
THE FOLLOWING DAY I WAS OFF WORK. TAKING AZT EVERY FOUR HOURS MADE ME FEEL LIKE I WAS SOMEHOW MAKING THIS SITUATION BETTER BUT IT ALSO MADE ME FEEL NAUSEOUS.
GETTING MY PRESCRIPTION FILLED WAS WEIRD TOO.
UM, MK? IS THERE AN MK HERE?
People
I HAVE NO RECORD OF YOU NEEDING THIS MEDICATION. YOU KNOW WHAT AZT IS FOR, DON'T YOU?
I'M A NURSE.

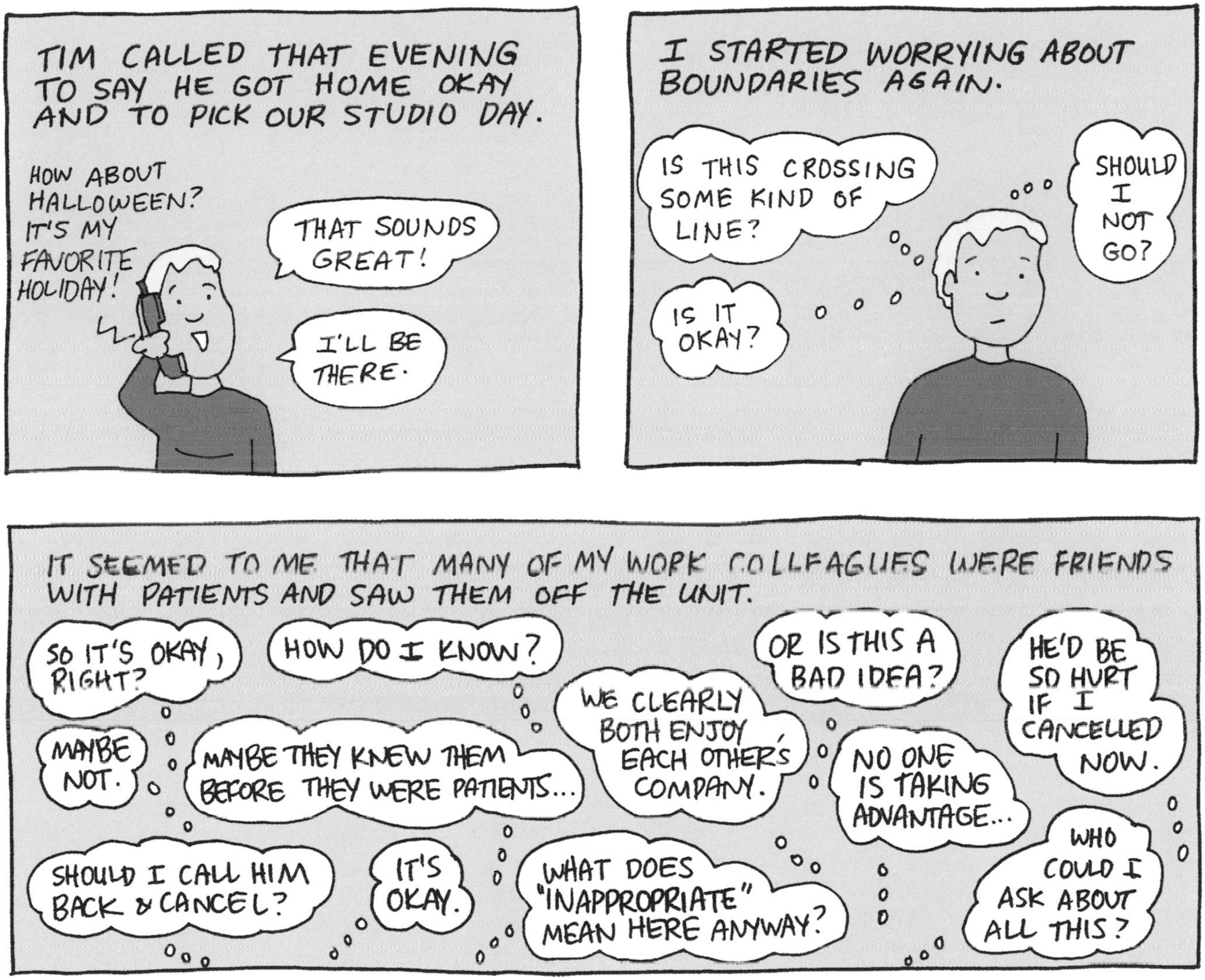
TIM CALLED THAT EVENING TO SAY HE GOT HOME OKAY AND TO PICK OUR STUDIO DAY.
HOW ABOUT HALLOWEEN? IT'S MY FAVORITE HOLIDAY!
THAT SOUNDS GREAT!
I'LL BE THERE.
I STARTED WORRYING ABOUT BOUNDARIES AGAIN.
IS THIS CROSSING SOME KIND OF LINE?
SHOULD I NOT GO?
IS IT OKAY?
IT SEEMED TO ME THAT MANY OF MY WORK COLLEAGUES WERE FRIENDS WITH PATIENTS AND SAW THEM OFF THE UNIT.
SO IT'S OKAY, RIGHT?
HOW DO I KNOW?
WE CLEARLY BOTH ENJOY EACH OTHER'S COMPANY.
OR IS THIS A BAD IDEA?
HE'D BE SO HURT IF I CANCELLED NOW.
MAYBE NOT.
MAYBE THEY KNEW THEM BEFORE THEY WERE PATIENTS...
NO ONE IS TAKING ADVANTAGE...
SHOULD I CALL HIM BACK & CANCEL?
IT'S OKAY.
WHAT DOES "INAPPROPRIATE" MEAN HERE ANYWAY?
WHO COULD I ASK ABOUT ALL THIS?

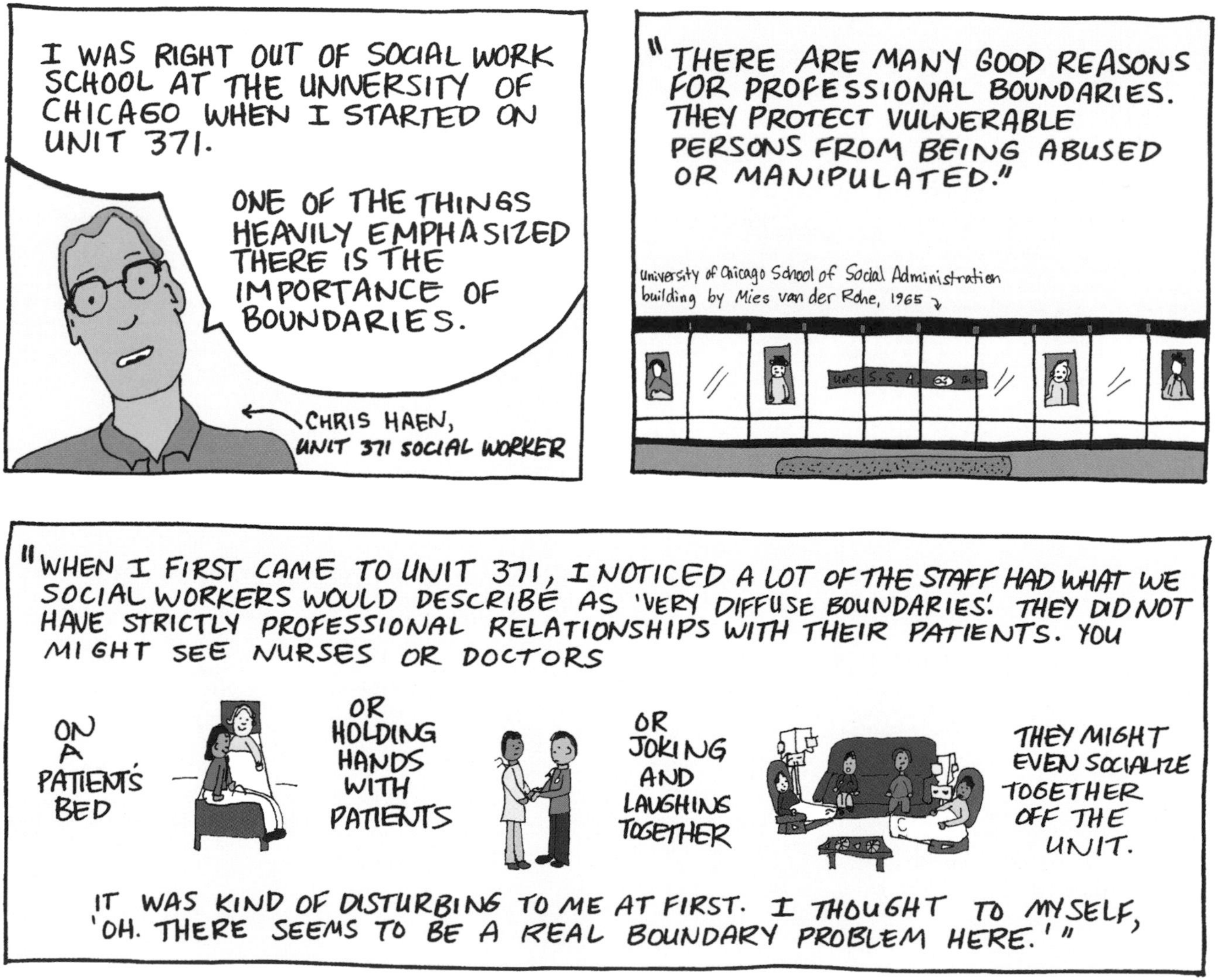
I WAS RIGHT OUT OF SOCIAL WORK SCHOOL AT THE UNIVERSITY OF CHICAGO WHEN I STARTED ON UNIT 371.
ONE OF THE THINGS HEAVILY EMPHASIZED THERE IS THE IMPORTANCE OF BOUNDARIES.
CHRIS HAEN, UNIT 371 SOCIAL WORKER
"THERE ARE MANY GOOD REASONS FOR PROFESSIONAL BOUNDARIES. THEY PROTECT VULNERABLE PERSONS FROM BEING ABUSED OR MANIPULATED."
University of Chicago School of Social Administration building by Mies van der Rohe, 1965
"WHEN I FIRST CAME TO UNIT 371, I NOTICED A LOT OF THE STAFF HAD WHAT WE SOCIAL WORKERS WOULD DESCRIBE AS 'VERY DIFFUSE BOUNDARIES'. THEY DID NOT HAVE STRICTLY PROFESSIONAL RELATIONSHIPS WITH THEIR PATIENTS. YOU MIGHT SEE NURSES OR DOCTORS
ON A PATIENT'S BED
OR HOLDING HANDS WITH PATIENTS
OR JOKING AND LAUGHING TOGETHER
THEY MIGHT EVEN SOCIALIZE TOGETHER OFF THE UNIT.
IT WAS KIND OF DISTURBING TO ME AT FIRST. I THOUGHT TO MYSELF, 'OH. THERE SEEMS TO BE A REAL BOUNDARY PROBLEM HERE.'"

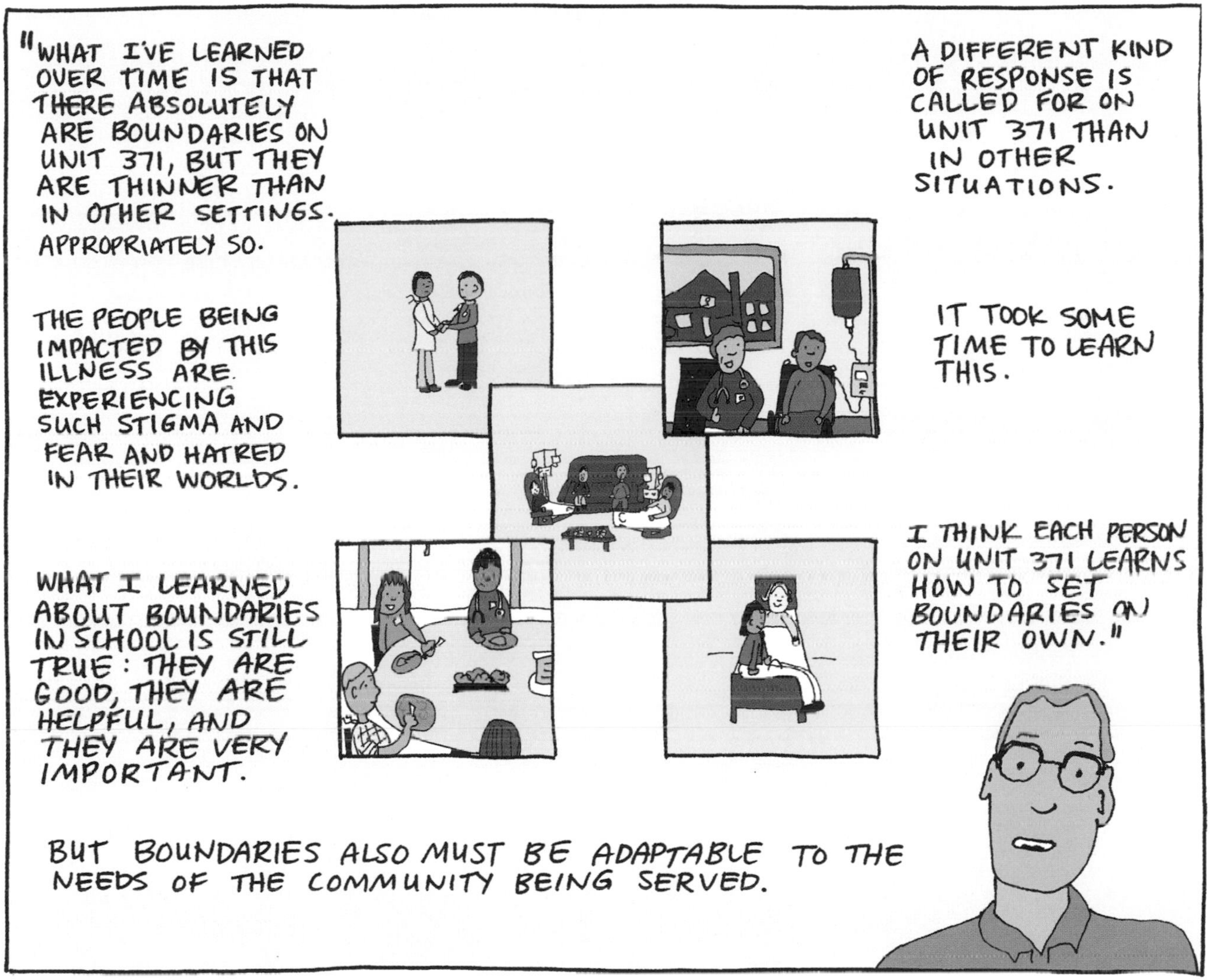
"WHAT I'VE LEARNED OVER TIME IS THAT THERE ABSOLUTELY ARE BOUNDARIES ON UNIT 371, BUT THEY ARE THINNER THAN IN OTHER SETTINGS. APPROPRIATELY SO.
THE PEOPLE BEING IMPACTED BY THIS ILLNESS ARE EXPERIENCING SUCH STIGMA AND FEAR AND HATRED IN THEIR WORLDS.
WHAT I LEARNED ABOUT BOUNDARIES IN SCHOOL IS STILL TRUE: THEY ARE GOOD, THEY ARE HELPFUL, AND THEY ARE VERY IMPORTANT.
A DIFFERENT KIND OF RESPONSE IS CALLED FOR ON UNIT 371 THAN IN OTHER SITUATIONS.
IT TOOK SOME TIME TO LEARN THIS.
I THINK EACH PERSON ON UNIT 371 LEARNS HOW TO SET BOUNDARIES ON THEIR OWN."
BUT BOUNDARIES ALSO MUST BE ADAPTABLE TO THE NEEDS OF THE COMMUNITY BEING SERVED.

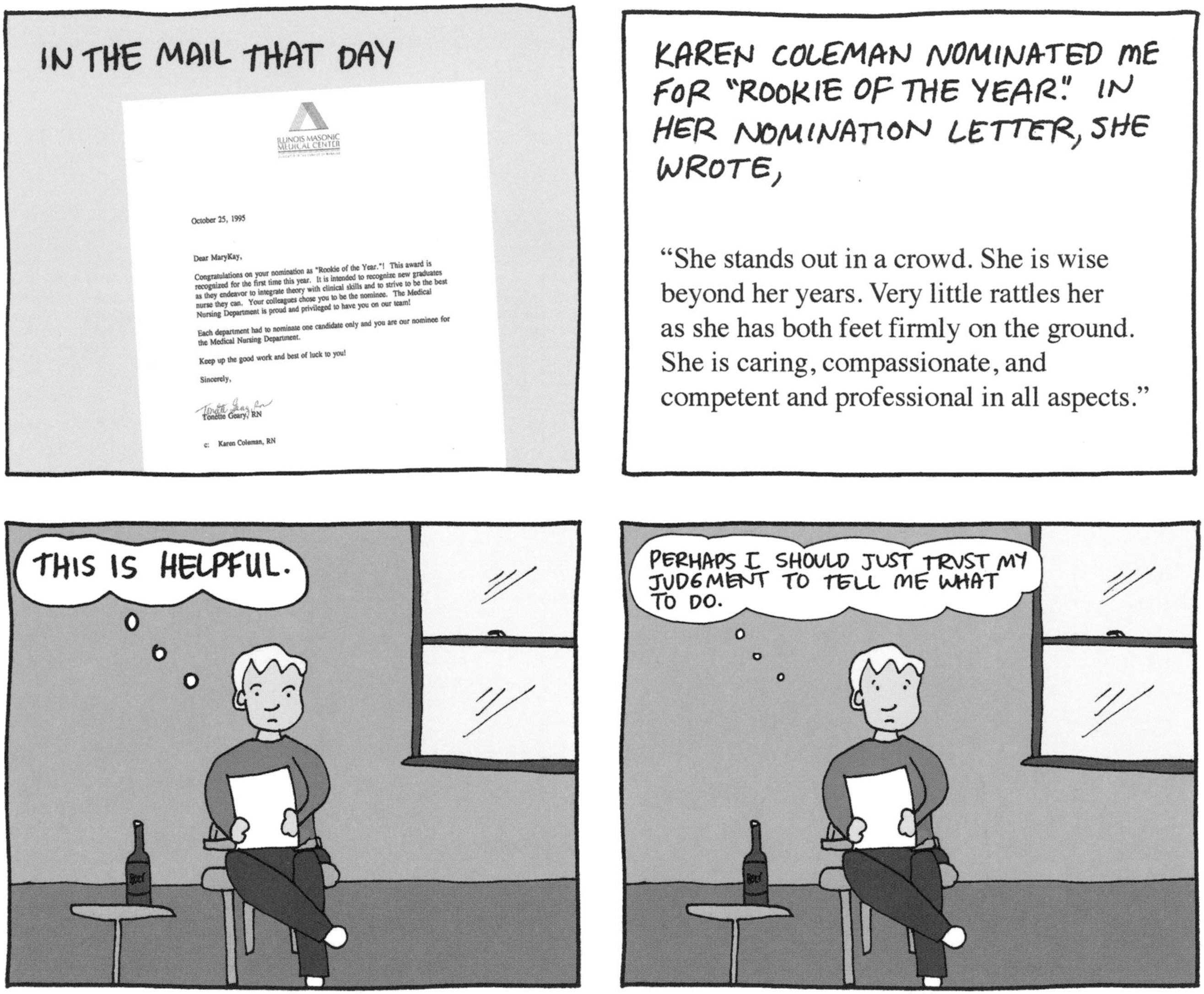

IN THE MAIL THAT DAY
ILLINOIS MASONIC MEDICAL CENTER
October 25, 1995
Dear MaryKay,
Congratulations on your nomination as "Rookie of the Year."! This award is recognized for the first time this year. It is intended to recognize new graduates as they endeavor to integrate theory with clinical skills and to strive to be the best nurse they can. Your colleagues chose you to be the nominee. The Medical Nursing Department is proud and privileged to have you on our team!
Each department had to nominate one candidate only and you are our nominee for the Medical Nursing Department.
Keep up the good work and best of luck to you!
Sincerely,
Tonette Geary, RN
c: Karen Coleman, RN
KAREN COLEMAN NOMINATED ME FOR "ROOKIE OF THE YEAR." IN HER NOMINATION LETTER, SHE WROTE,
"She stands out in a crowd. She is wise beyond her years. Very little rattles her as she has both feet firmly on the ground. She is caring, compassionate, and competent and professional in all aspects."
THIS IS HELPFUL.
PERHAPS I SHOULD JUST TRUST MY JUDGEMENT TO TELL ME WHAT TO DO.

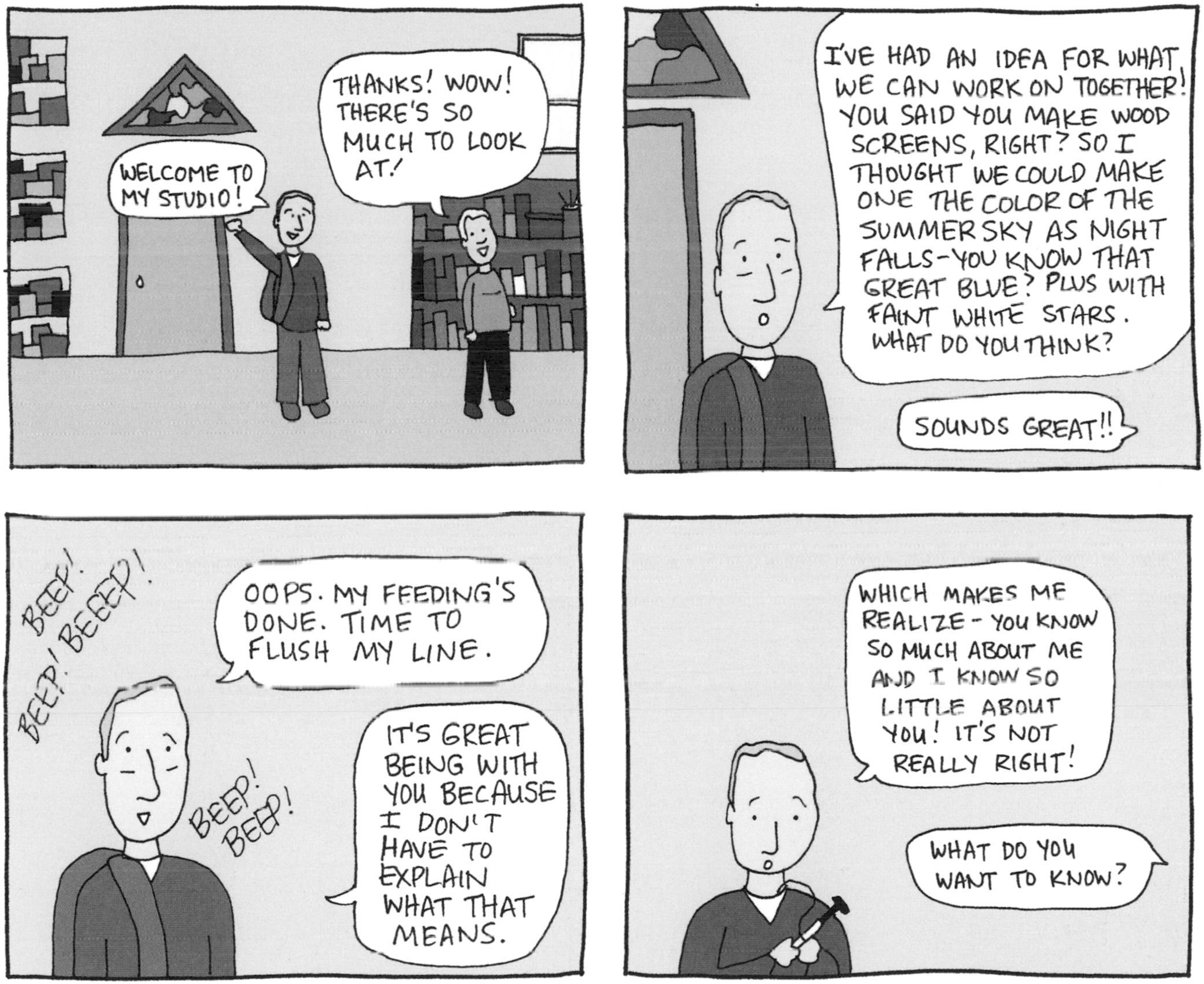
WELCOME TO MY STUDIO!
THANKS! WOW! THERE'S SO MUCH TO LOOK AT!
I'VE HAD AN IDEA FOR WHAT WE CAN WORK ON TOGETHER! YOU SAID YOU MAKE WOOD SCREENS, RIGHT? SO I THOUGHT WE COULD MAKE ONE THE COLOR OF THE SUMMER SKY AS NIGHT FALLS-YOU KNOW THAT GREAT BLUE? PLUS WITH FAINT WHITE STARS. WHAT DO YOU THINK?
SOUNDS GREAT!!
BEEP! BEEP! BEEEP!
OOPS. MY FEEDING'S DONE. TIME TO FLUSH MY LINE.
BEEP! BEEP!
IT'S GREAT BEING WITH YOU BECAUSE I DON'T HAVE TO EXPLAIN WHAT THAT MEANS.
WHICH MAKES ME REALIZE - YOU KNOW SO MUCH ABOUT ME AND I KNOW SO LITTLE ABOUT YOU! IT'S NOT REALLY RIGHT!
WHAT DO YOU WANT TO KNOW?

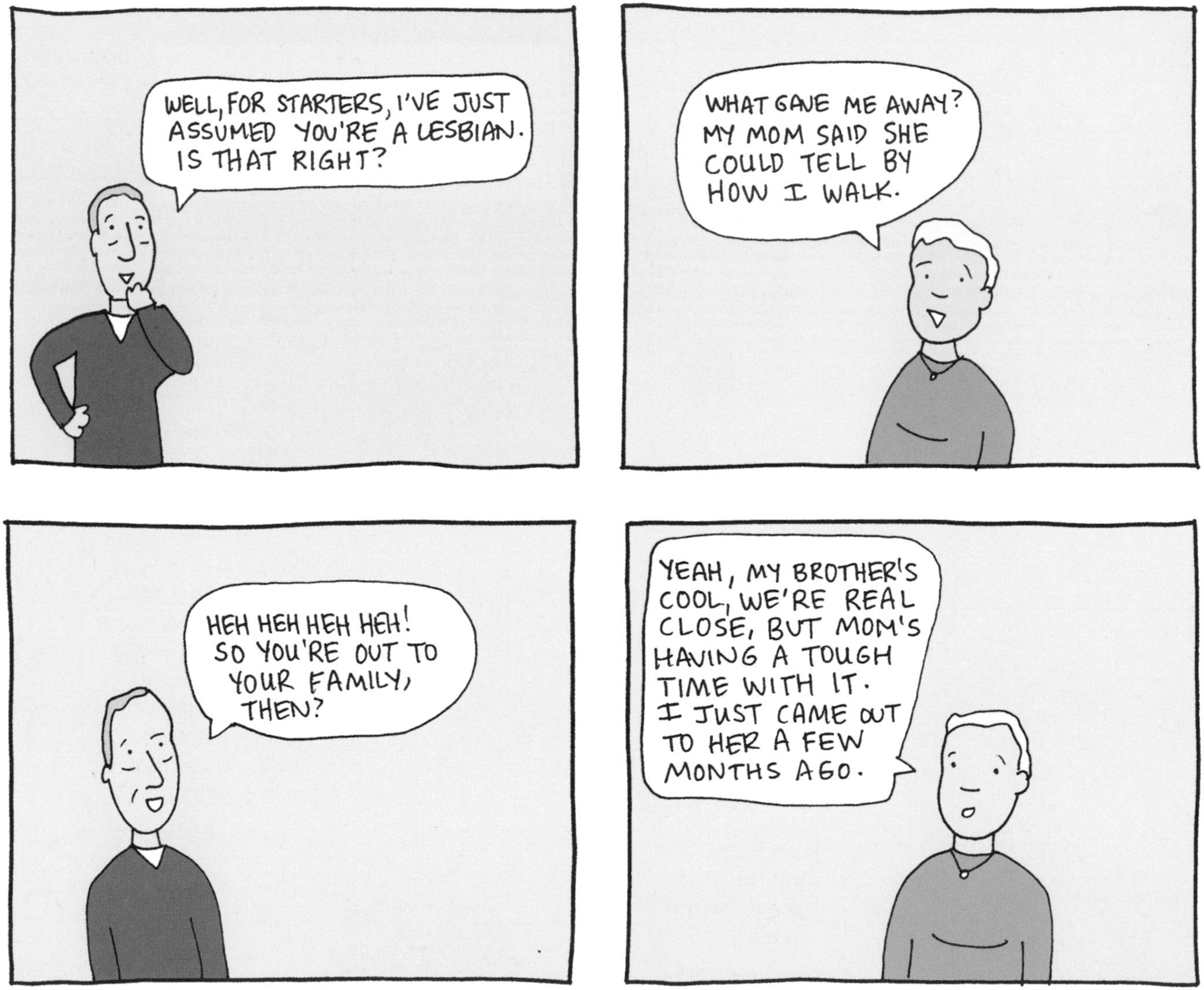
WELL, FOR STARTERS, I'VE JUST ASSUMED YOU'RE A LESBIAN. IS THAT RIGHT?
WHAT GAVE ME AWAY? MY MOM SAID SHE COULD TELL BY HOW I WALK.
HEH HEH HEH HEH! SO YOU'RE OUT TO YOUR FAMILY, THEN?
YEAH, MY BROTHER'S COOL, WE'RE REAL CLOSE, BUT MOM'S HAVING A TOUGH TIME WITH IT. I JUST CAME OUT TO HER A FEW MONTHS AGO.

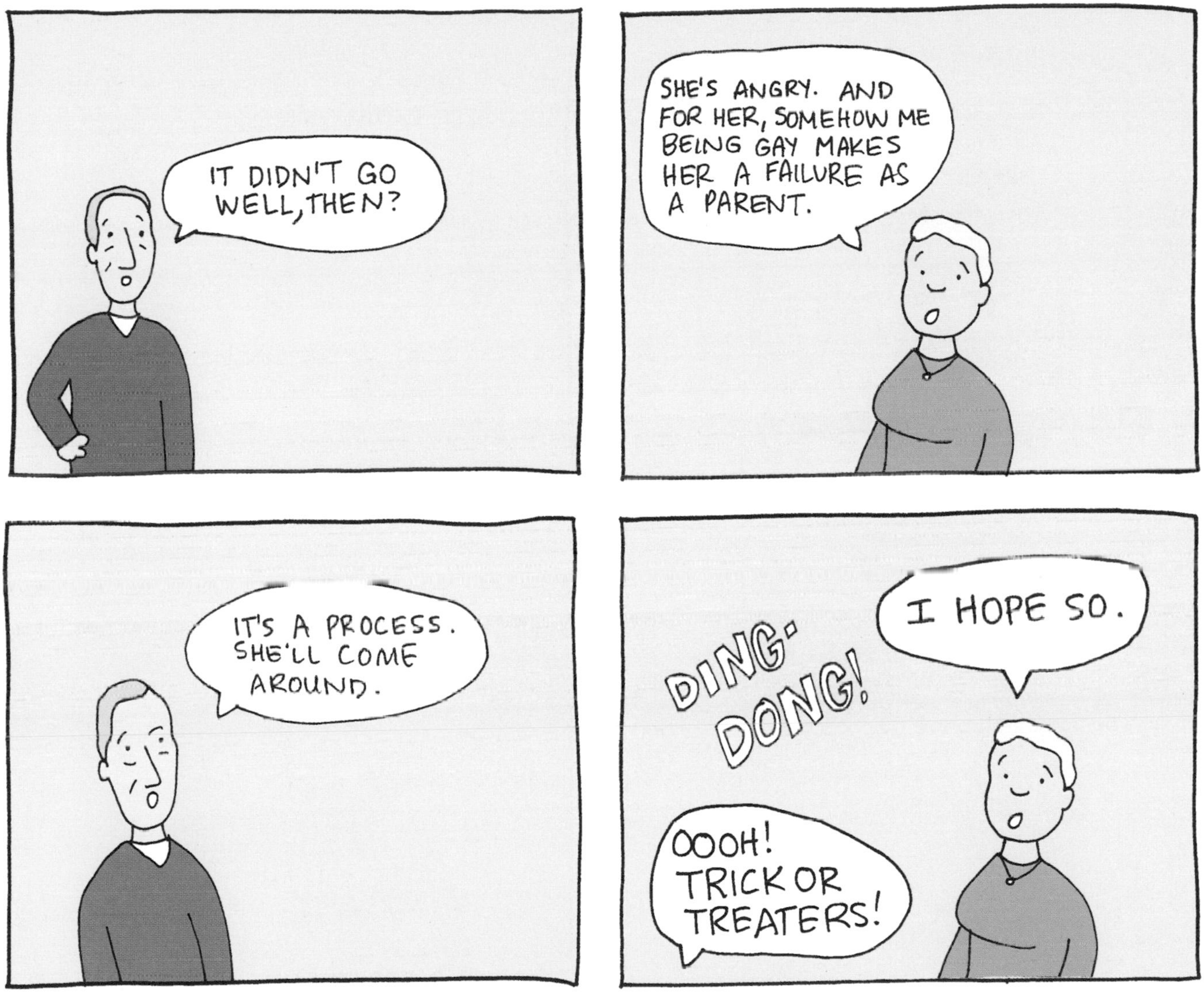
IT DIDN'T GO WELL, THEN?
SHE'S ANGRY. AND FOR HER, SOMEHOW ME BEING GAY MAKES HER A FAILURE AS A PARENT.
IT'S A PROCESS. SHE'LL COME AROUND.
DING-DONG!
I HOPE SO.
OOOH! TRICK OR TREATERS!

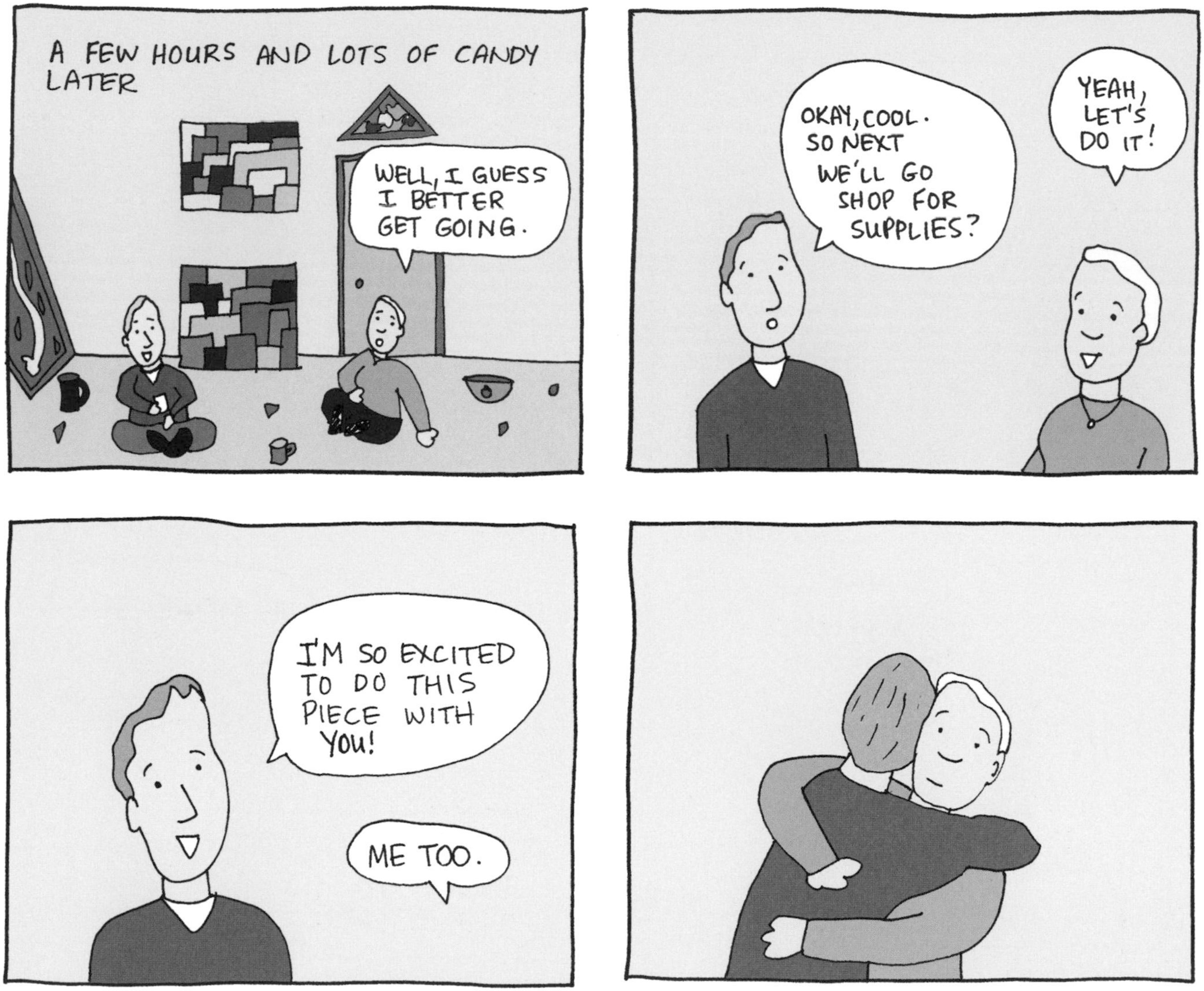
A FEW HOURS AND LOTS OF CANDY LATER
WELL, I GUESS I BETTER GET GOING.
OKAY, COOL. SO NEXT WE'LL GO SHOP FOR SUPPLIES?
YEAH, LET'S DO IT!
I'M SO EXCITED TO DO THIS PIECE WITH YOU!
ME TOO.

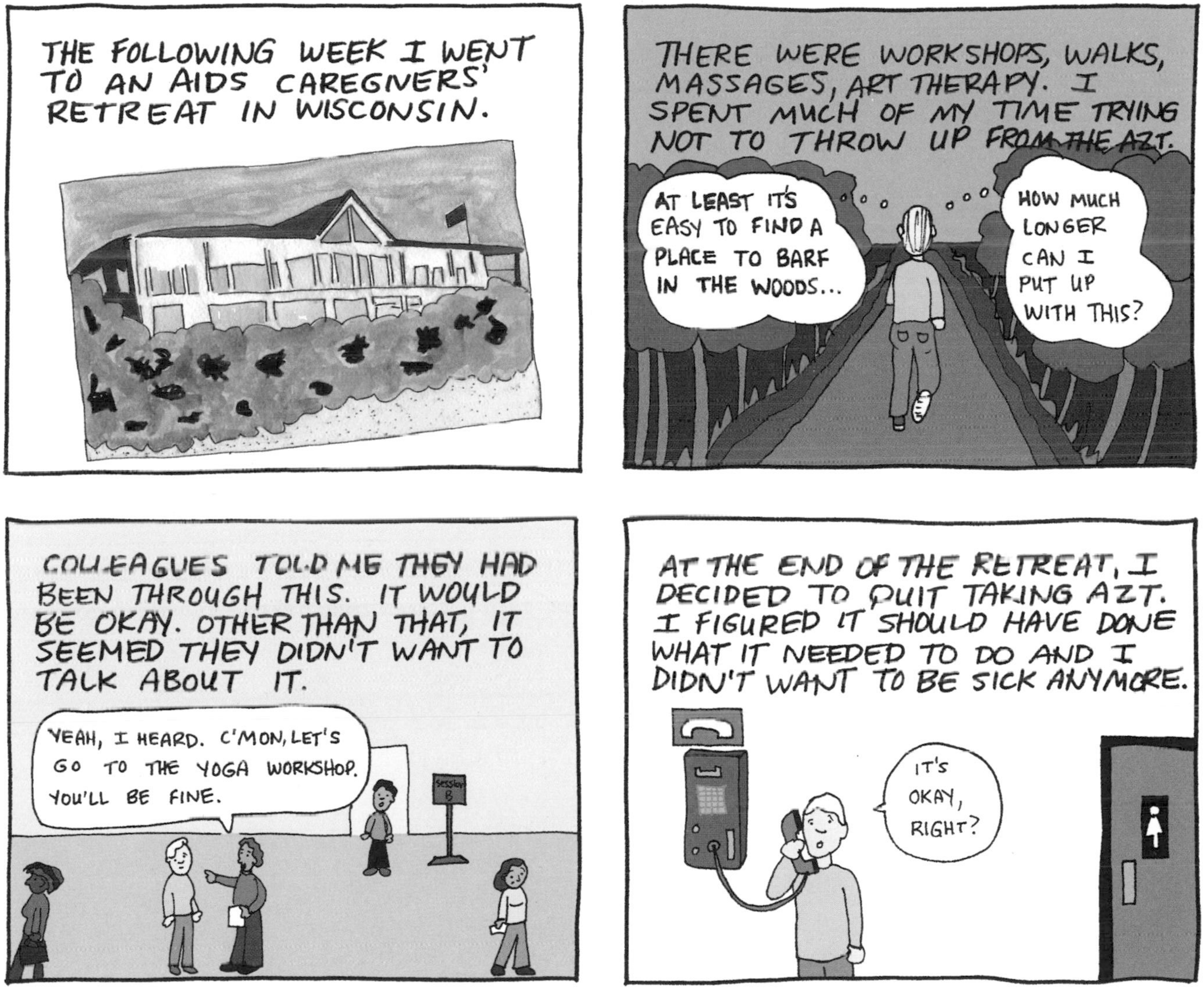
THE FOLLOWING WEEK I WENT TO AN AIDS CAREGIVERS' RETREAT IN WISCONSIN.
THERE WERE WORKSHOPS, WALKS, MASSAGES, ART THERAPY. I SPENT MUCH OF MY TIME TRYING NOT TO THROW UP FROM THE AZT.
AT LEAST IT'S EASY TO FIND A PLACE TO BARF IN THE WOODS...
HOW MUCH LONGER CAN I PUT UP WITH THIS?
COLLEAGUES TOLD ME THEY HAD BEEN THROUGH THIS. IT WOULD BE OKAY. OTHER THAN THAT, IT SEEMED THEY DIDN'T WANT TO TALK ABOUT IT.
YEAH, I HEARD. C'MON, LET'S GO TO THE YOGA WORKSHOP. YOU'LL BE FINE.
SESSION B
AT THE END OF THE RETREAT, I DECIDED TO QUIT TAKING AZT. I FIGURED IT SHOULD HAVE DONE WHAT IT NEEDED TO DO AND I DIDN'T WANT TO BE SICK ANYMORE.
IT'S OKAY, RIGHT?

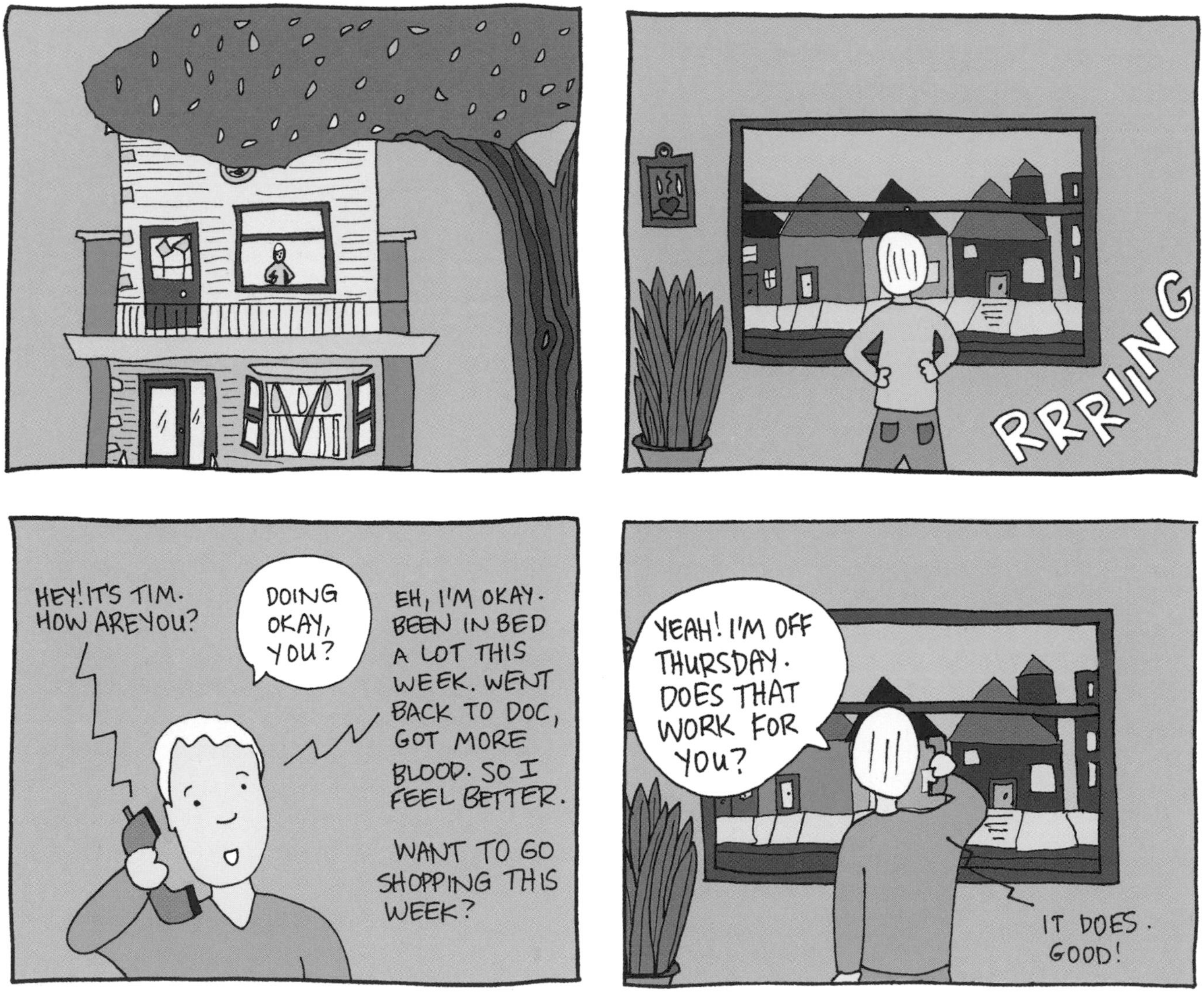
RRRING
HEY! IT'S TIM. HOW ARE YOU?
DOING OKAY, YOU?
EH, I'M OKAY. BEEN IN BED A LOT THIS WEEK. WENT BACK TO DOC, GOT MORE BLOOD. SO I FEEL BETTER.
WANT TO GO SHOPPING THIS WEEK?
YEAH! I'M OFF THURSDAY. DOES THAT WORK FOR YOU?
IT DOES. GOOD!

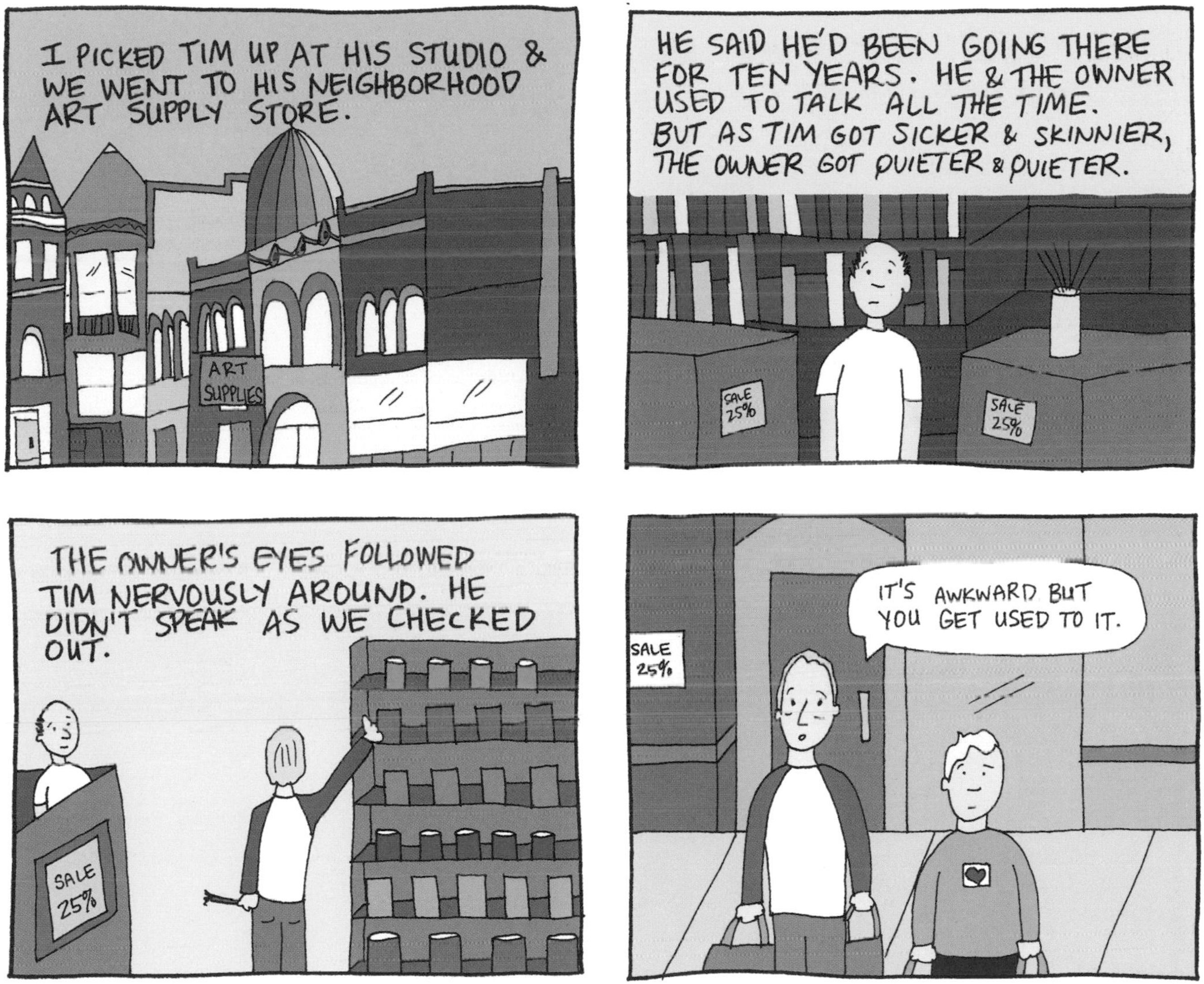
I PICKED TIM UP AT HIS STUDIO & WE WENT TO HIS NEIGHBORHOOD ART SUPPLY STORE.
ART SUPPLIES
HE SAID HE'D BEEN GOING THERE FOR TEN YEARS. HE & THE OWNER USED TO TALK ALL THE TIME. BUT AS TIM GOT SICKER & SKINNIER, THE OWNER GOT QUIETER & QUIETER.
SALE 25%
SALE 25%
THE OWNER'S EYES FOLLOWED TIM NERVOUSLY AROUND. HE DIDN'T SPEAK AS WE CHECKED OUT.
SALE 25%
SALE 25%
IT'S AWKWARD BUT YOU GET USED TO IT.

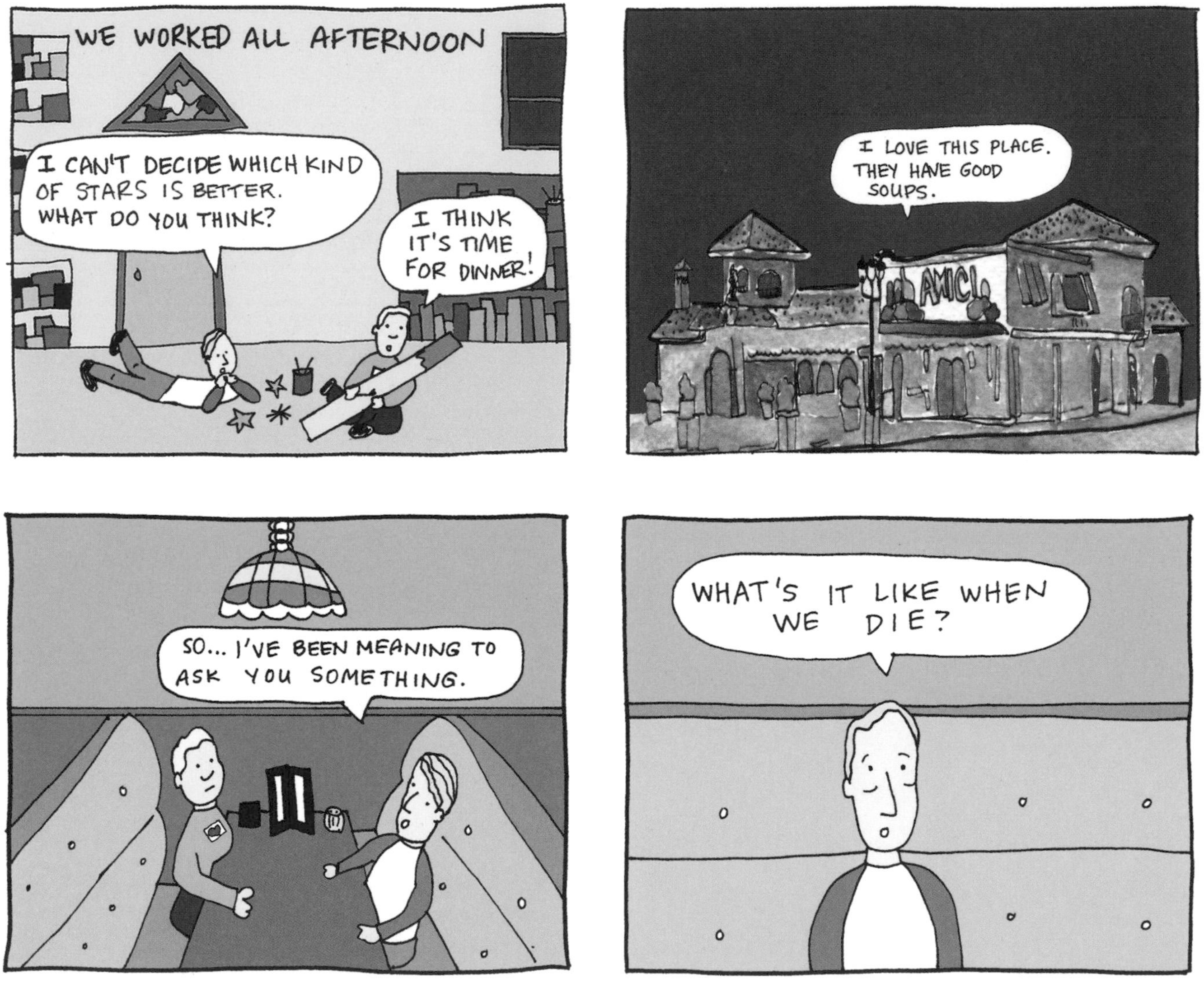
WE WORKED ALL AFTERNOON
I CAN'T DECIDE WHICH KIND OF STARS IS BETTER. WHAT DO YOU THINK?
I THINK IT'S TIME FOR DINNER!
I LOVE THIS PLACE. THEY HAVE GOOD SOUPS.
AMICI
SO... I'VE BEEN MEANING TO ASK YOU SOMETHING.
WHAT'S IT LIKE WHEN WE DIE?

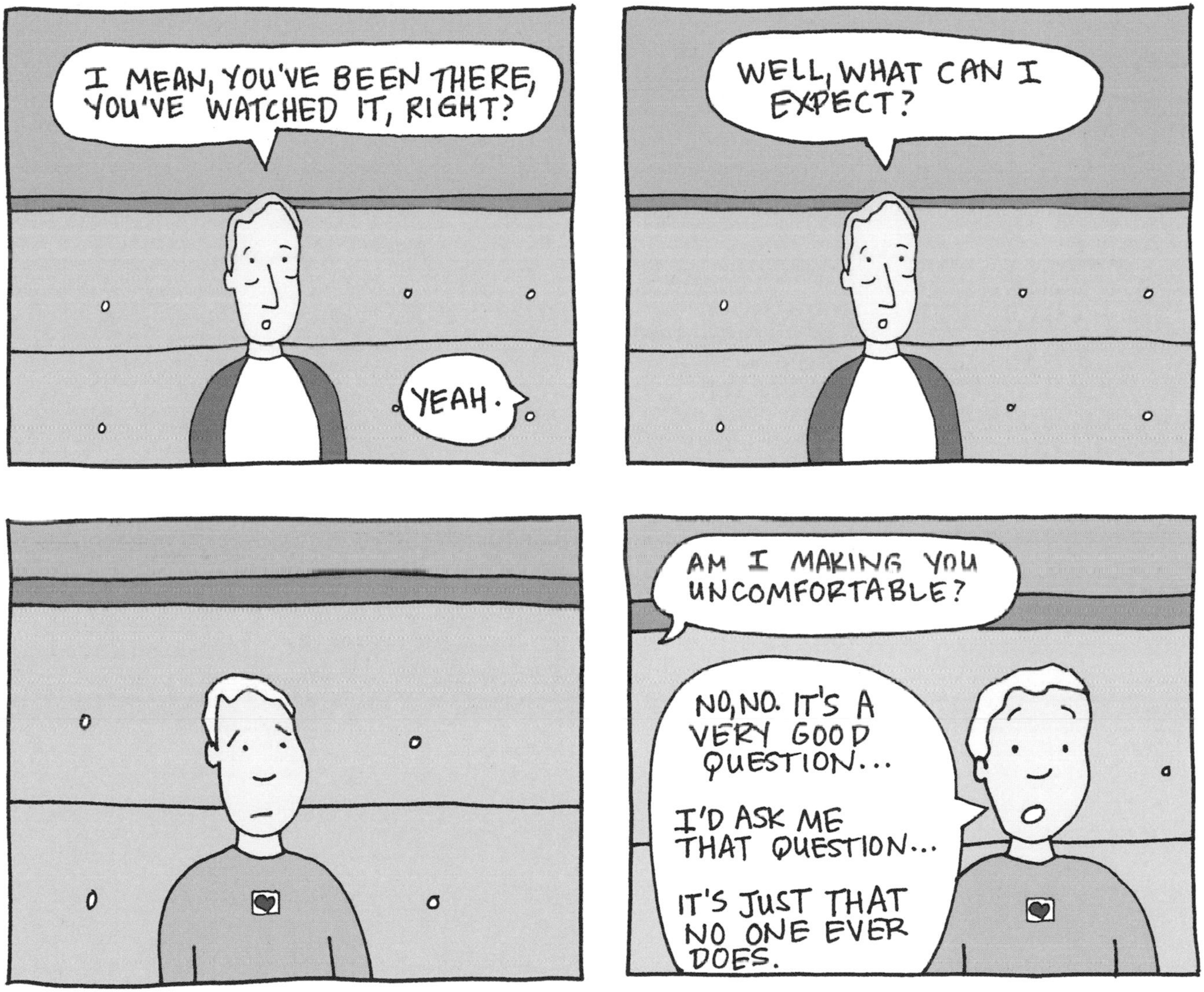
I MEAN, YOU'VE BEEN THERE, YOU'VE WATCHED IT, RIGHT?
YEAH.
WELL, WHAT CAN I EXPECT?
AM I MAKING YOU UNCOMFORTABLE?
NO, NO. IT'S A VERY GOOD QUESTION...
I'D ASK ME THAT QUESTION...
IT'S JUST THAT NO ONE EVER DOES.

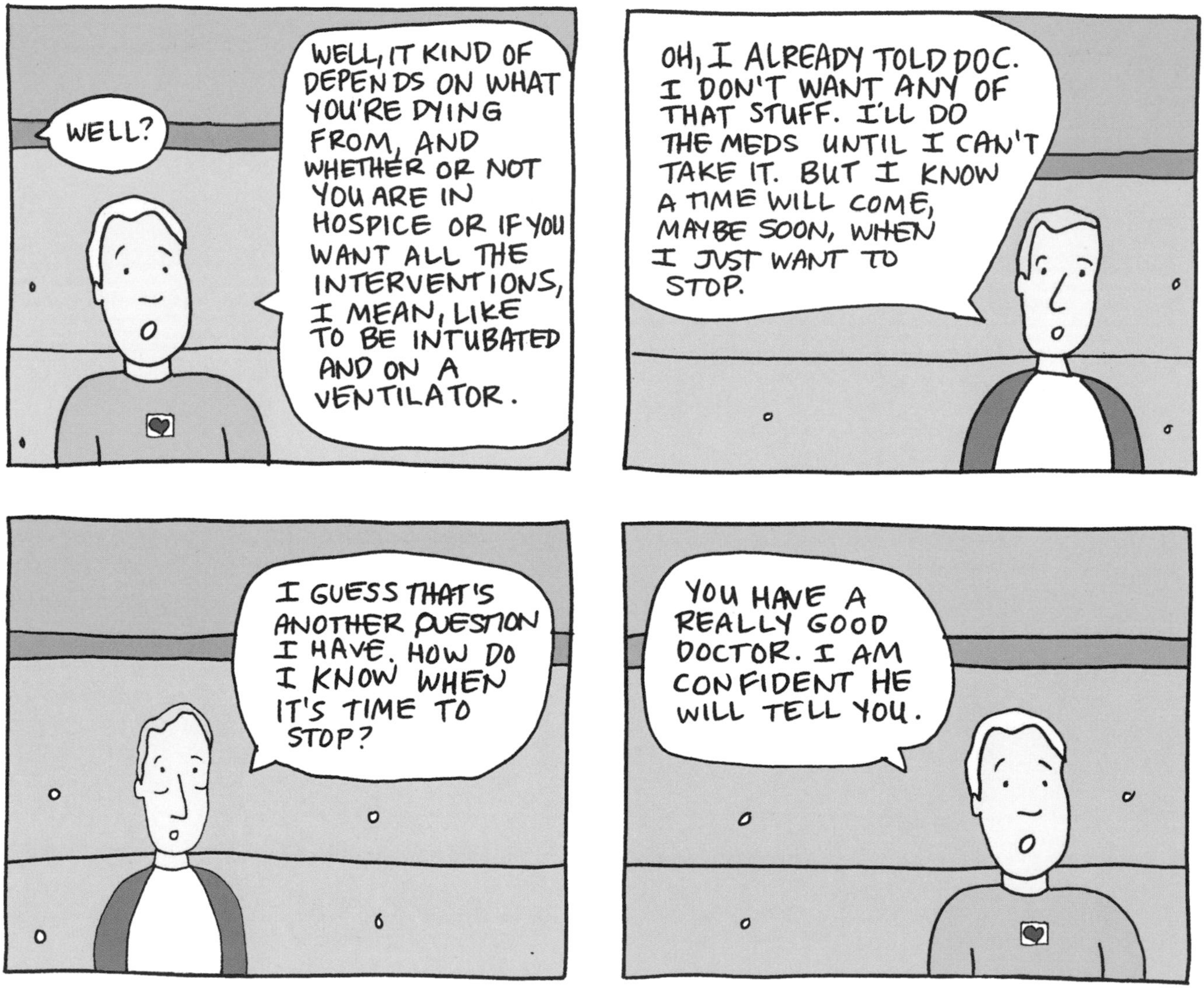
WELL?
WELL, IT KIND OF DEPENDS ON WHAT YOU'RE DYING FROM, AND WHETHER OR NOT YOU ARE IN HOSPICE OR IF YOU WANT ALL THE INTERVENTIONS, I MEAN, LIKE TO BE INTUBATED AND ON A VENTILATOR.
OH, I ALREADY TOLD DOC. I DON'T WANT ANY OF THAT STUFF. I'LL DO THE MEDS UNTIL I CAN'T TAKE IT. BUT I KNOW A TIME WILL COME, MAYBE SOON, WHEN I JUST WANT TO STOP.
I GUESS THAT'S ANOTHER QUESTION I HAVE. HOW DO I KNOW WHEN IT'S TIME TO STOP?
YOU HAVE A REALLY GOOD DOCTOR. I AM CONFIDENT HE WILL TELL YOU.

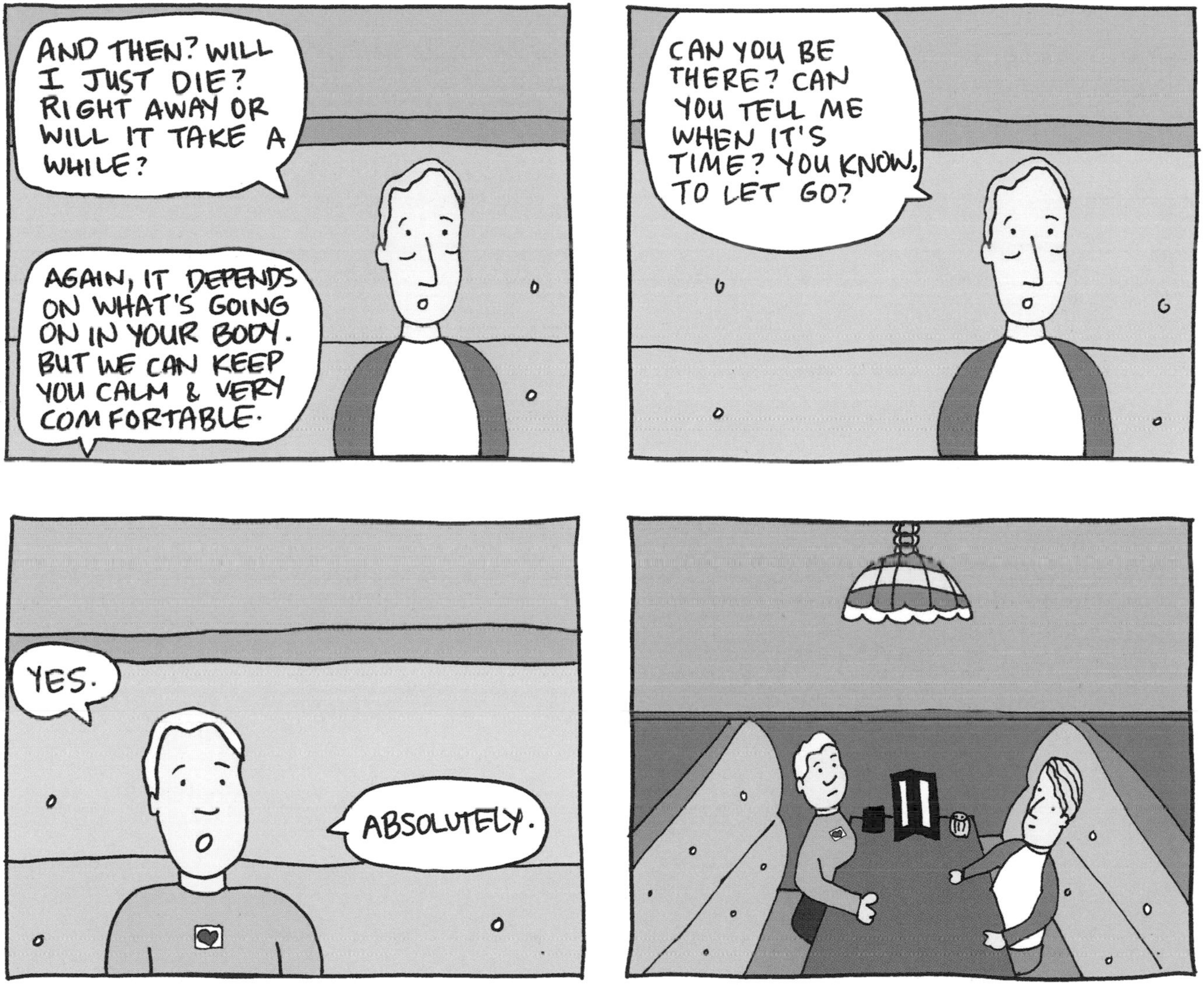
AND THEN? WILL I JUST DIE? RIGHT AWAY OR WILL IT TAKE A WHILE?
AGAIN, IT DEPENDS ON WHAT'S GOING ON IN YOUR BODY. BUT WE CAN KEEP YOU CALM & VERY COMFORTABLE.
CAN YOU BE THERE? CAN YOU TELL ME WHEN IT'S TIME? YOU KNOW, TO LET GO?
YES.
ABSOLUTELY.

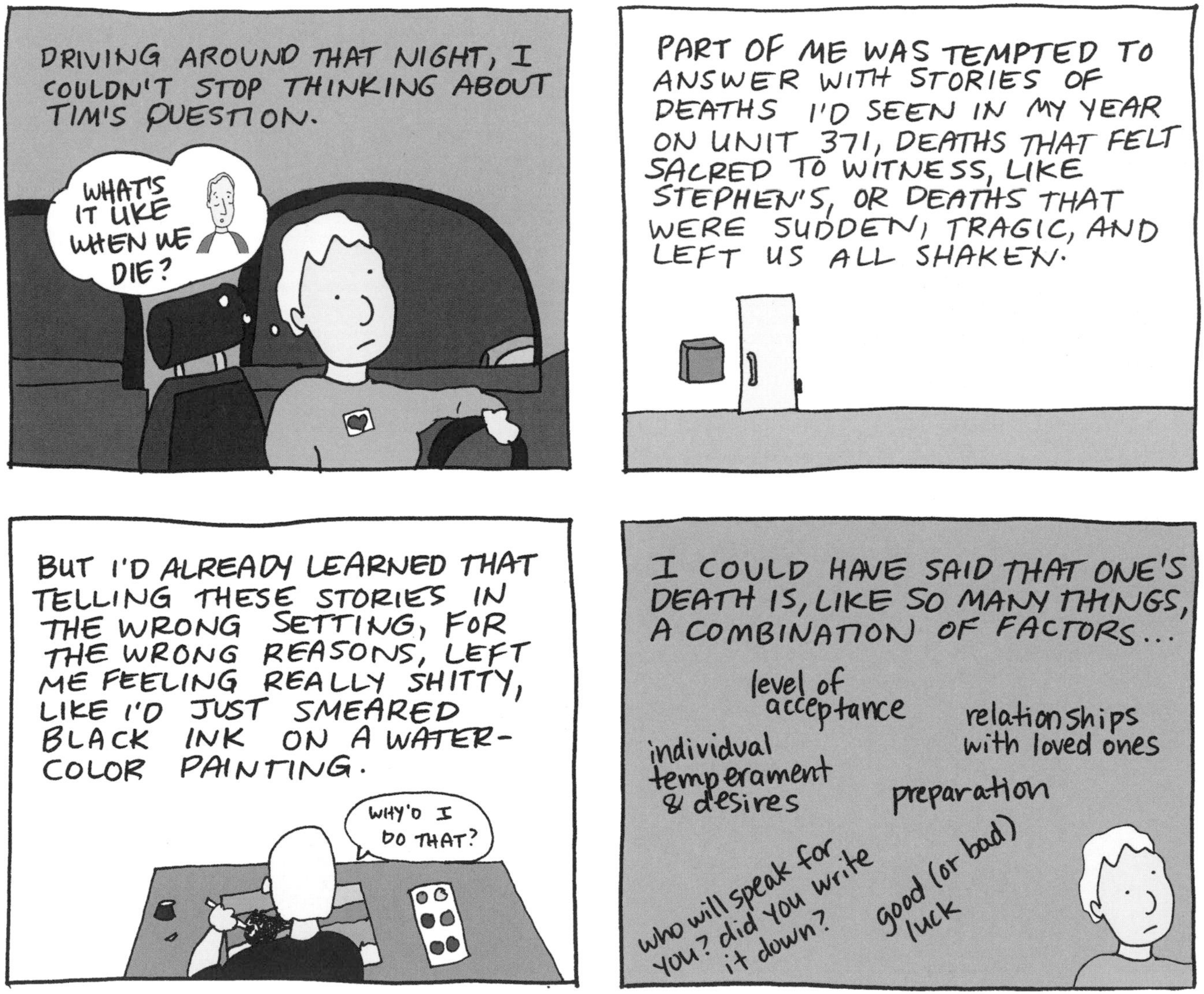
DRIVING AROUND THAT NIGHT, I COULDN'T STOP THINKING ABOUT TIM'S QUESTION.
WHAT'S IT LIKE WHEN WE DIE?
PART OF ME WAS TEMPTED TO ANSWER WITH STORIES OF DEATHS I'D SEEN IN MY YEAR ON UNIT 371, DEATHS THAT FELT SACRED TO WITNESS, LIKE STEPHEN'S, OR DEATHS THAT WERE SUDDEN, TRAGIC, AND LEFT US ALL SHAKEN.
BUT I'D ALREADY LEARNED THAT TELLING THESE STORIES IN THE WRONG SETTING, FOR THE WRONG REASONS, LEFT ME FEELING REALLY SHITTY, LIKE I'D JUST SMEARED BLACK INK ON A WATER-COLOR PAINTING.
WHY'D I DO THAT?
I COULD HAVE SAID THAT ONE'S DEATH IS, LIKE SO MANY THINGS, A COMBINATION OF FACTORS...
level of acceptance
relationships with loved ones
individual temperament & desires
preparation
who will speak for you? did you write it down?
good (or bad) luck

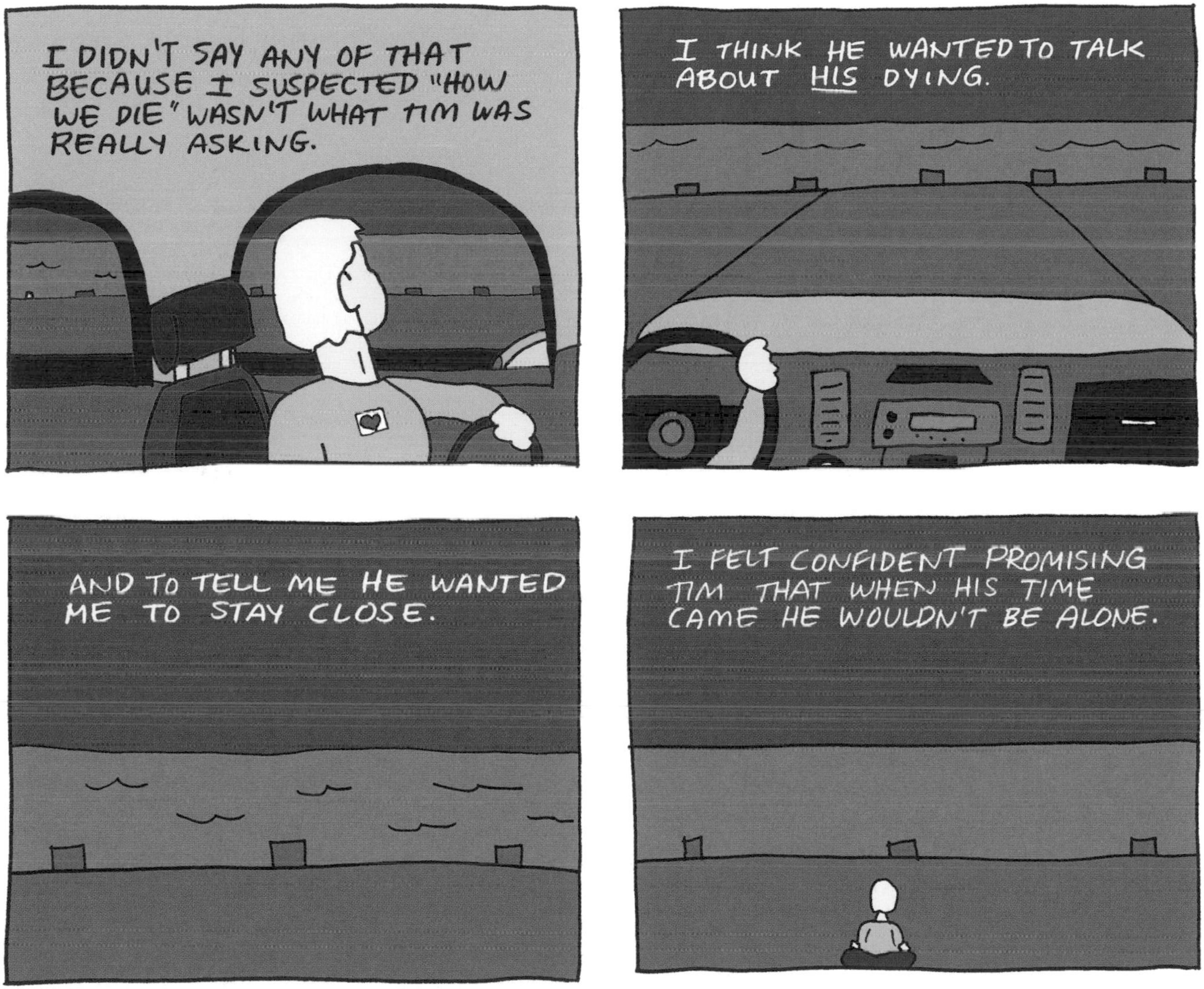
I DIDN'T SAY ANY OF THAT BECAUSE I SUSPECTED "HOW WE DIE" WASN'T WHAT TIM WAS REALLY ASKING.
I THINK HE WANTED TO TALK ABOUT HIS DYING.
AND TO TELL ME HE WANTED ME TO STAY CLOSE.
I FELT CONFIDENT PROMISING TIM THAT WHEN HIS TIME CAME HE WOULDN'T BE ALONE.

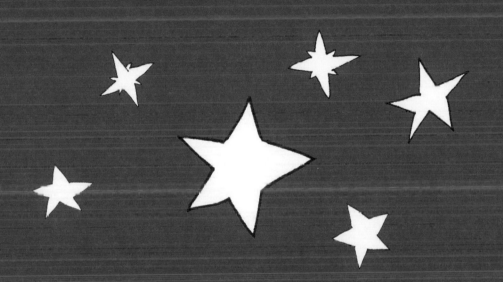

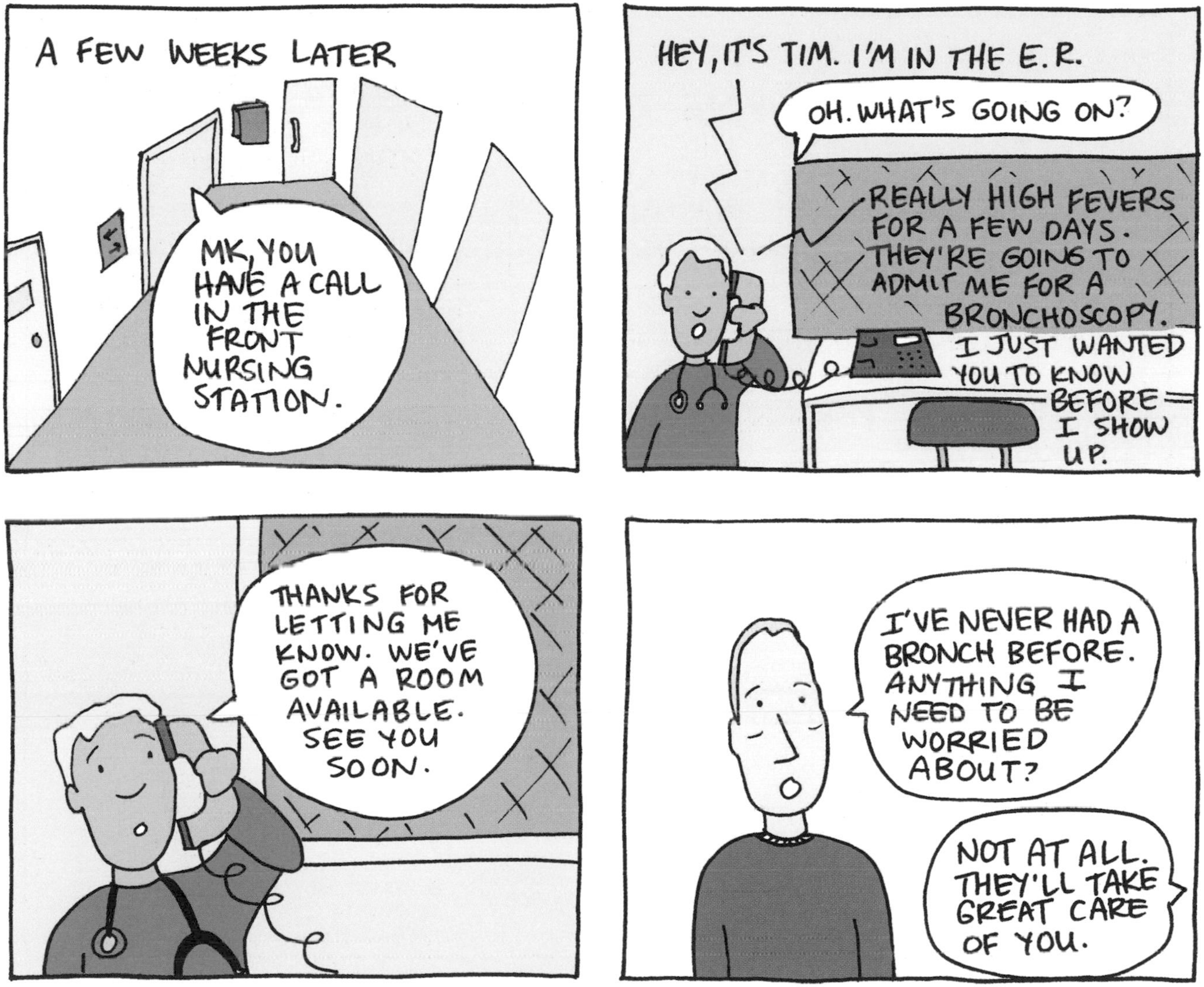
A FEW WEEKS LATER
MK, YOU HAVE A CALL IN THE FRONT NURSING STATION.
HEY, IT'S TIM. I'M IN THE E.R.
OH. WHAT'S GOING ON?
REALLY HIGH FEVERS FOR A FEW DAYS. THEY'RE GOING TO ADMIT ME FOR A BRONCHOSCOPY.
I JUST WANTED YOU TO KNOW BEFORE I SHOW UP.
THANKS FOR LETTING ME KNOW. WE'VE GOT A ROOM AVAILABLE. SEE YOU SOON.
I'VE NEVER HAD A BRONCH BEFORE. ANYTHING I NEED TO BE WORRIED ABOUT?
NOT AT ALL. THEY'LL TAKE GREAT CARE OF YOU.

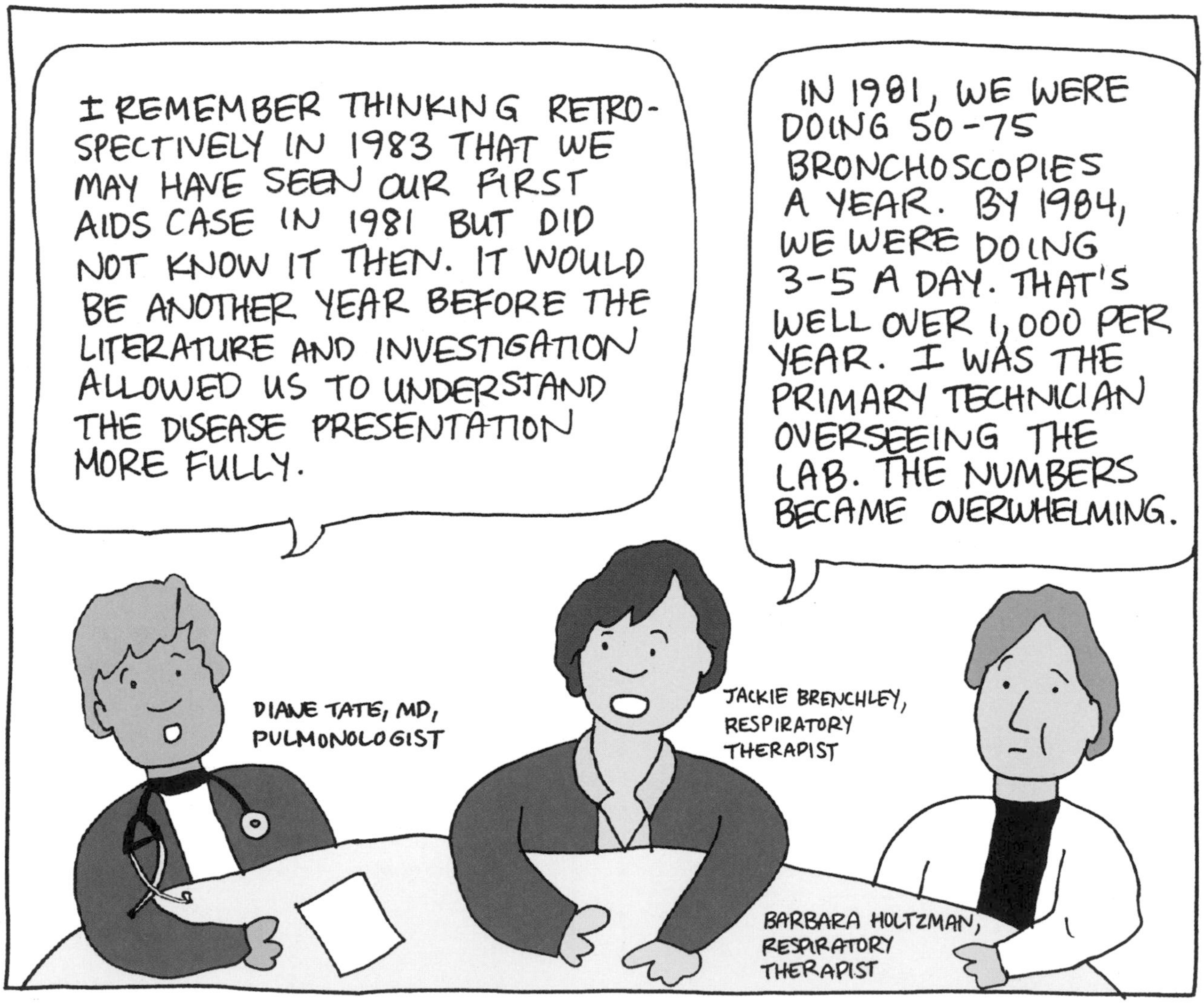
I REMEMBER THINKING RETROSPECTIVELY IN 1983 THAT WE MAY HAVE SEEN OUR FIRST AIDS CASE IN 1981 BUT DID NOT KNOW IT THEN. IT WOULD BE ANOTHER YEAR BEFORE THE LITERATURE AND INVESTIGATION ALLOWED US TO UNDERSTAND THE DISEASE PRESENTATION MORE FULLY.
IN 1981, WE WERE DOING 50-75 BRONCHOSCOPIES A YEAR. BY 1984, WE WERE DOING 3-5 A DAY. THAT'S WELL OVER 1,000 PER YEAR. I WAS THE PRIMARY TECHNICIAN OVERSEEING THE LAB. THE NUMBERS BECAME OVERWHELMING.
DIANE TATE, MD, PULMONOLOGIST
JACKIE BRENCHLEY, RESPIRATORY THERAPIST
BARBARA HOLTZMAN, RESPIRATORY THERAPIST

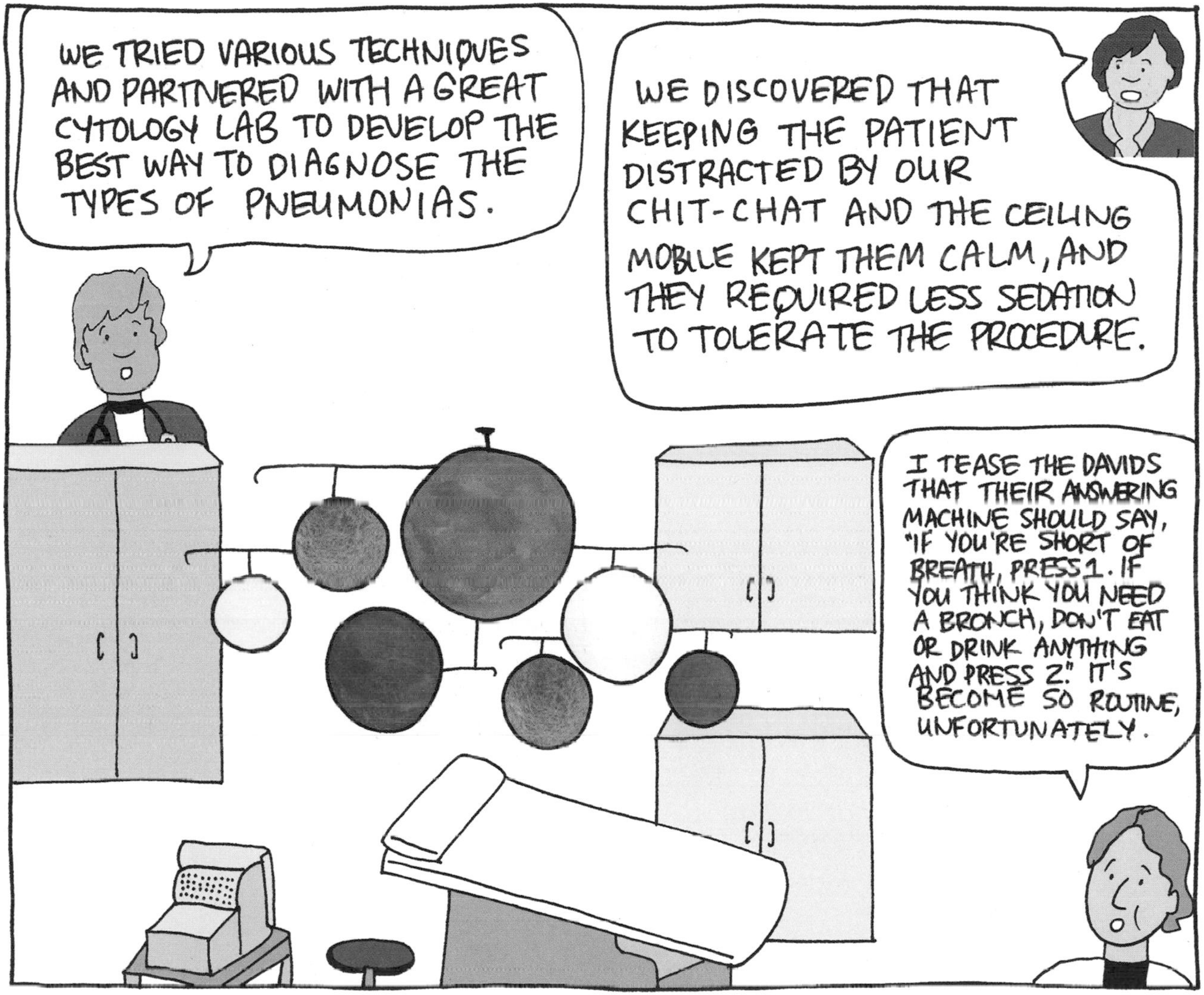
WE TRIED VARIOUS TECHNIQUES AND PARTNERED WITH A GREAT CYTOLOGY LAB TO DEVELOP THE BEST WAY TO DIAGNOSE THE TYPES OF PNEUMONIAS.
WE DISCOVERED THAT KEEPING THE PATIENT DISTRACTED BY OUR CHIT-CHAT AND THE CEILING MOBILE KEPT THEM CALM, AND THEY REQUIRED LESS SEDATION TO TOLERATE THE PROCEDURE.
I TEASE THE DAVIDS THAT THEIR ANSWERING MACHINE SHOULD SAY, "IF YOU'RE SHORT OF BREATH, PRESS 1. IF YOU THINK YOU NEED A BRONCH, DON'T EAT OR DRINK ANYTHING AND PRESS 2." IT'S BECOME SO ROUTINE, UNFORTUNATELY.

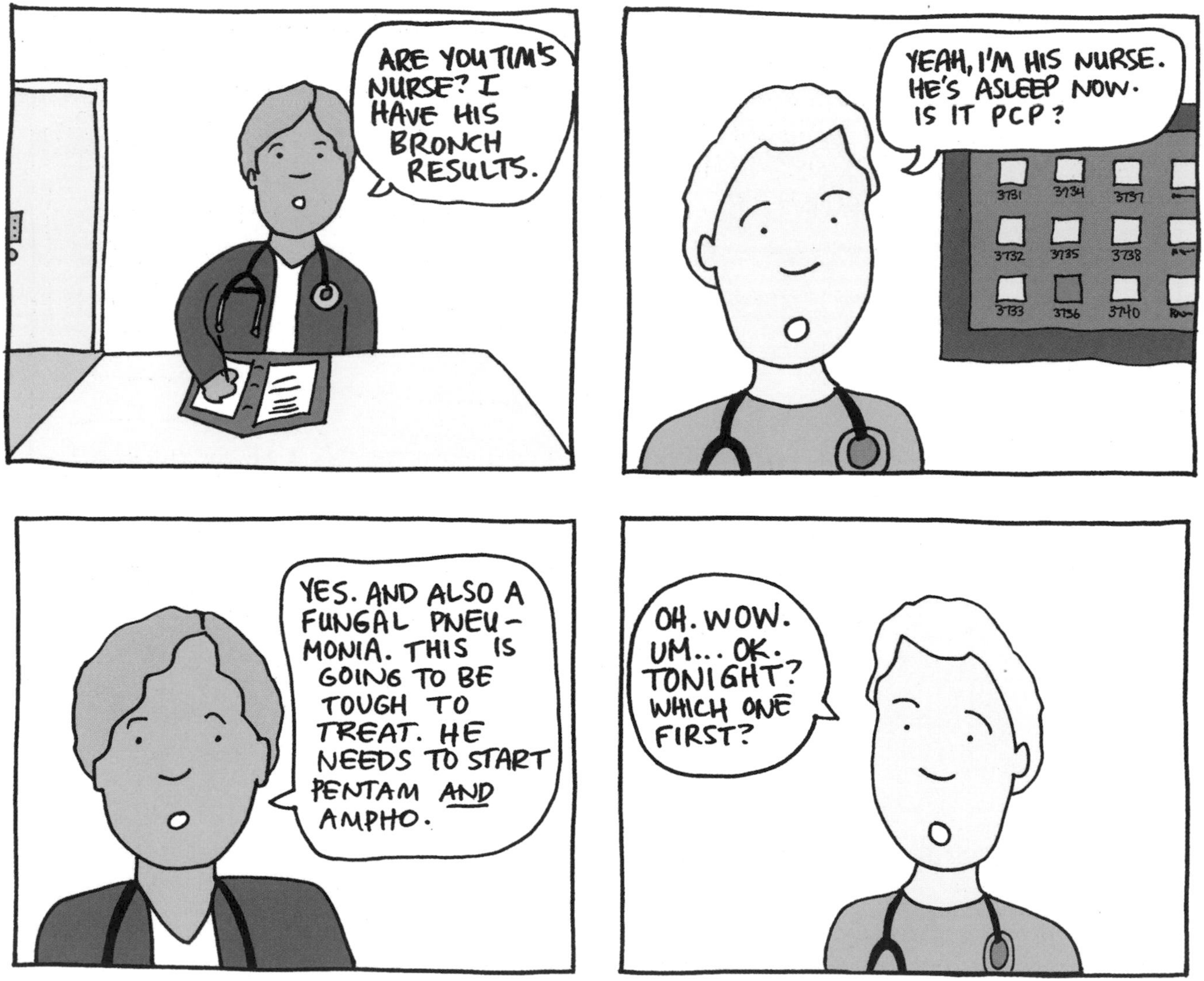
ARE YOU TIM'S NURSE? I HAVE HIS BRONCH RESULTS.
YEAH, I'M HIS NURSE. HE'S ASLEEP NOW. IS IT PCP?
YES. AND ALSO A FUNGAL PNEU-MONIA. THIS IS GOING TO BE TOUGH TO TREAT. HE NEEDS TO START PENTAM AND AMPHO.
OH. WOW. UM... OK. TONIGHT? WHICH ONE FIRST?

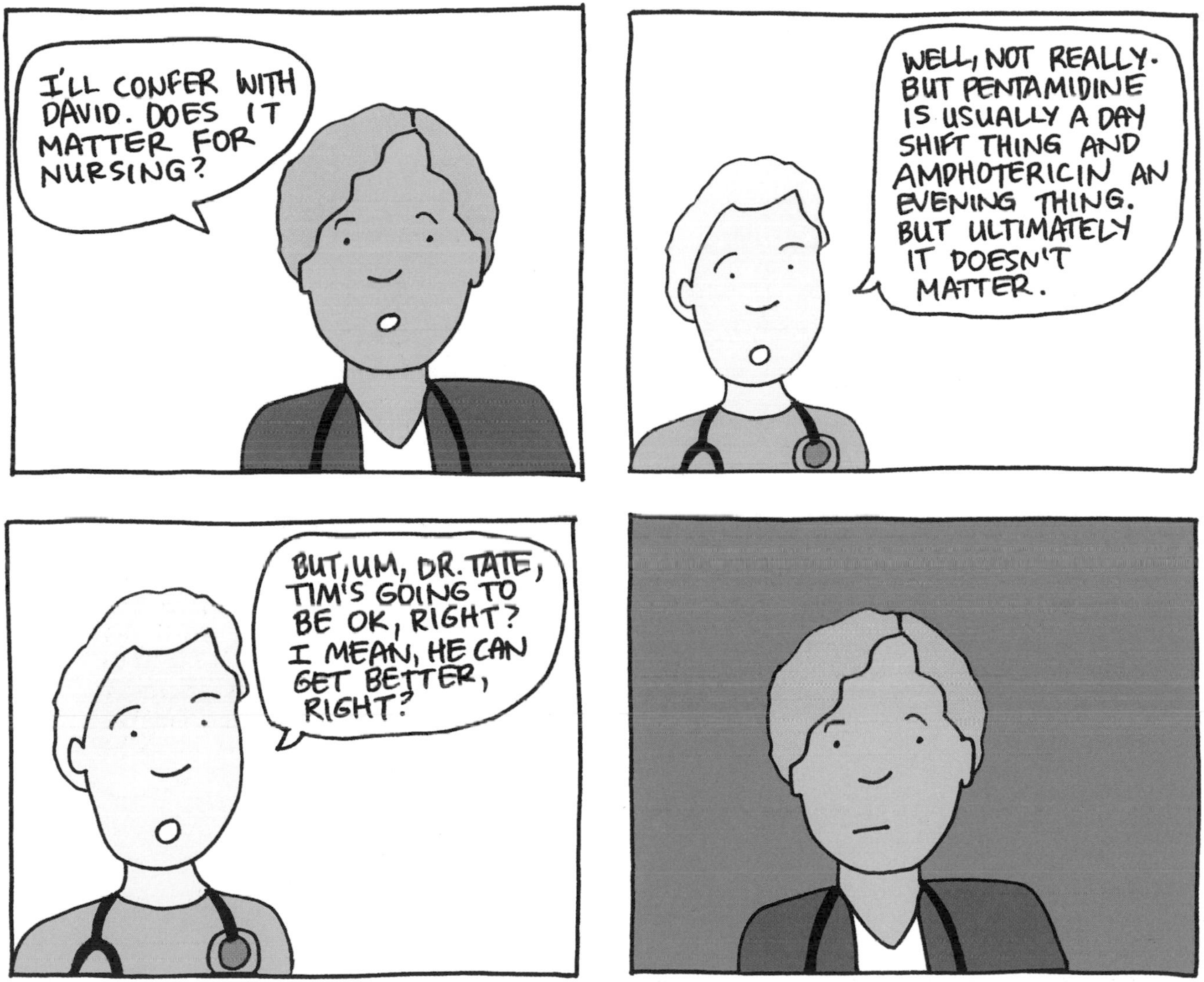
I'LL CONFER WITH DAVID. DOES IT MATTER FOR NURSING?
WELL, NOT REALLY. BUT PENTAMIDINE IS USUALLY A DAY SHIFT THING AND AMPHOTERICIN AN EVENING THING. BUT ULTIMATELY IT DOESN'T MATTER.
BUT, UM, DR. TATE, TIM'S GOING TO BE OK, RIGHT? I MEAN, HE CAN GET BETTER, RIGHT?

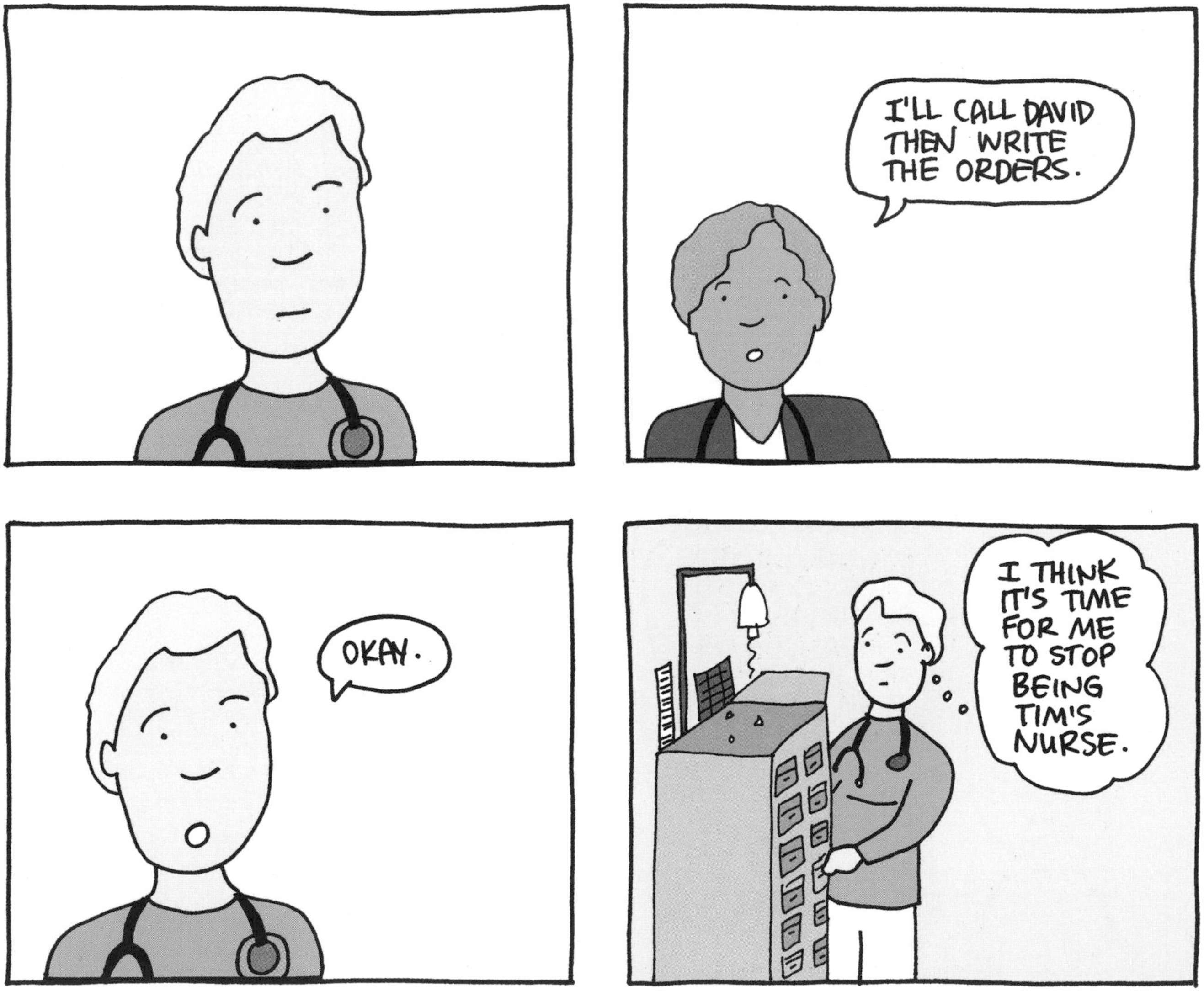
I'LL CALL DAVID THEN WRITE THE ORDERS.
OKAY.
I THINK IT'S TIME FOR ME TO STOP BEING TIM'S NURSE.

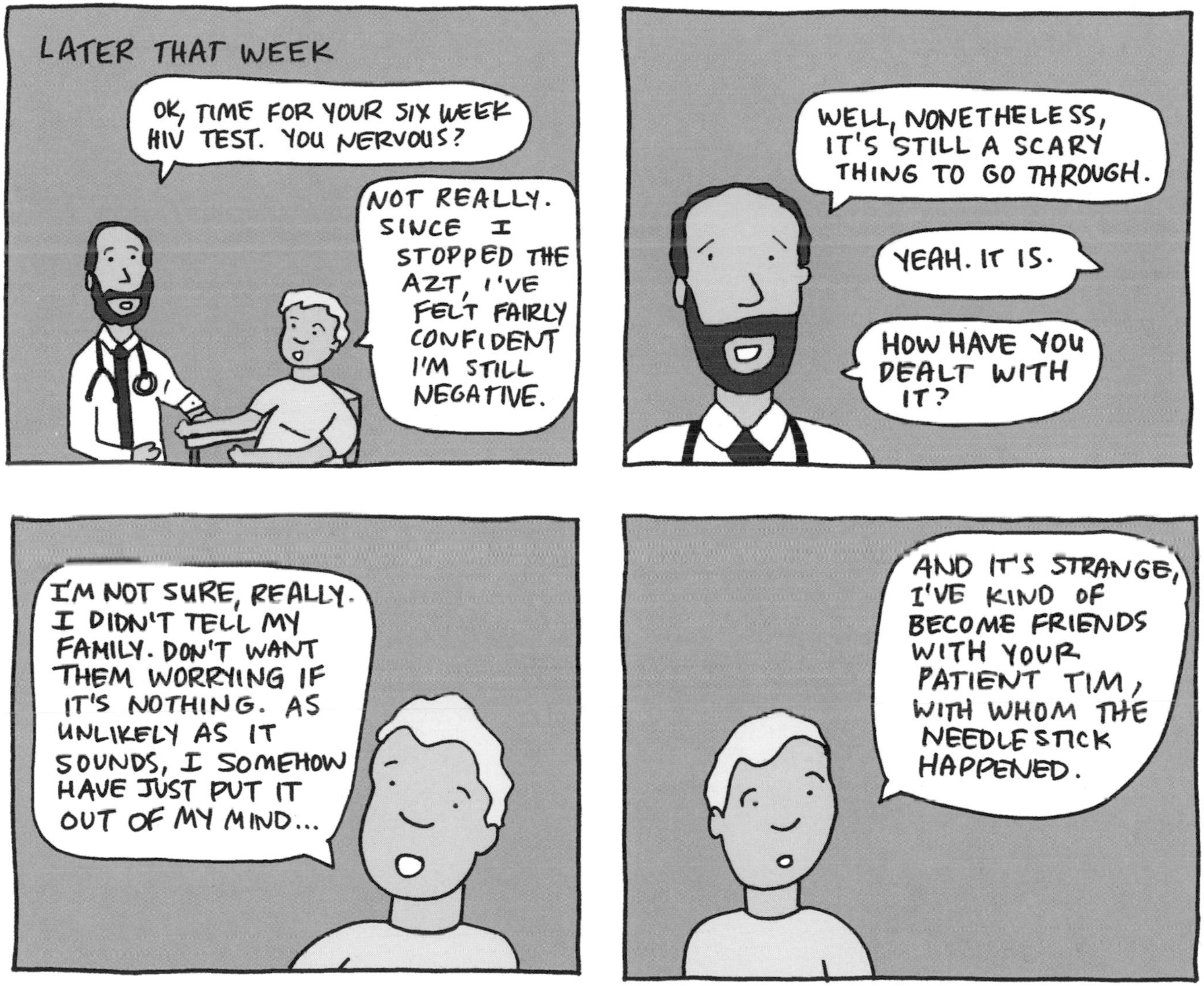

LATER THAT WEEK
OK, TIME FOR YOUR SIX WEEK HIV TEST. YOU NERVOUS?
NOT REALLY. SINCE I STOPPED THE AZT, I'VE FELT FAIRLY CONFIDENT I'M STILL NEGATIVE.
WELL, NONETHELESS, IT'S STILL A SCARY THING TO GO THROUGH.
YEAH. IT IS.
HOW HAVE YOU DEALT WITH IT?
I'M NOT SURE, REALLY. I DIDN'T TELL MY FAMILY. DON'T WANT THEM WORRYING IF IT'S NOTHING. AS UNLIKELY AS IT SOUNDS, I SOMEHOW HAVE JUST PUT IT OUT OF MY MIND...
AND IT'S STRANGE, I'VE KIND OF BECOME FRIENDS WITH YOUR PATIENT TIM, WITH WHOM THE NEEDLESTICK HAPPENED.

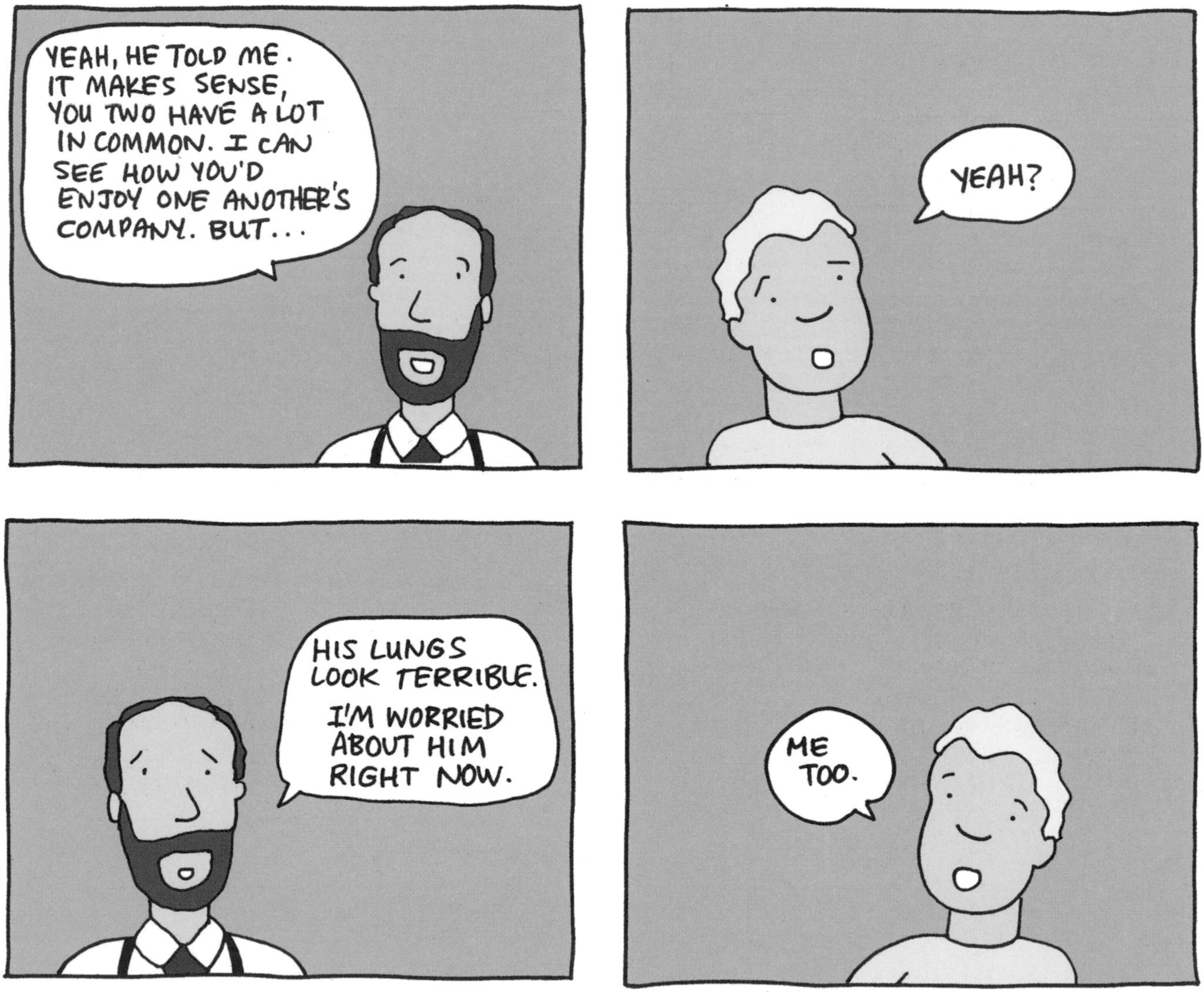
YEAH, HE TOLD ME. IT MAKES SENSE, YOU TWO HAVE A LOT IN COMMON. I CAN SEE HOW YOU'D ENJOY ONE ANOTHER'S COMPANY. BUT...
YEAH?
HIS LUNGS LOOK TERRIBLE.
I'M WORRIED ABOUT HIM RIGHT NOW.
ME TOO.

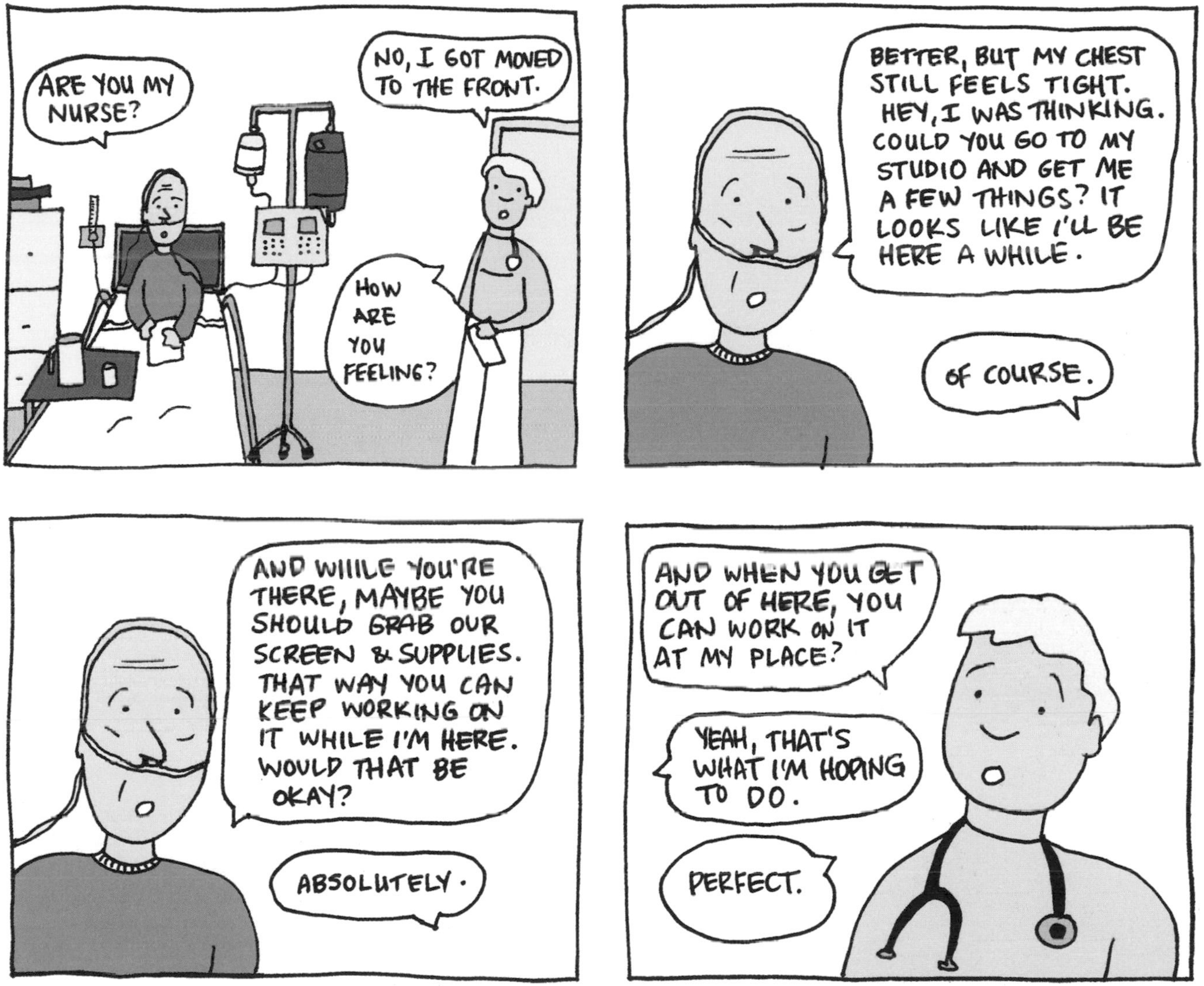
ARE YOU MY NURSE?
NO, I GOT MOVED TO THE FRONT.
HOW ARE YOU FEELING?
BETTER, BUT MY CHEST STILL FEELS TIGHT. HEY, I WAS THINKING. COULD YOU GO TO MY STUDIO AND GET ME A FEW THINGS? IT LOOKS LIKE I'LL BE HERE A WHILE.
OF COURSE.
AND WHILE YOU'RE THERE, MAYBE YOU SHOULD GRAB OUR SCREEN & SUPPLIES. THAT WAY YOU CAN KEEP WORKING ON IT WHILE I'M HERE. WOULD THAT BE OKAY?
ABSOLUTELY.
AND WHEN YOU GET OUT OF HERE, YOU CAN WORK ON IT AT MY PLACE?
YEAH, THAT'S WHAT I'M HOPING TO DO.
PERFECT.

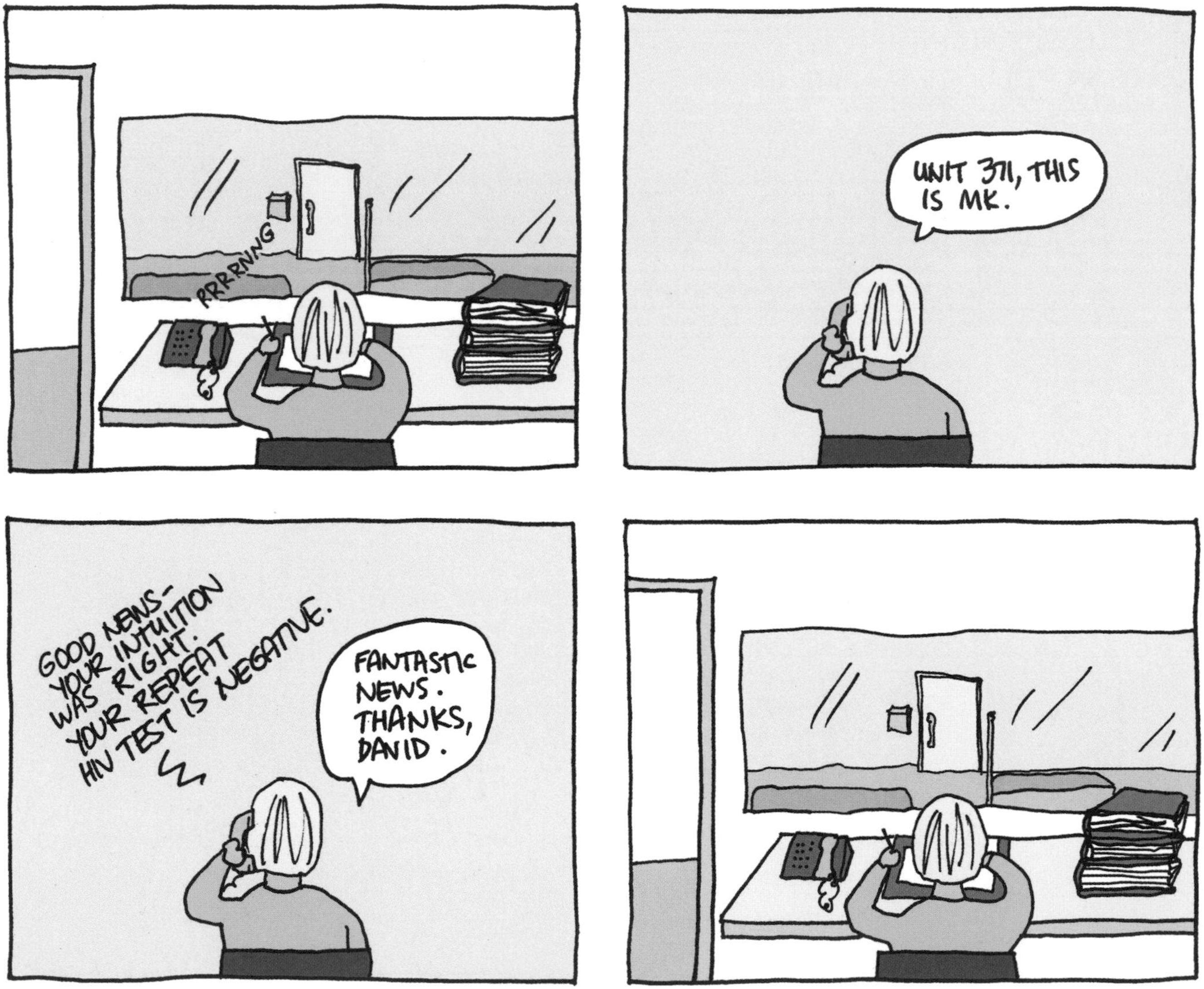
RRRRNNG
UNIT 371, THIS IS MK.
GOOD NEWS- YOUR INTUITION WAS RIGHT. YOUR REPEAT HIV TEST IS NEGATIVE.
FANTASTIC NEWS. THANKS, DAVID.

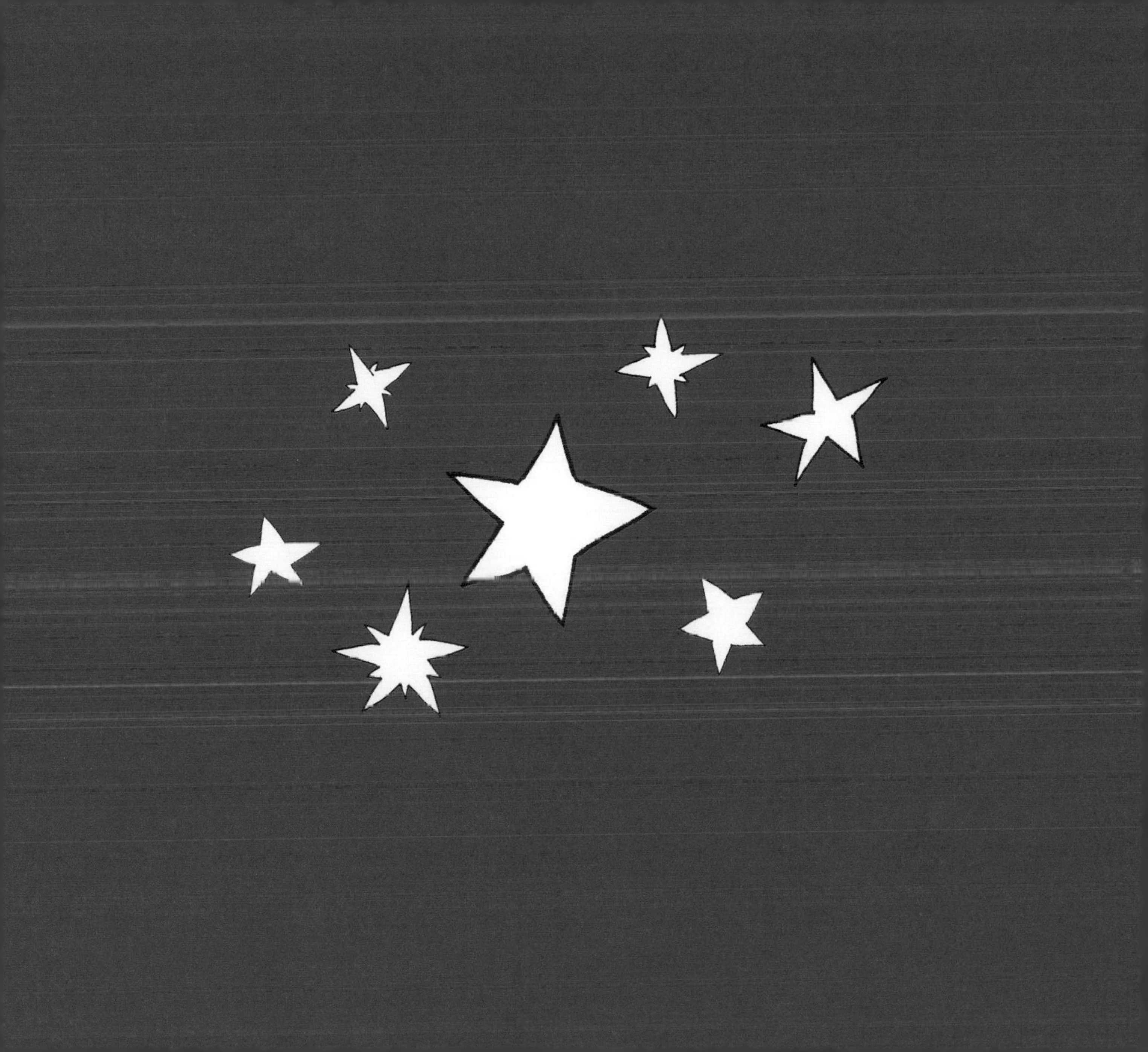

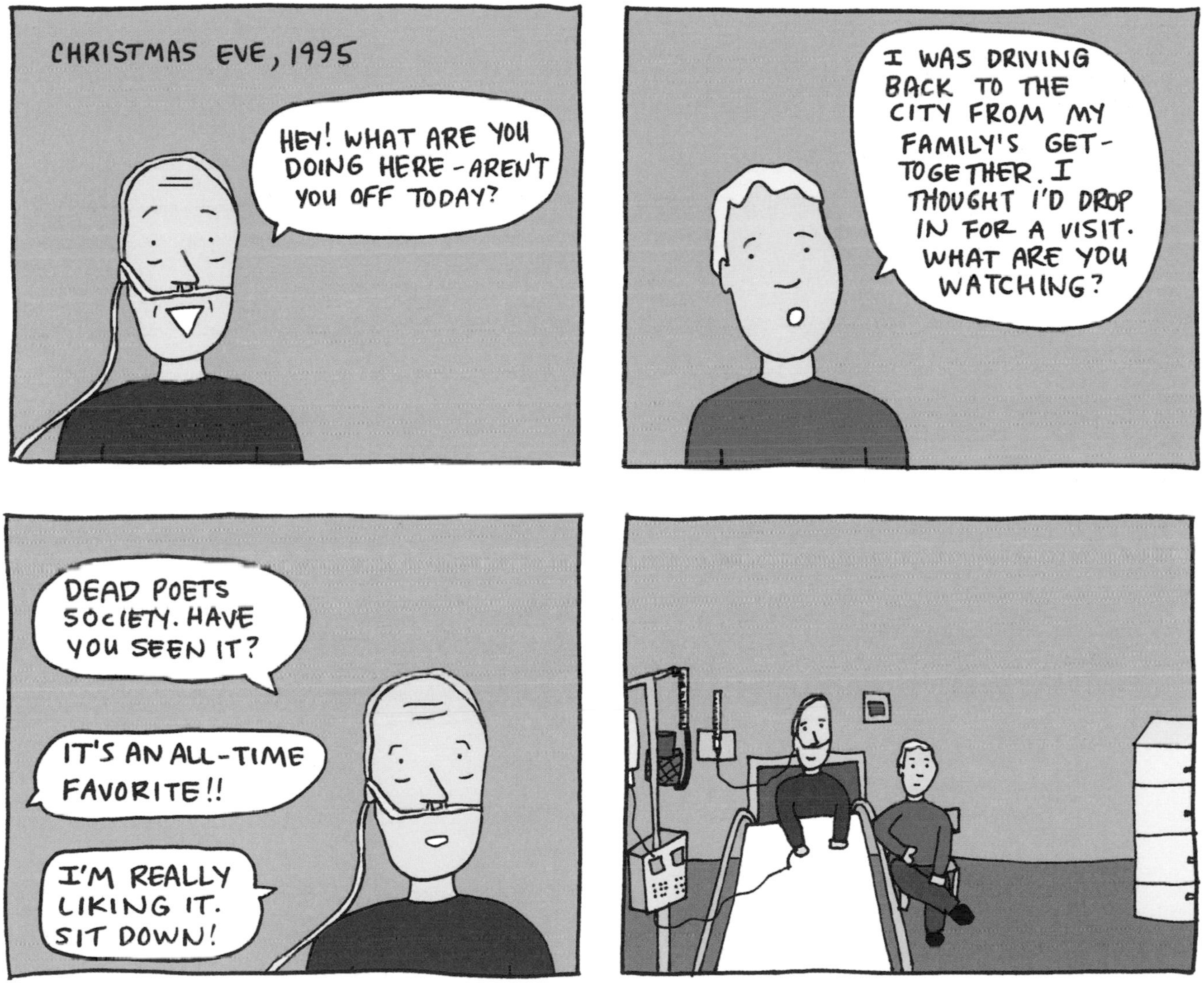
CHRISTMAS EVE, 1995
HEY! WHAT ARE YOU DOING HERE - AREN'T YOU OFF TODAY?
I WAS DRIVING BACK TO THE CITY FROM MY FAMILY'S GET-TOGETHER. I THOUGHT I'D DROP IN FOR A VISIT. WHAT ARE YOU WATCHING?
DEAD POETS SOCIETY. HAVE YOU SEEN IT?
IT'S AN ALL-TIME FAVORITE!!
I'M REALLY LIKING IT. SIT DOWN!

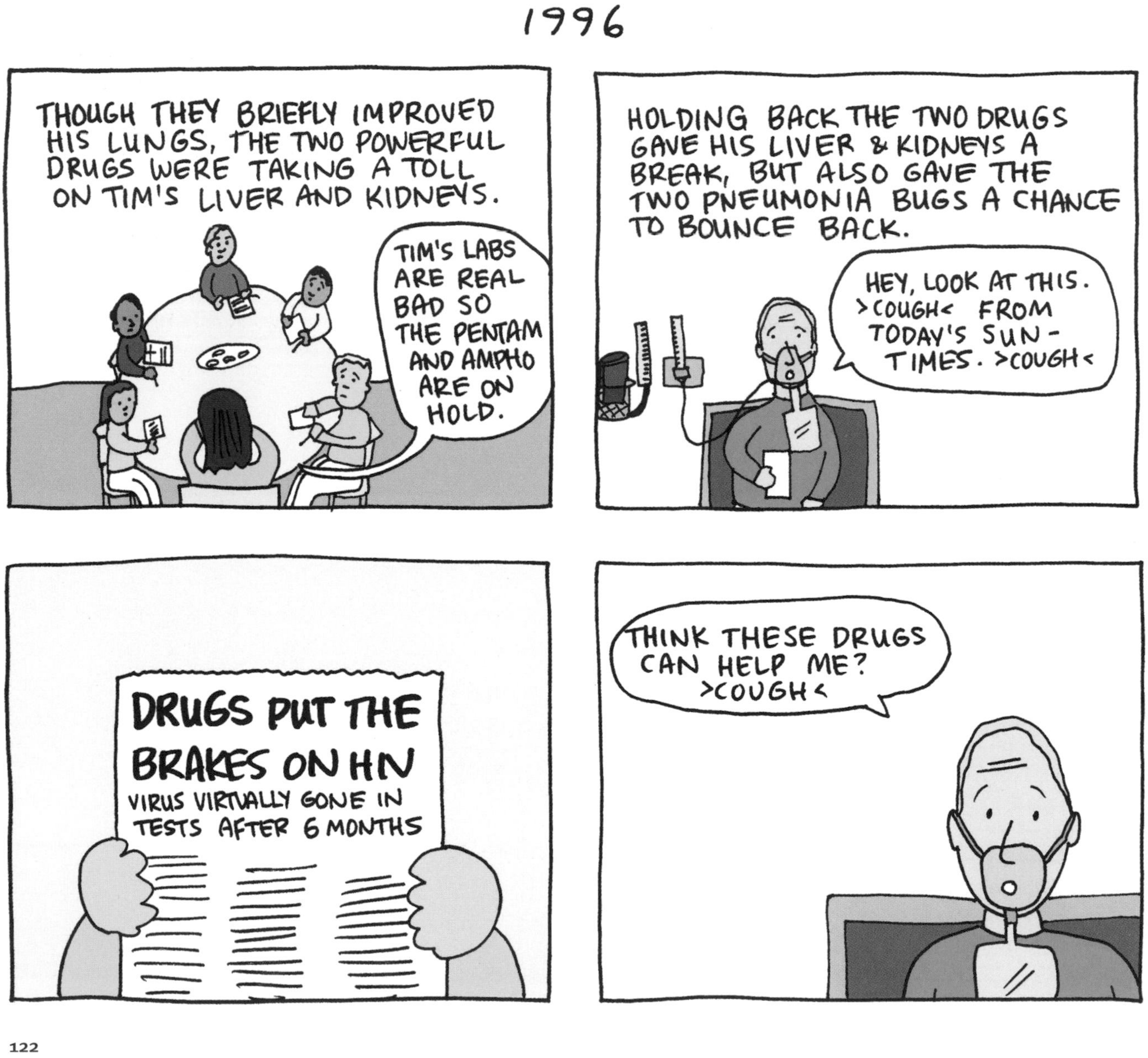
1996
THOUGH THEY BRIEFLY IMPROVED HIS LUNGS, THE TWO POWERFUL DRUGS WERE TAKING A TOLL ON TIM'S LIVER AND KIDNEYS.
TIM'S LABS ARE REAL BAD SO THE PENTAM AND AMPHO ARE ON HOLD.
HOLDING BACK THE TWO DRUGS GAVE HIS LIVER & KIDNEYS A BREAK, BUT ALSO GAVE THE TWO PNEUMONIA BUGS A CHANCE TO BOUNCE BACK.
HEY, LOOK AT THIS. >COUGH< FROM TODAY'S SUN-TIMES. >COUGH<
DRUGS PUT THE BRAKES ON HIV
VIRUS VIRTUALLY GONE IN TESTS AFTER 6 MONTHS
THINK THESE DRUGS CAN HELP ME? >COUGH<

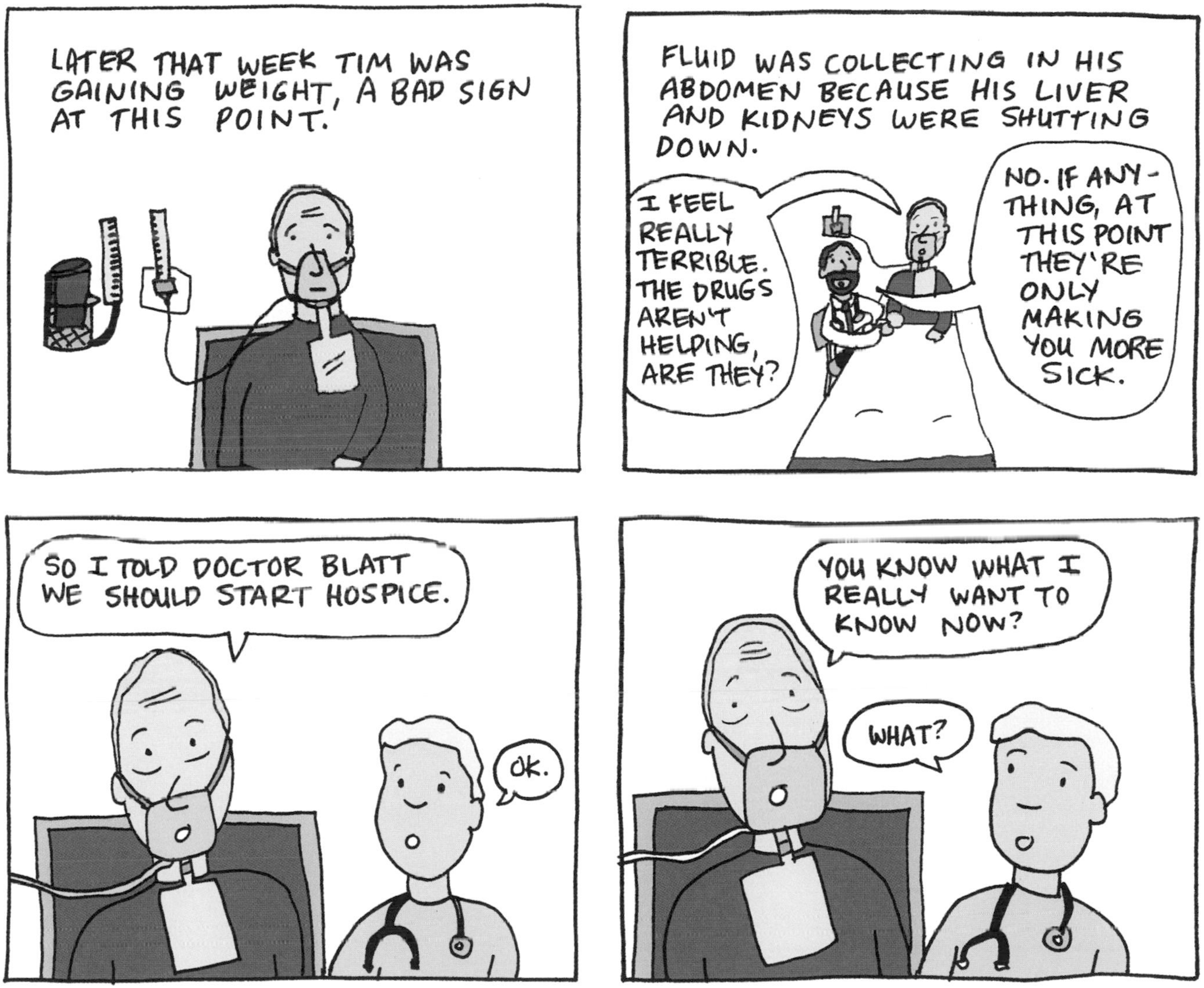
LATER THAT WEEK TIM WAS GAINING WEIGHT, A BAD SIGN AT THIS POINT.
FLUID WAS COLLECTING IN HIS ABDOMEN BECAUSE HIS LIVER AND KIDNEYS WERE SHUTTING DOWN.
I FEEL REALLY TERRIBLE. THE DRUGS AREN'T HELPING, ARE THEY?
NO. IF ANYTHING, AT THIS POINT THEY'RE ONLY MAKING YOU MORE SICK.
SO I TOLD DOCTOR BLATT WE SHOULD START HOSPICE.
OK.
YOU KNOW WHAT I REALLY WANT TO KNOW NOW?
WHAT?

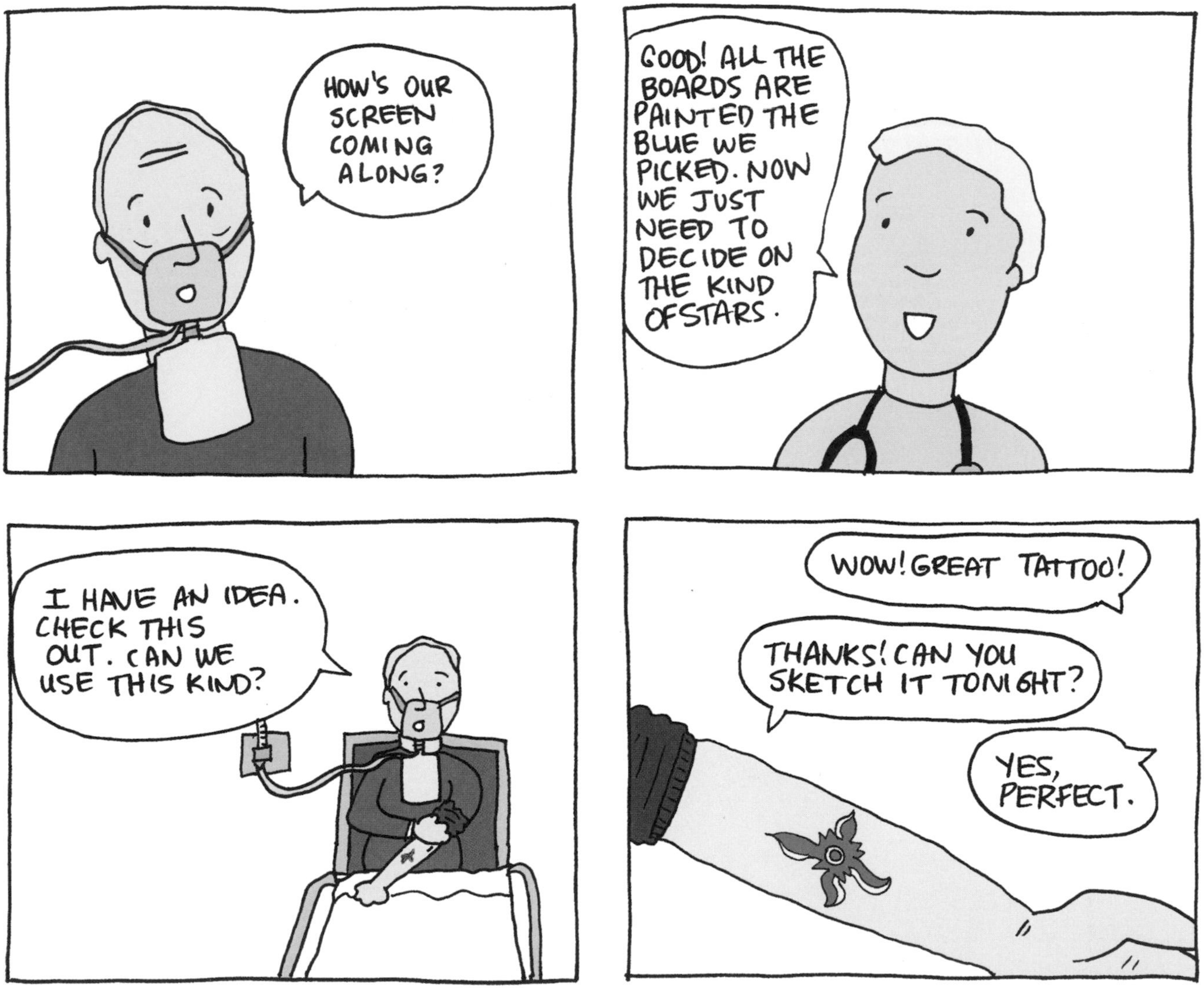
HOW'S OUR SCREEN COMING ALONG?
GOOD! ALL THE BOARDS ARE PAINTED THE BLUE WE PICKED. NOW WE JUST NEED TO DECIDE ON THE KIND OFSTARS.
I HAVE AN IDEA. CHECK THIS OUT. CAN WE USE THIS KIND?
WOW! GREAT TATTOO!
THANKS! CAN YOU SKETCH IT TONIGHT?
YES, PERFECT.

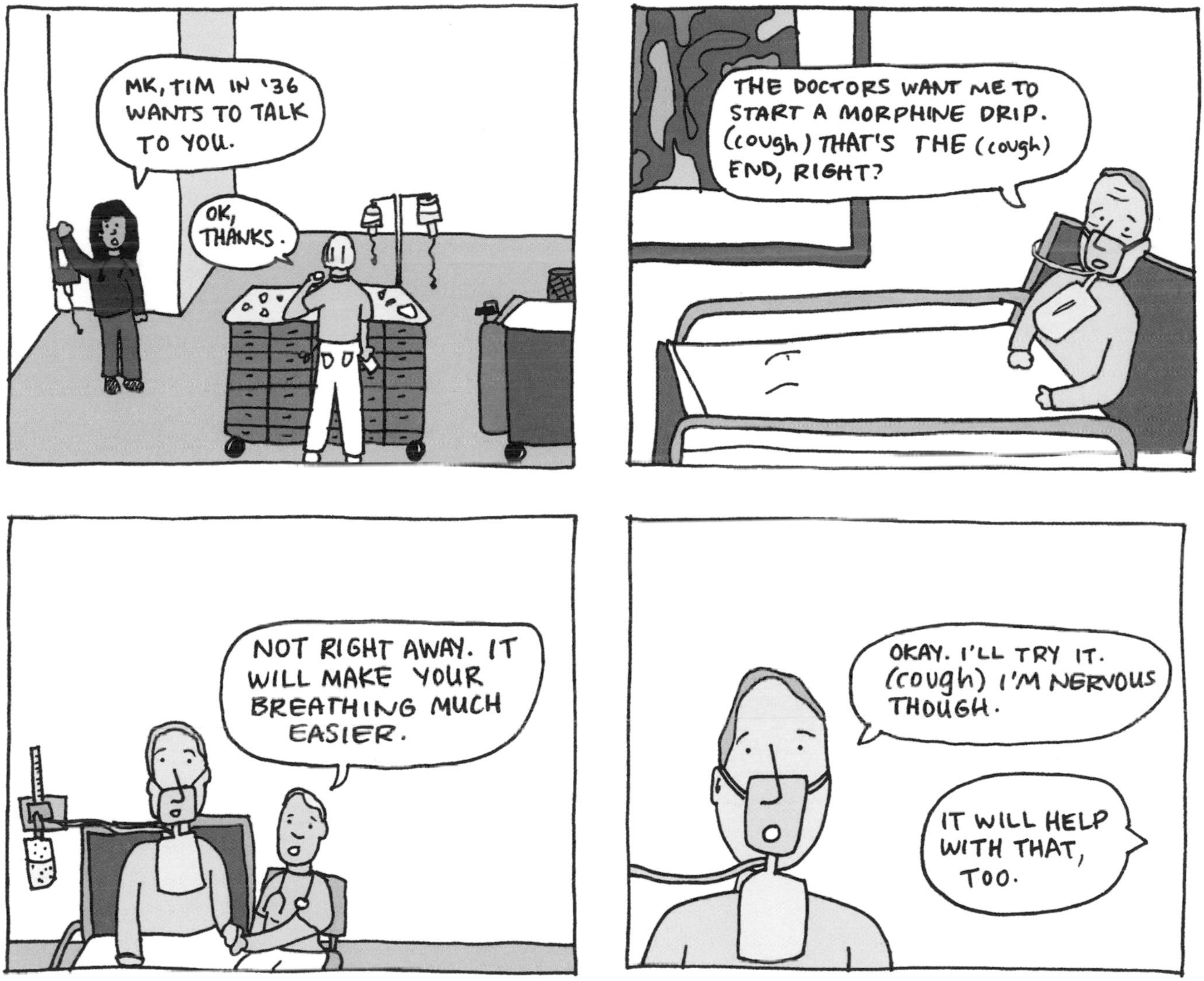
MK, TIM IN '36 WANTS TO TALK TO YOU.
OK, THANKS.
THE DOCTORS WANT ME TO START A MORPHINE DRIP. (cough) THAT'S THE (cough) END, RIGHT?
NOT RIGHT AWAY. IT WILL MAKE YOUR BREATHING MUCH EASIER.
OKAY. I'LL TRY IT. (cough) I'M NERVOUS THOUGH.
IT WILL HELP WITH THAT, TOO.

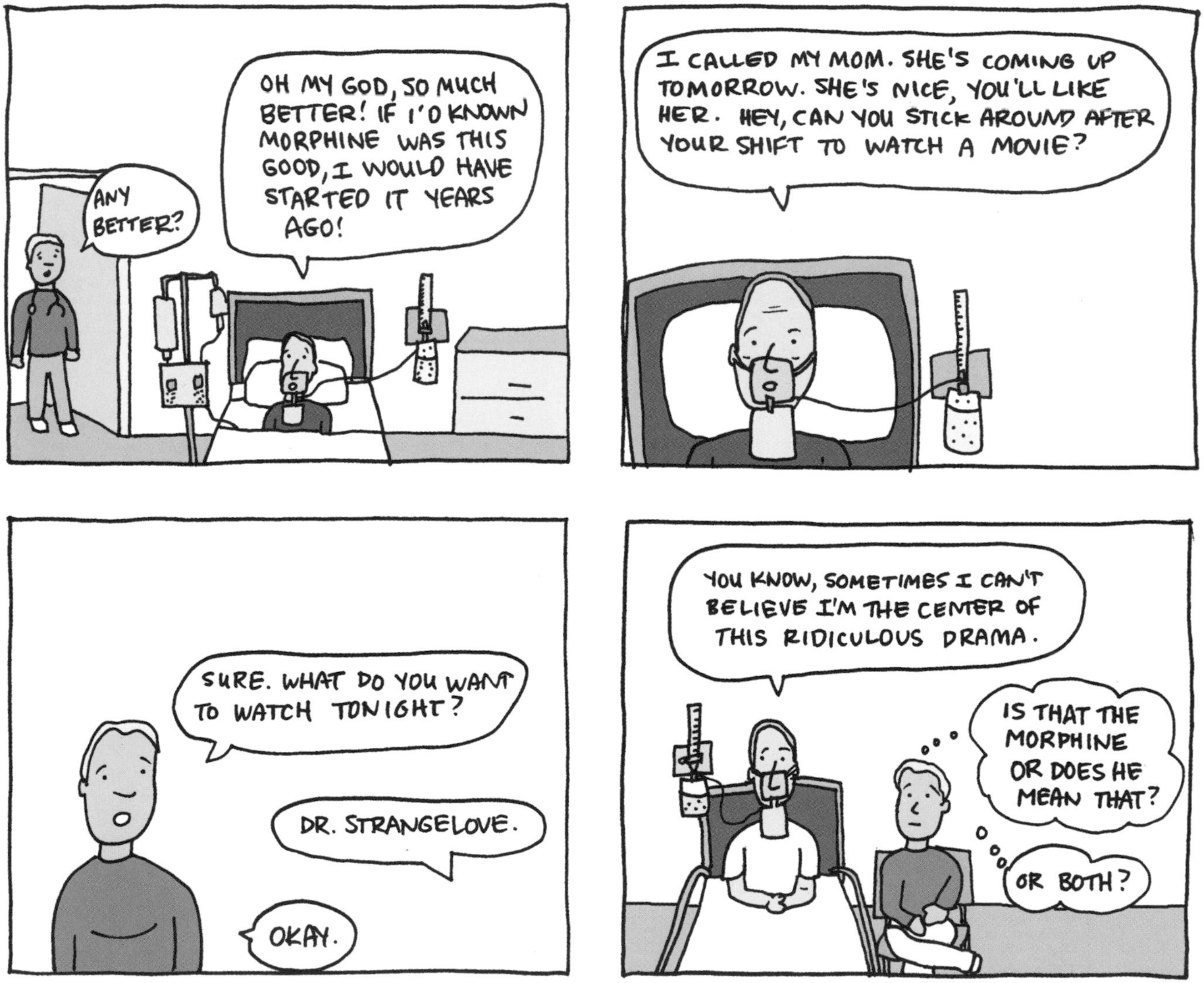
ANY BETTER?
OH MY GOD, SO MUCH BETTER! IF I'D KNOWN MORPHINE WAS THIS GOOD, I WOULD HAVE STARTED IT YEARS AGO!
I CALLED MY MOM. SHE'S COMING UP TOMORROW. SHE'S NICE, YOU'LL LIKE HER. HEY, CAN YOU STICK AROUND AFTER YOUR SHIFT TO WATCH A MOVIE?
SURE. WHAT DO YOU WANT TO WATCH TONIGHT?
DR. STRANGELOVE.
OKAY.
YOU KNOW, SOMETIMES I CAN'T BELIEVE I'M THE CENTER OF THIS RIDICULOUS DRAMA.
IS THAT THE MORPHINE OR DOES HE MEAN THAT?
OR BOTH?

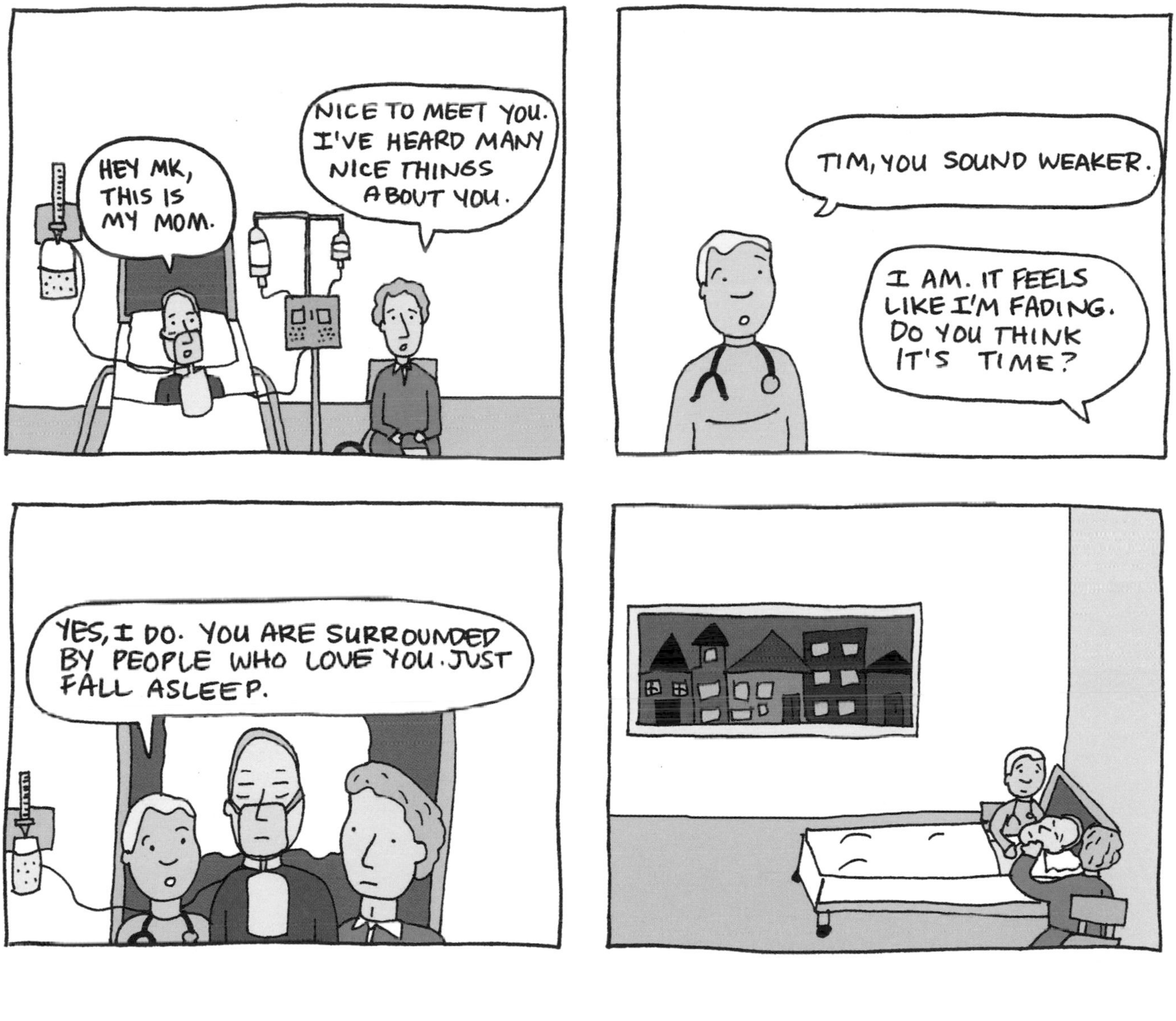
HEY MK, THIS IS MY MOM.
NICE TO MEET YOU. I'VE HEARD MANY NICE THINGS ABOUT YOU.
TIM, YOU SOUND WEAKER.
I AM. IT FEELS LIKE I'M FADING. DO YOU THINK IT'S TIME?
YES, I DO. YOU ARE SURROUNDED BY PEOPLE WHO LOVE YOU. JUST FALL ASLEEP.

THAT LAST PAGE IS A LIE.
IT'S NOT WHAT HAPPENED.
IT'S WHAT I WISH HAD HAPPENED.

WHAT REALLY HAPPENED IS
THAT TIM HAD A PANIC
ATTACK. HIS DAY NURSE
CALLED ME IN.
HE WAS INCOHERENT, A WILD
LOOK IN HIS EYES.
I'M NOT SURE HE SAW ME.
HIS MOTHER WAS CRYING.

HIS NURSE PUSHED A DOSE
OF ATIVAN INTO THE I.V.
HE VISIBLY RELAXED.
HIS BLUE EYES CLOSED,
NEVER TO REOPEN. HIS
VOICE STILLED, NEVER
TO BE HEARD AGAIN.

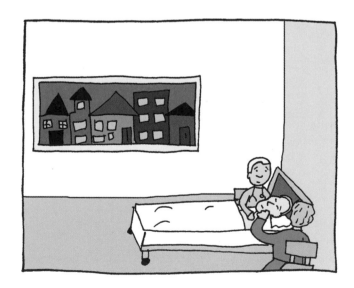

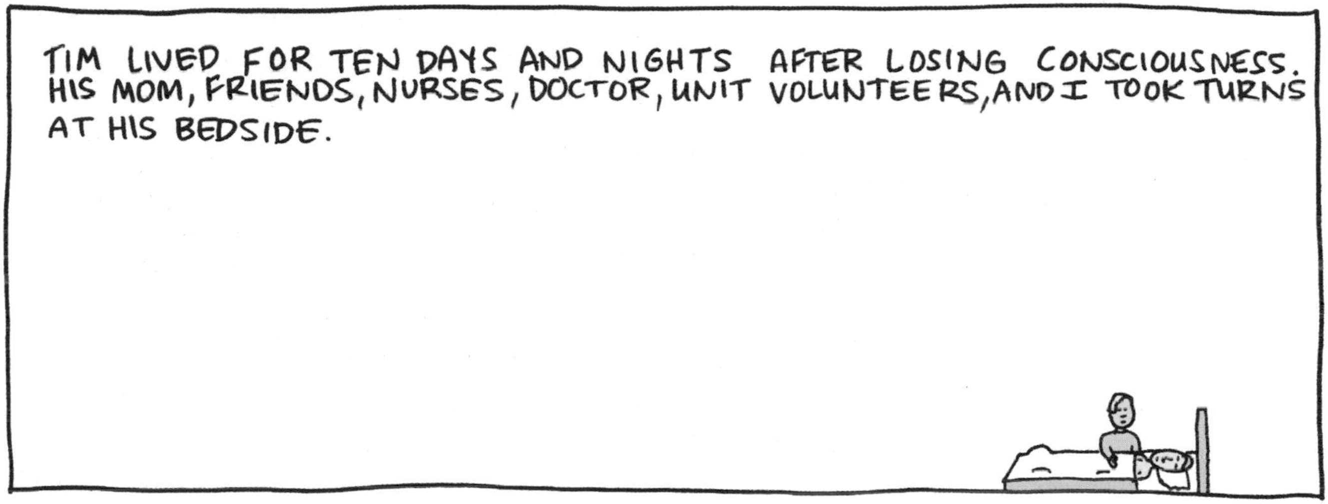
TIM LIVED FOR TEN DAYS AND NIGHTS AFTER LOSING CONSCIOUSNESS. HIS MOM, FRIENDS, NURSES, DOCTOR, UNIT VOLUNTEERS, AND I TOOK TURNS AT HIS BEDSIDE.

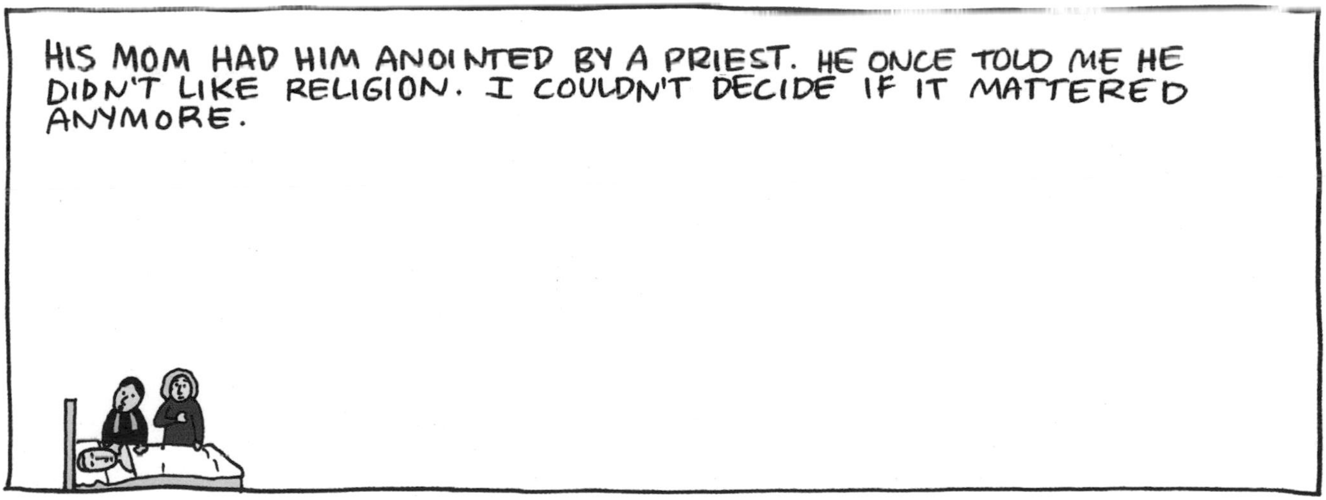
HIS MOM HAD HIM ANOINTED BY A PRIEST. HE ONCE TOLD ME HE DIDN'T LIKE RELIGION. I COULDN'T DECIDE IF IT MATTERED ANYMORE.

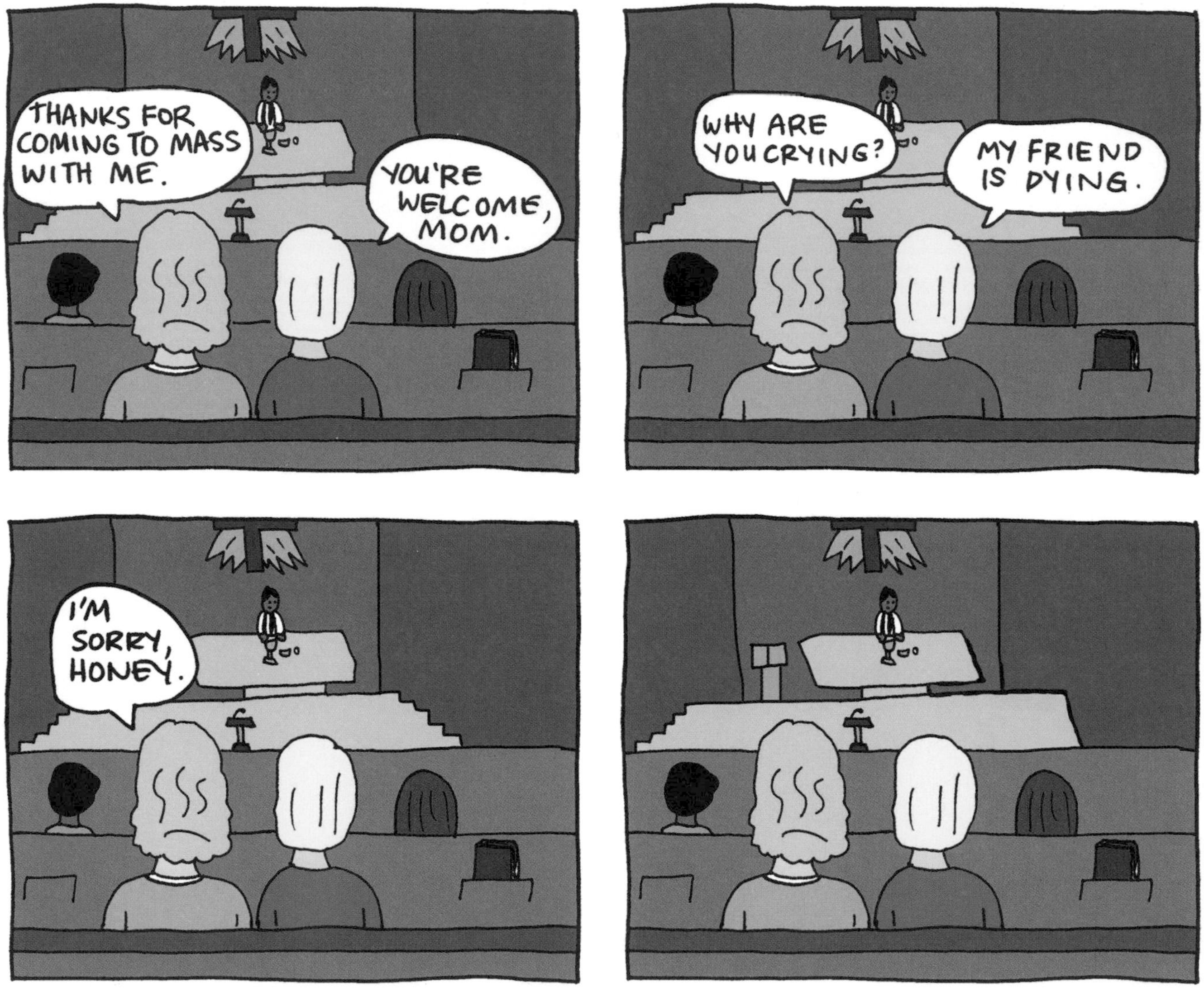
THANKS FOR COMING TO MASS WITH ME.
YOU'RE WELCOME, MOM.
WHY ARE YOU CRYING?
MY FRIEND IS DYING.
I'M SORRY, HONEY.

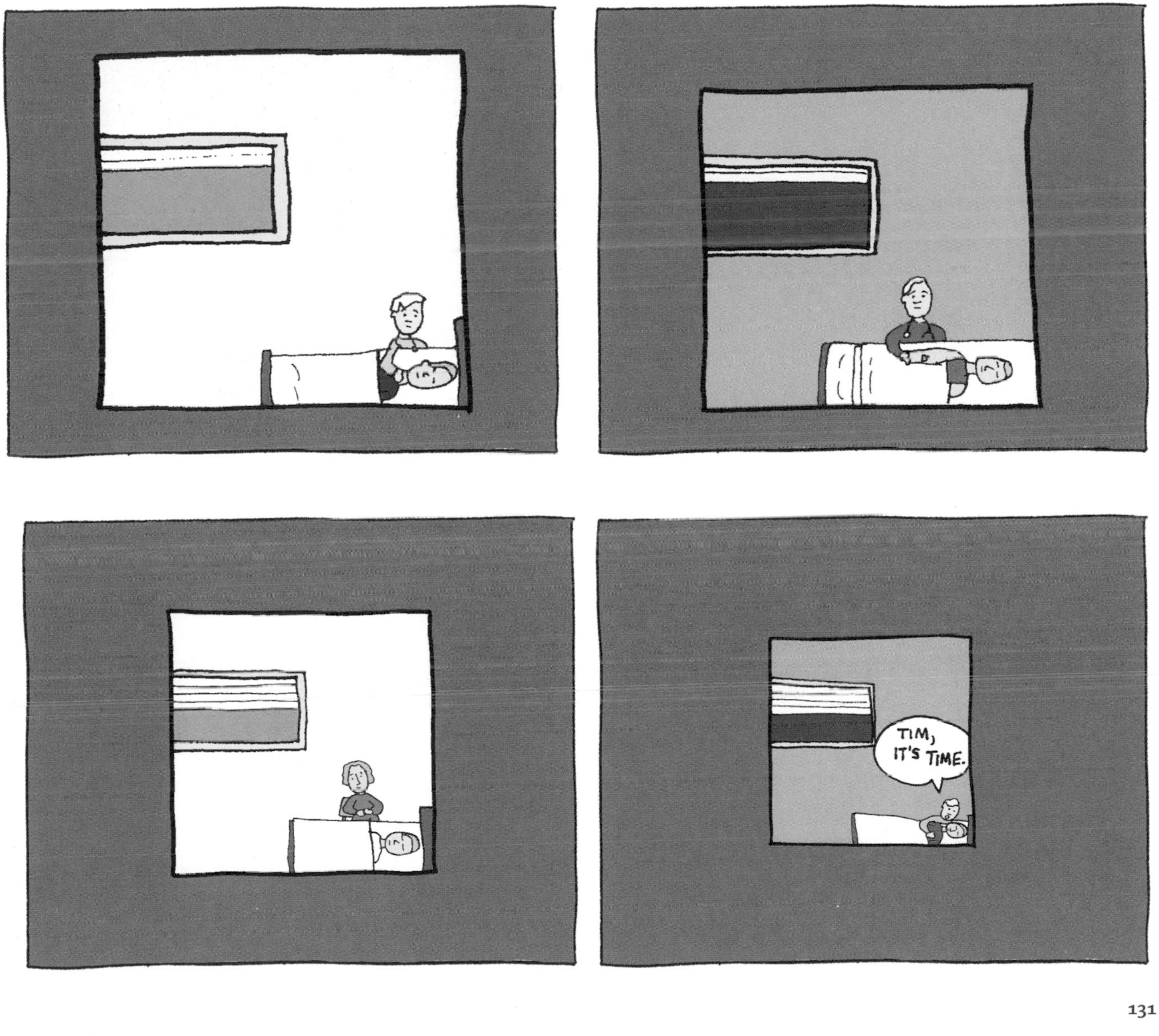
TIM,
IT'S TIME.

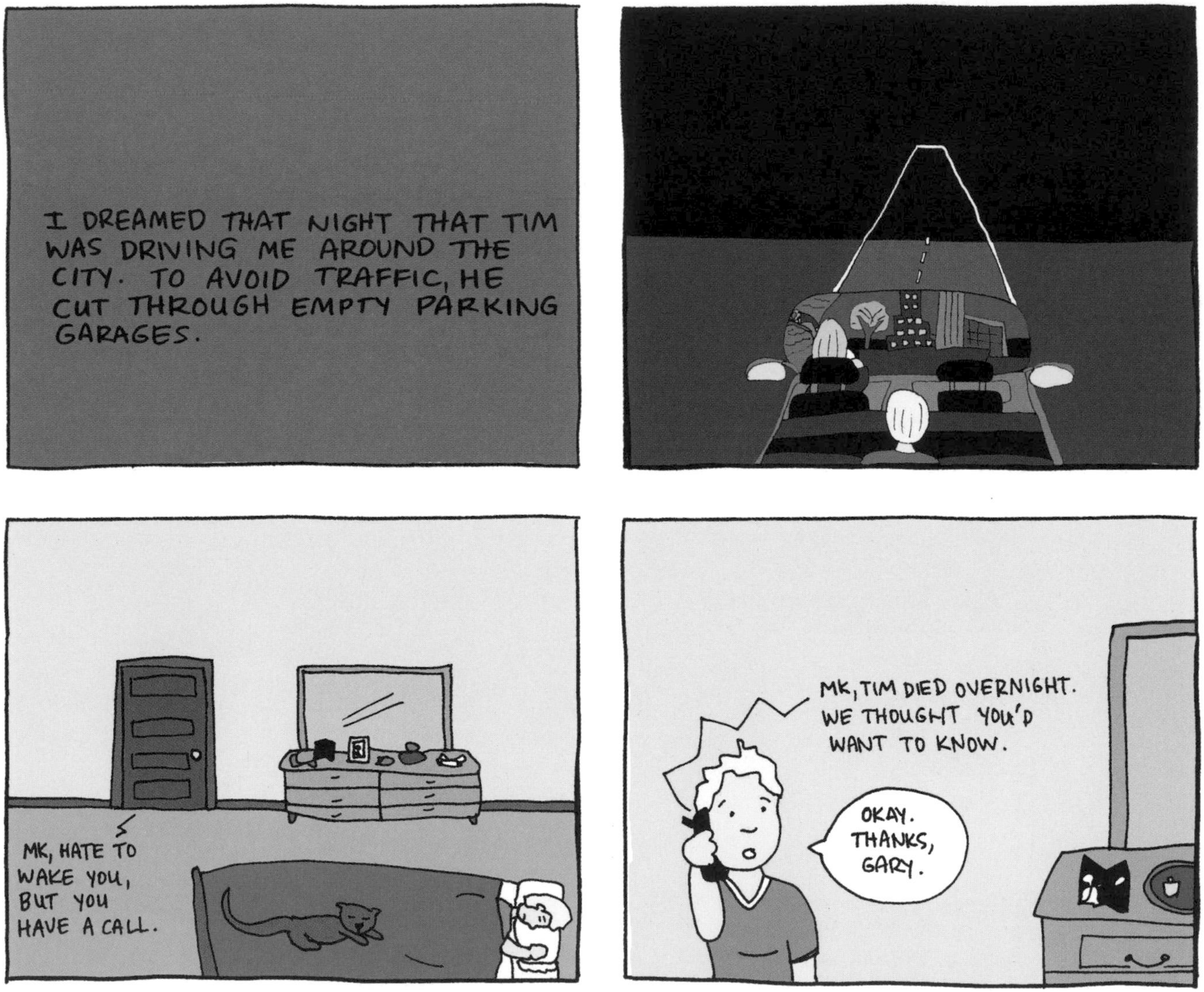
I DREAMED THAT NIGHT THAT TIM WAS DRIVING ME AROUND THE CITY. TO AVOID TRAFFIC, HE CUT THROUGH EMPTY PARKING GARAGES.
MK, HATE TO WAKE YOU, BUT YOU HAVE A CALL.
MK, TIM DIED OVERNIGHT. WE THOUGHT YOU'D WANT TO KNOW.
OKAY. THANKS, GARY.

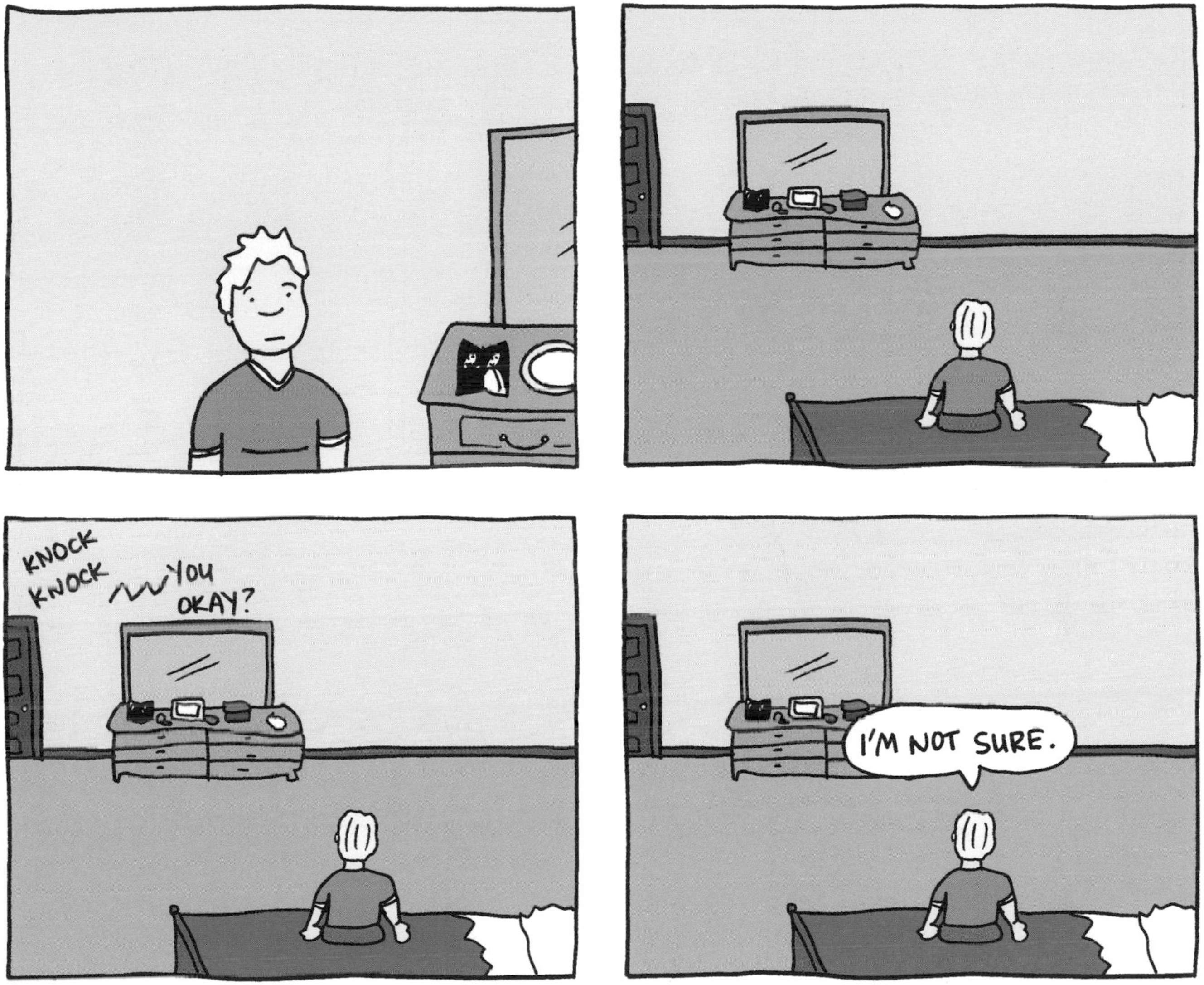
KNOCK
KNOCK
YOU OKAY?
I'M NOT SURE.

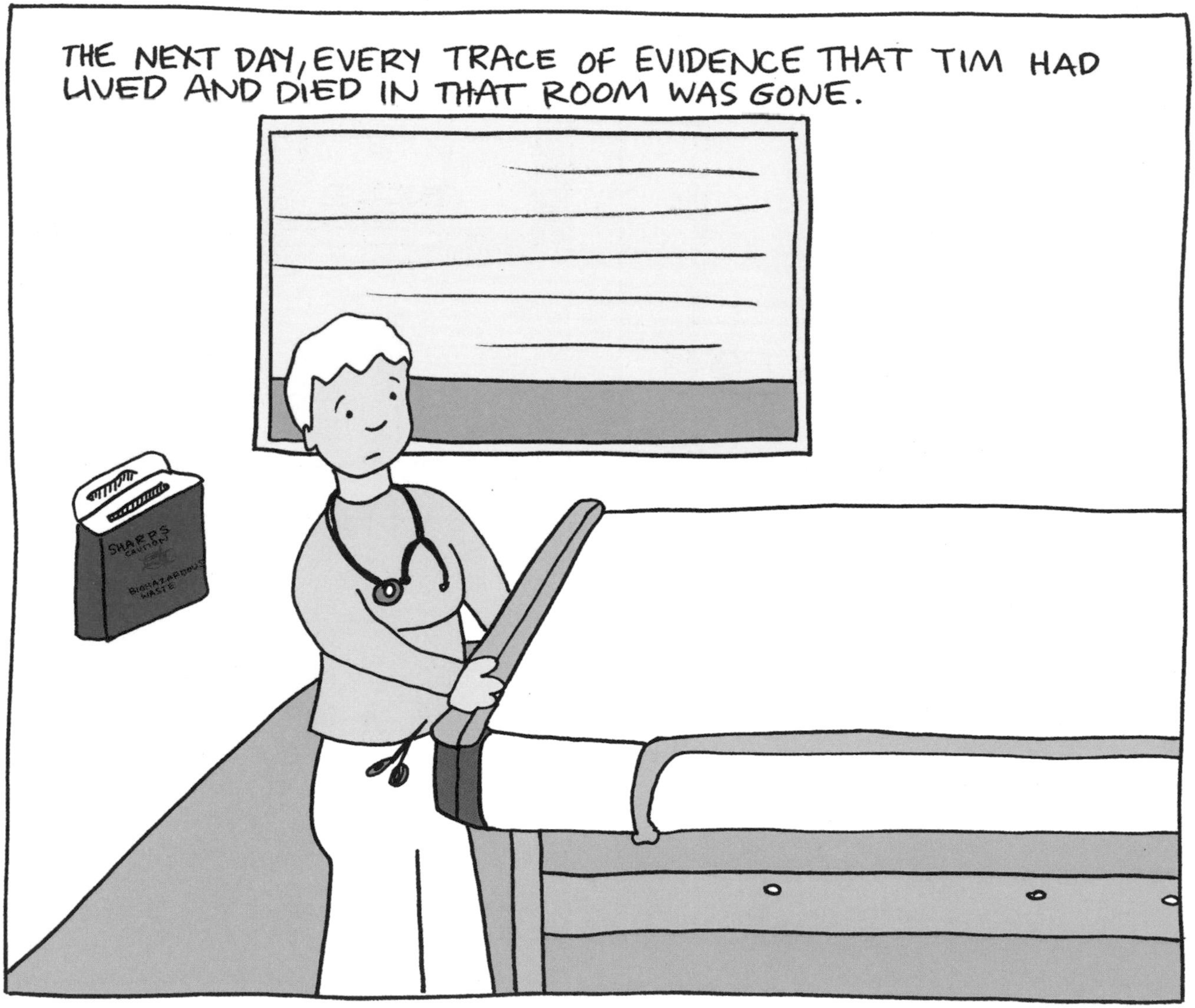
THE NEXT DAY, EVERY TRACE OF EVIDENCE THAT TIM HAD LIVED AND DIED IN THAT ROOM WAS GONE.
SHARPS
CAUTION
BIOHAZARDOUS
WASTE

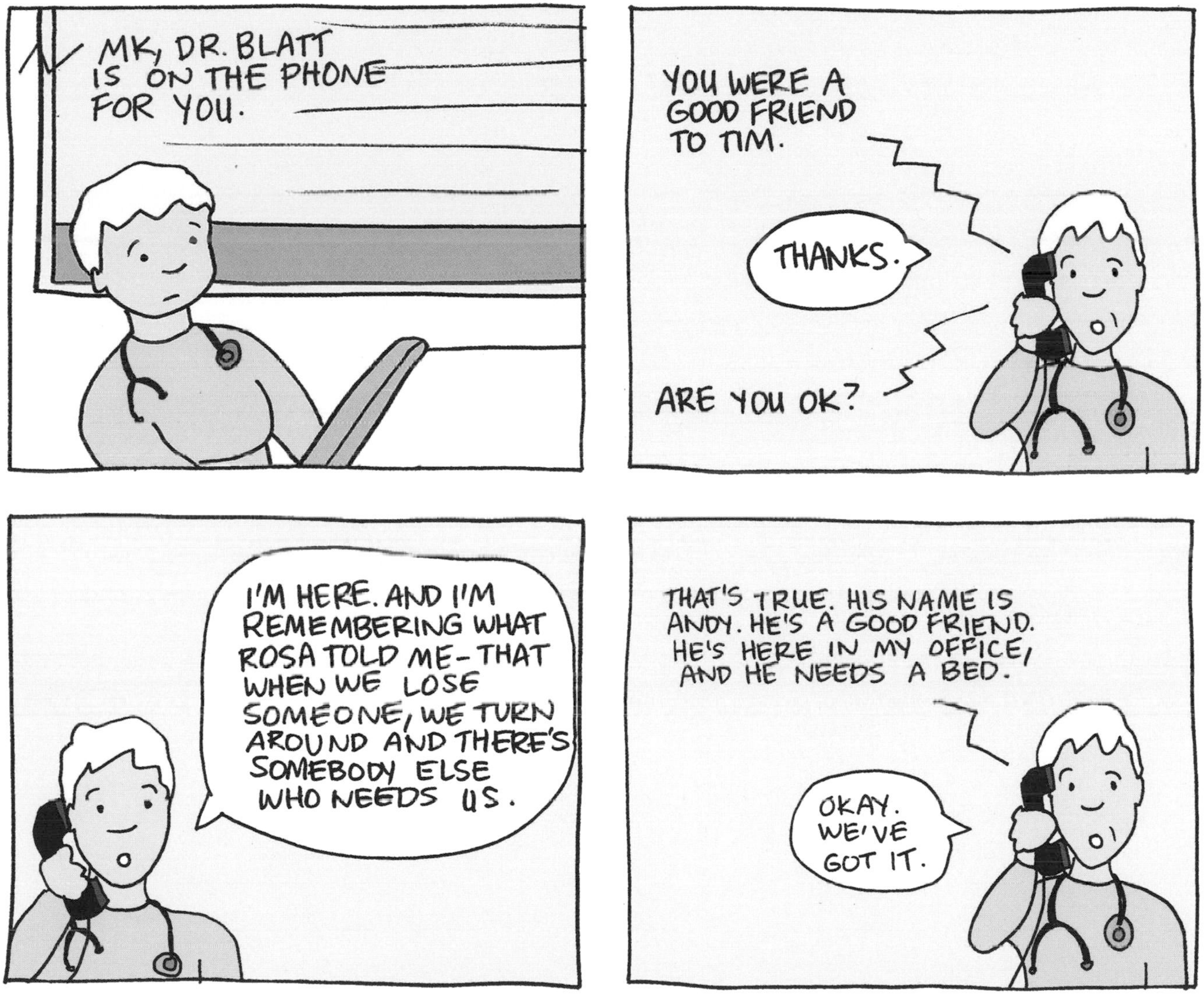
MK, DR. BLATT IS ON THE PHONE FOR YOU.
YOU WERE A GOOD FRIEND TO TIM.
THANKS.
ARE YOU OK?
I'M HERE. AND I'M REMEMBERING WHAT ROSA TOLD ME—THAT WHEN WE LOSE SOMEONE, WE TURN AROUND AND THERE'S SOMEBODY ELSE WHO NEEDS US.
THAT'S TRUE. HIS NAME IS ANDY. HE'S A GOOD FRIEND. HE'S HERE IN MY OFFICE, AND HE NEEDS A BED.
OKAY. WE'VE GOT IT.

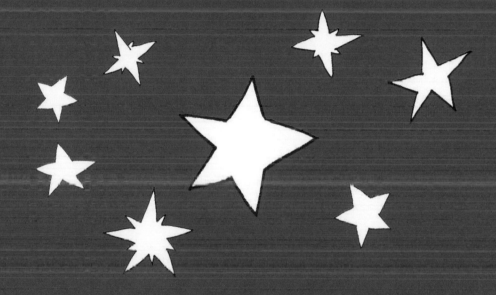

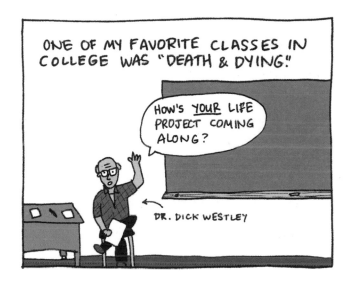

ONE OF MY FAVORITE CLASSES IN COLLEGE WAS "DEATH & DYING!"

HOW'S YOUR LIFE PROJECT COMING ALONG?

DR. DICK WESTLEY

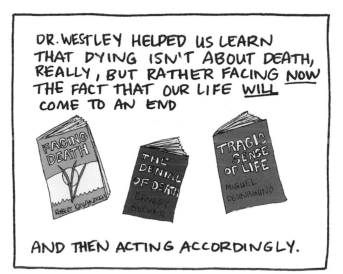

DR. WESTLEY HELPED US LEARN THAT DYING ISN'T ABOUT DEATH, REALLY, BUT RATHER FACING NOW THE FACT THAT OUR LIFE WILL COME TO AN END

FACING DEATH
ROBERT KAVANAUGH

THE DENIAL OF DEATH
ERNEST BECKER

TRAGIC SENSE OF LIFE
MIGUEL DEUNAMUNO

AND THEN ACTING ACCORDINGLY.

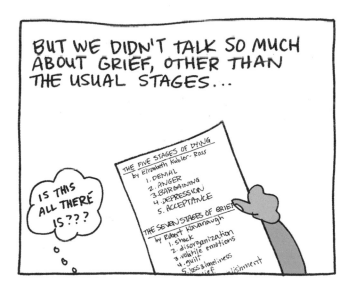

BUT WE DIDN'T TALK SO MUCH ABOUT GRIEF, OTHER THAN THE USUAL STAGES...

IS THIS ALL THERE IS???

THE FIVE STAGES OF DYING
by Elizabeth Kübler-Ross
1. DENIAL
2. ANGER
3. BARGAINING
4. DEPRESSION
5. ACCEPTANCE

THE SEVEN STAGES OF GRIEF
by Robert Kavanaugh
1. shock
2. disorganization
3. volatile emotions
4. guilt
5. loss & loneliness

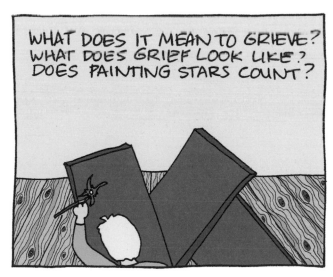

WHAT DOES IT MEAN TO GRIEVE? WHAT DOES GRIEF LOOK LIKE? DOES PAINTING STARS COUNT?

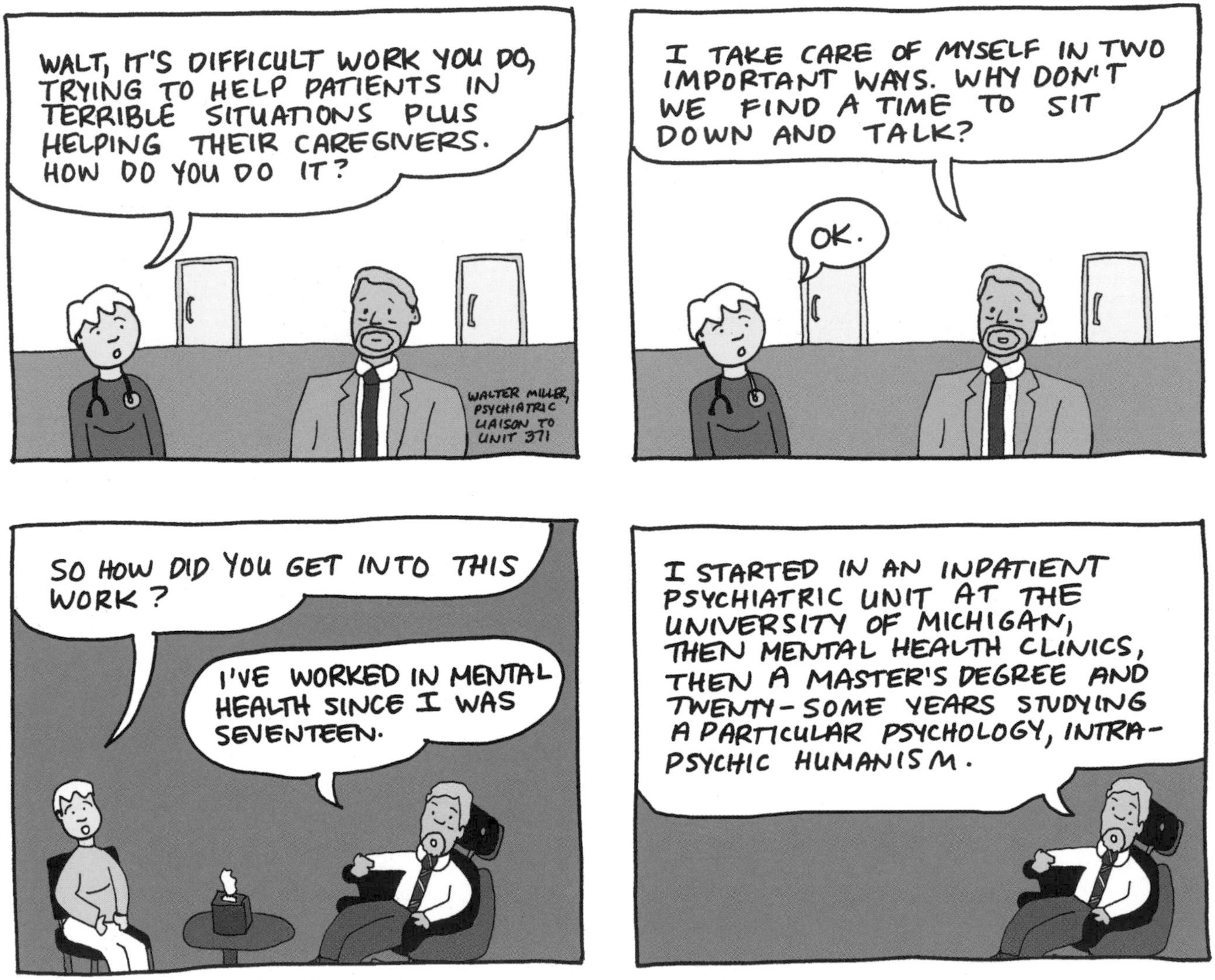
WALT, IT'S DIFFICULT WORK YOU DO, TRYING TO HELP PATIENTS IN TERRIBLE SITUATIONS PLUS HELPING THEIR CAREGIVERS. HOW DO YOU DO IT?
WALTER MILLER, PSYCHIATRIC LIAISON TO UNIT 371
I TAKE CARE OF MYSELF IN TWO IMPORTANT WAYS. WHY DON'T WE FIND A TIME TO SIT DOWN AND TALK?
OK.
SO HOW DID YOU GET INTO THIS WORK?
I'VE WORKED IN MENTAL HEALTH SINCE I WAS SEVENTEEN.
I STARTED IN AN INPATIENT PSYCHIATRIC UNIT AT THE UNIVERSITY OF MICHIGAN, THEN MENTAL HEALTH CLINICS, THEN A MASTER'S DEGREE AND TWENTY-SOME YEARS STUDYING A PARTICULAR PSYCHOLOGY, INTRA-PSYCHIC HUMANISM.

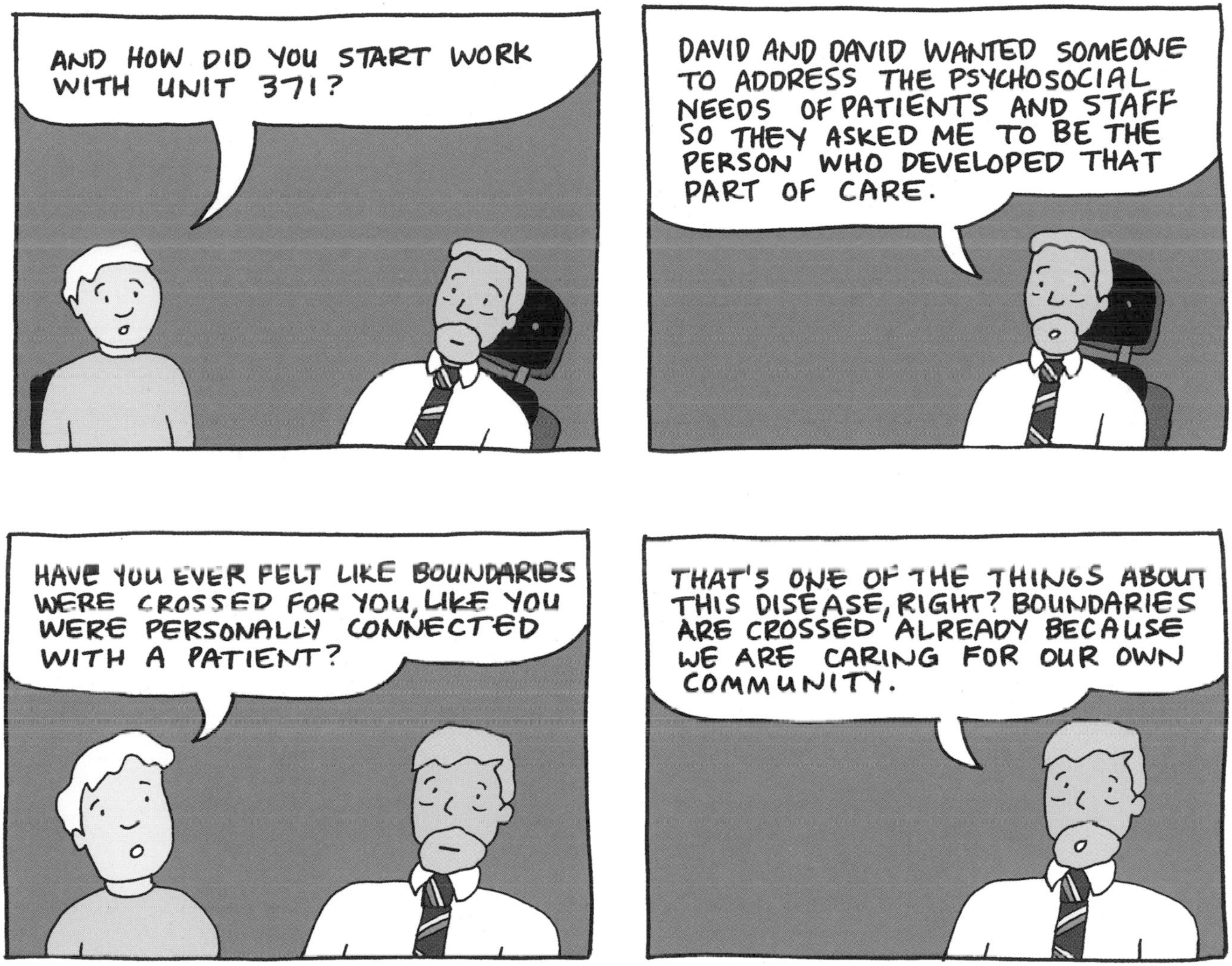
AND HOW DID YOU START WORK WITH UNIT 371?
DAVID AND DAVID WANTED SOMEONE TO ADDRESS THE PSYCHOSOCIAL NEEDS OF PATIENTS AND STAFF SO THEY ASKED ME TO BE THE PERSON WHO DEVELOPED THAT PART OF CARE.
HAVE YOU EVER FELT LIKE BOUNDARIES WERE CROSSED FOR YOU, LIKE YOU WERE PERSONALLY CONNECTED WITH A PATIENT?
THAT'S ONE OF THE THINGS ABOUT THIS DISEASE, RIGHT? BOUNDARIES ARE CROSSED ALREADY BECAUSE WE ARE CARING FOR OUR OWN COMMUNITY.

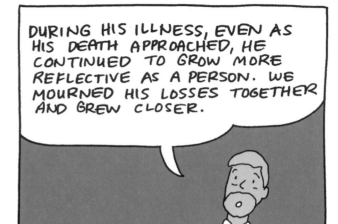

ONE SITUATION THAT COMES TO MIND IS A GUY I HAD KNOWN FOR YEARS BUT HAD NOT SEEN UNTIL HE WAS IN THE HOSPITAL. HE WAS MY FRIEND, AND HIS DIAGNOSIS WAS A PERSONAL SHOCK.

DURING HIS ILLNESS, EVEN AS HIS DEATH APPROACHED, HE CONTINUED TO GROW MORE REFLECTIVE AS A PERSON. WE MOURNED HIS LOSSES TOGETHER AND GREW CLOSER.

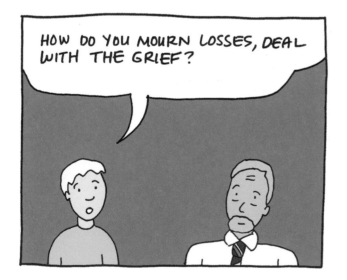

HOW DO YOU MOURN LOSSES, DEAL WITH THE GRIEF?

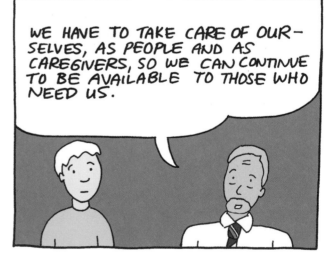

WE HAVE TO TAKE CARE OF OUR-SELVES, AS PEOPLE AND AS CAREGIVERS, SO WE CAN CONTINUE TO BE AVAILABLE TO THOSE WHO NEED US.

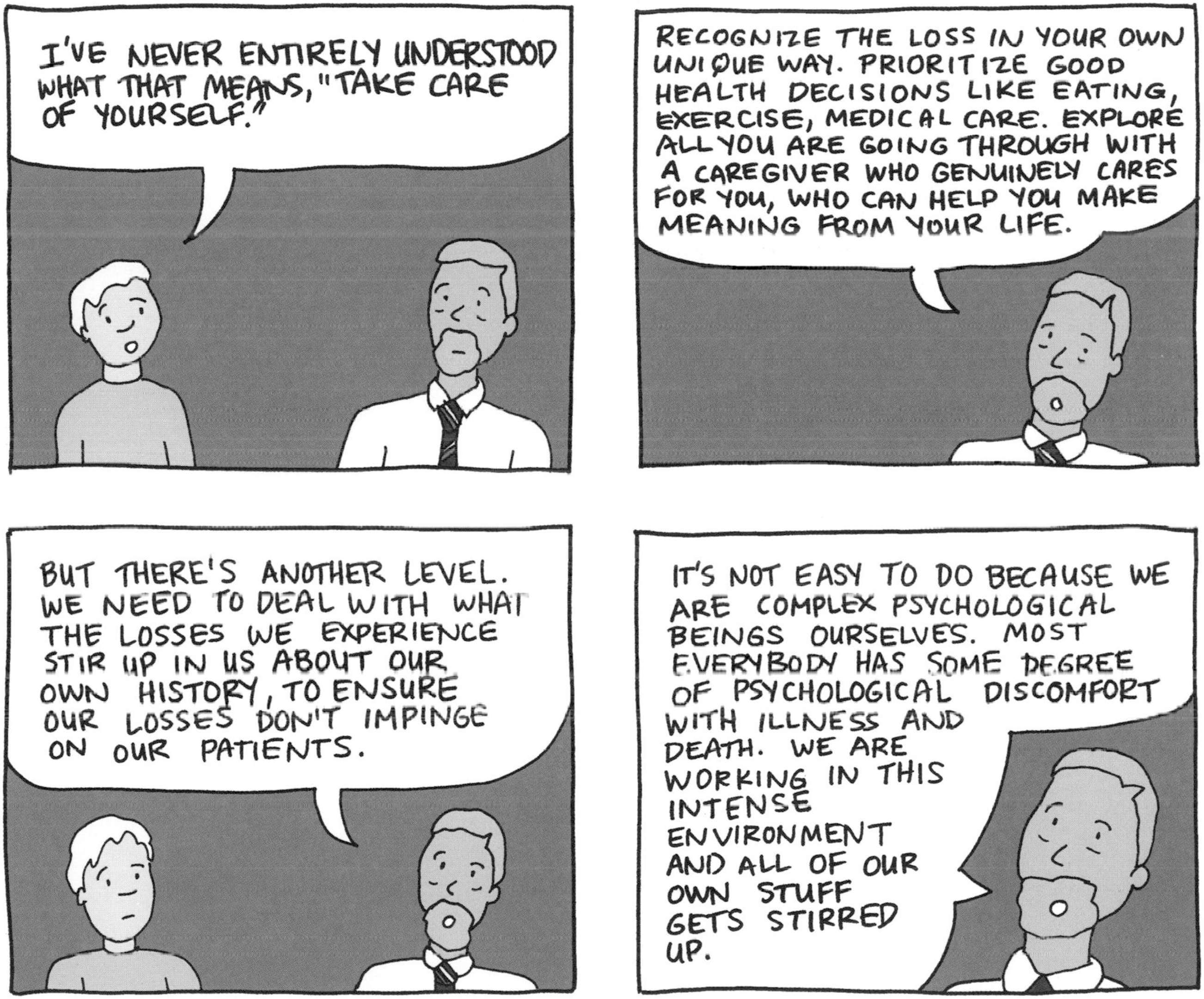
I'VE NEVER ENTIRELY UNDERSTOOD WHAT THAT MEANS, "TAKE CARE OF YOURSELF."
RECOGNIZE THE LOSS IN YOUR OWN UNIQUE WAY. PRIORITIZE GOOD HEALTH DECISIONS LIKE EATING, EXERCISE, MEDICAL CARE. EXPLORE ALL YOU ARE GOING THROUGH WITH A CAREGIVER WHO GENUINELY CARES FOR YOU, WHO CAN HELP YOU MAKE MEANING FROM YOUR LIFE.
BUT THERE'S ANOTHER LEVEL. WE NEED TO DEAL WITH WHAT THE LOSSES WE EXPERIENCE STIR UP IN US ABOUT OUR OWN HISTORY, TO ENSURE OUR LOSSES DON'T IMPINGE ON OUR PATIENTS.
IT'S NOT EASY TO DO BECAUSE WE ARE COMPLEX PSYCHOLOGICAL BEINGS OURSELVES. MOST EVERYBODY HAS SOME DEGREE OF PSYCHOLOGICAL DISCOMFORT WITH ILLNESS AND DEATH. WE ARE WORKING IN THIS INTENSE ENVIRONMENT AND ALL OF OUR OWN STUFF GETS STIRRED UP.

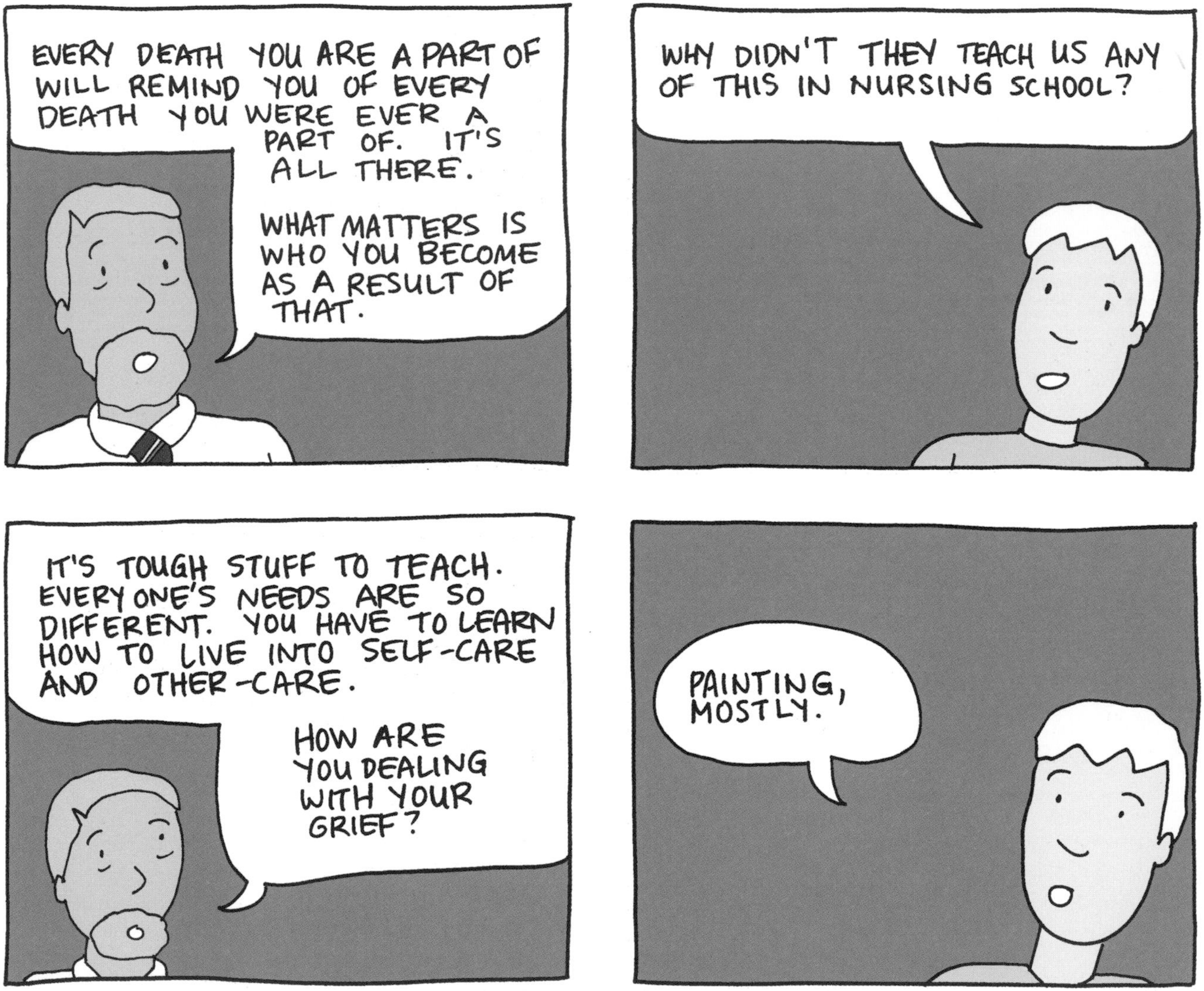
EVERY DEATH YOU ARE A PART OF WILL REMIND YOU OF EVERY DEATH YOU WERE EVER A PART OF. IT'S ALL THERE.
WHAT MATTERS IS WHO YOU BECOME AS A RESULT OF THAT.
WHY DIDN'T THEY TEACH US ANY OF THIS IN NURSING SCHOOL?
IT'S TOUGH STUFF TO TEACH. EVERYONE'S NEEDS ARE SO DIFFERENT. YOU HAVE TO LEARN HOW TO LIVE INTO SELF-CARE AND OTHER-CARE.
HOW ARE YOU DEALING WITH YOUR GRIEF?
PAINTING, MOSTLY.

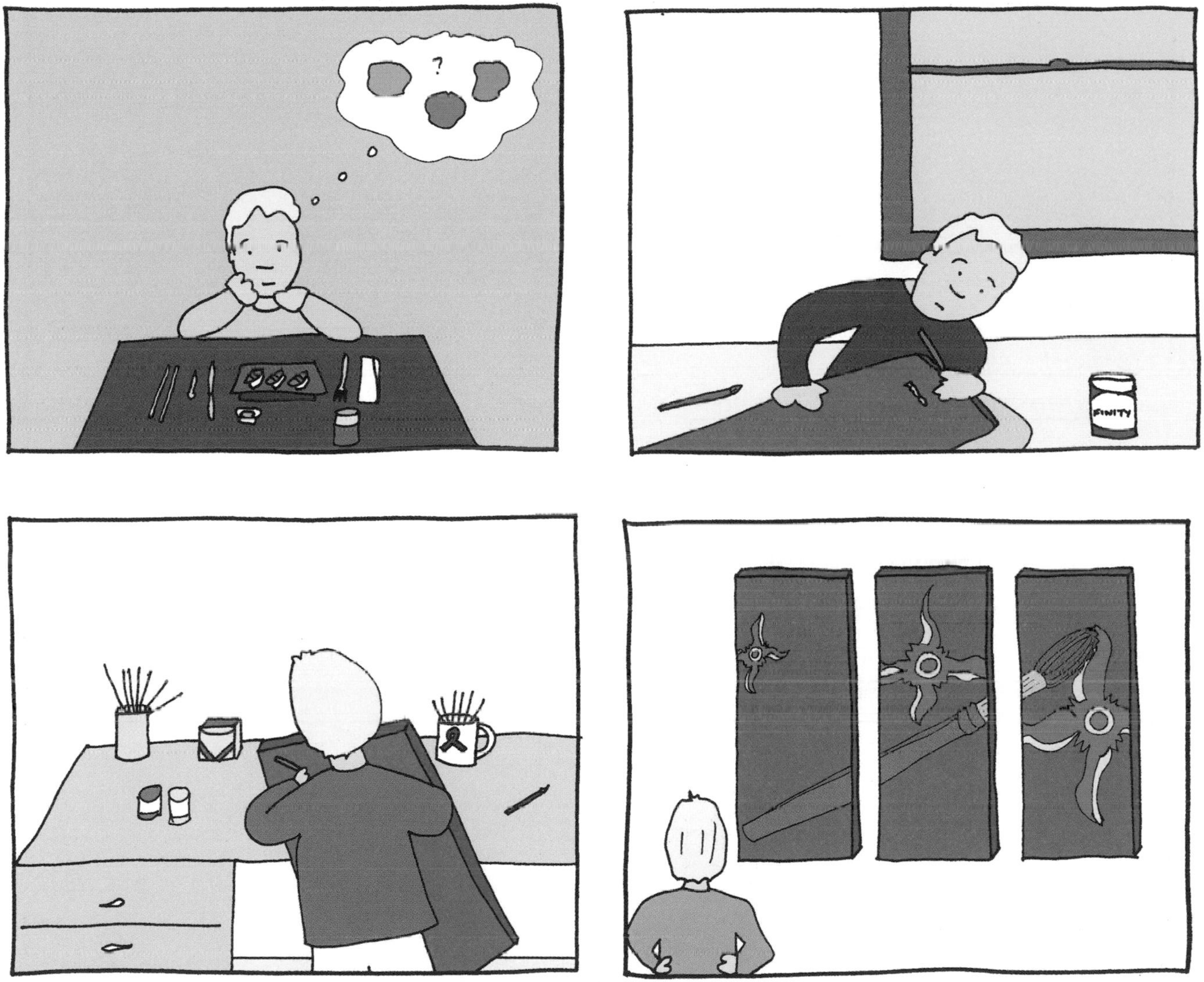
?
FINITY

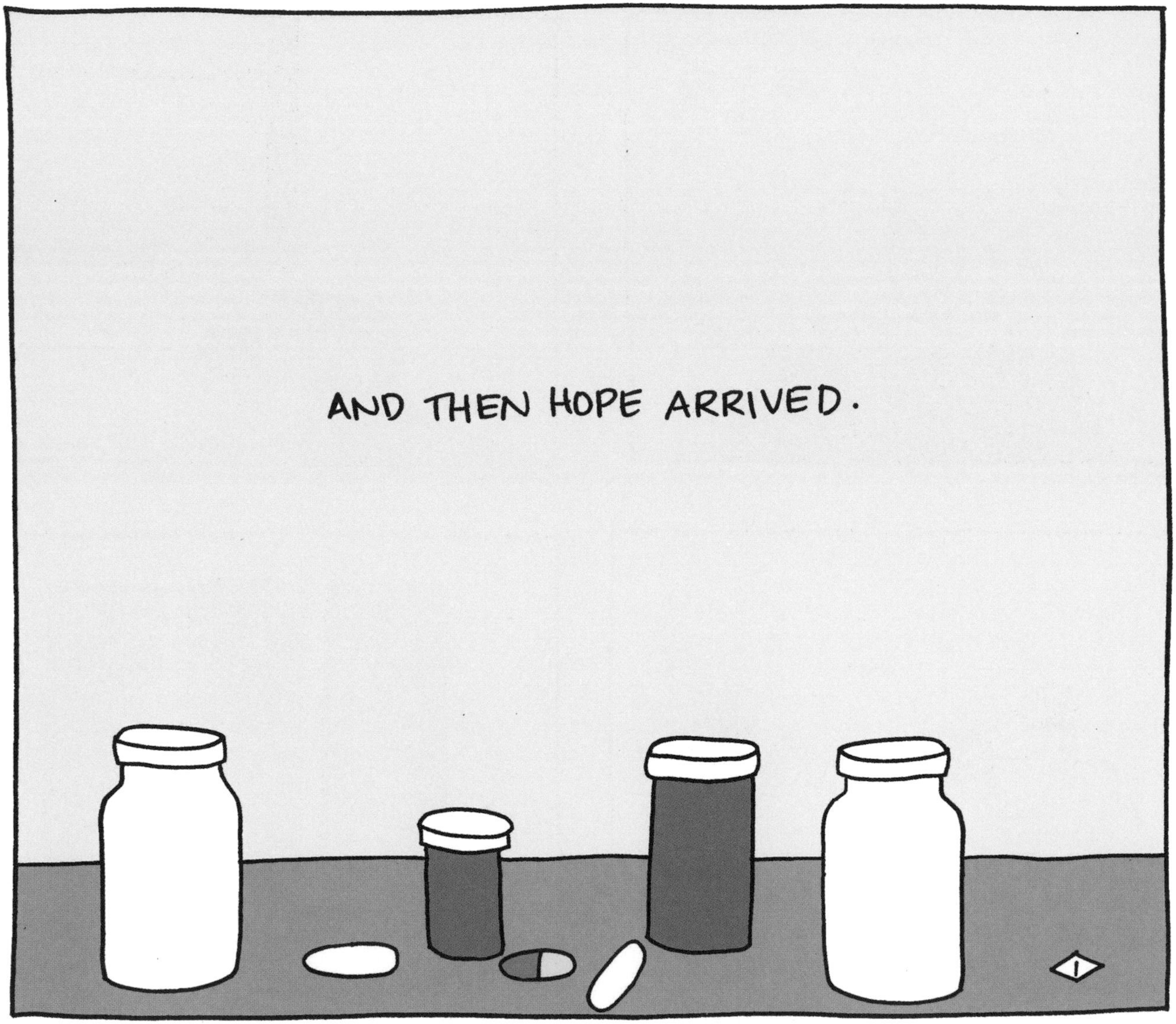
AND THEN HOPE ARRIVED.

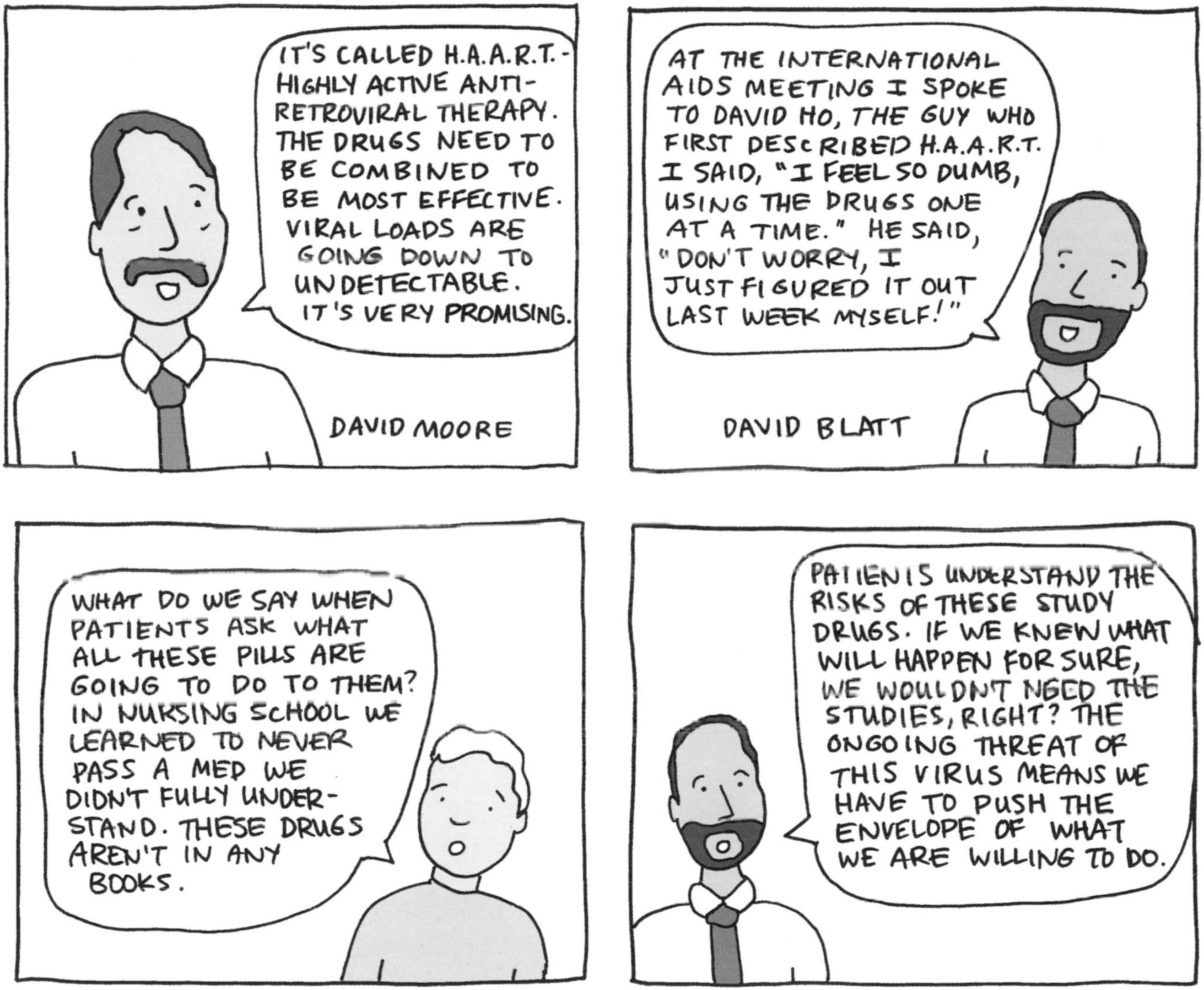
IT'S CALLED H.A.A.R.T.- HIGHLY ACTIVE ANTI-RETROVIRAL THERAPY. THE DRUGS NEED TO BE COMBINED TO BE MOST EFFECTIVE. VIRAL LOADS ARE GOING DOWN TO UNDETECTABLE. IT'S VERY PROMISING.
DAVID MOORE
AT THE INTERNATIONAL AIDS MEETING I SPOKE TO DAVID HO, THE GUY WHO FIRST DESCRIBED H.A.A.R.T. I SAID, "I FEEL SO DUMB, USING THE DRUGS ONE AT A TIME." HE SAID, "DON'T WORRY, I JUST FIGURED IT OUT LAST WEEK MYSELF!"
DAVID BLATT
WHAT DO WE SAY WHEN PATIENTS ASK WHAT ALL THESE PILLS ARE GOING TO DO TO THEM? IN NURSING SCHOOL WE LEARNED TO NEVER PASS A MED WE DIDN'T FULLY UNDER-STAND. THESE DRUGS AREN'T IN ANY BOOKS.
PATIENTS UNDERSTAND THE RISKS OF THESE STUDY DRUGS. IF WE KNEW WHAT WILL HAPPEN FOR SURE, WE WOULDN'T NEED THE STUDIES, RIGHT? THE ONGOING THREAT OF THIS VIRUS MEANS WE HAVE TO PUSH THE ENVELOPE OF WHAT WE ARE WILLING TO DO.

REMEMBER THAT BRILLIANT BUT JERKY MOVE WHERE HIV TURNS T-CELLS INTO FACTORIES FOR MORE HIV?

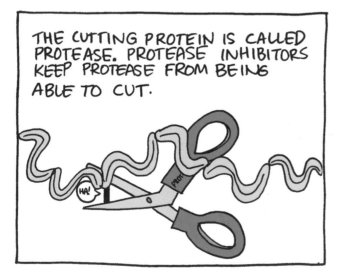

WELL, TO DO THAT, LONG CHAINS OF HIV RNA ARE ASSEMBLED AND NEED TO BE CUT BEFORE RELEASE.

THE CUTTING PROTEIN IS CALLED PROTEASE. PROTEASE INHIBITORS KEEP PROTEASE FROM BEING ABLE TO CUT.

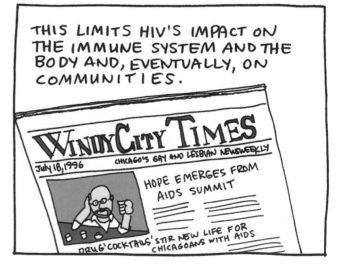

HA!

PROT.

THIS LIMITS HIV'S IMPACT ON THE IMMUNE SYSTEM AND THE BODY AND, EVENTUALLY, ON COMMUNITIES.

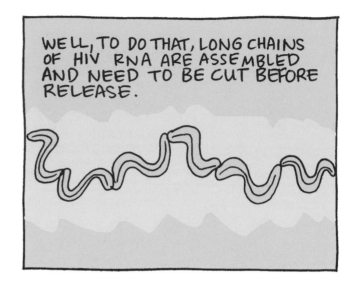

WINDY CITY TIMES

CHICAGO'S GAY AND LESBIAN NEWSWEEKLY

JULY 18, 1996

HOPE EMERGES FROM AIDS SUMMIT

DRUG 'COCKTAILS' STIR NEW LIFE FOR CHICAGOANS WITH AIDS

1997

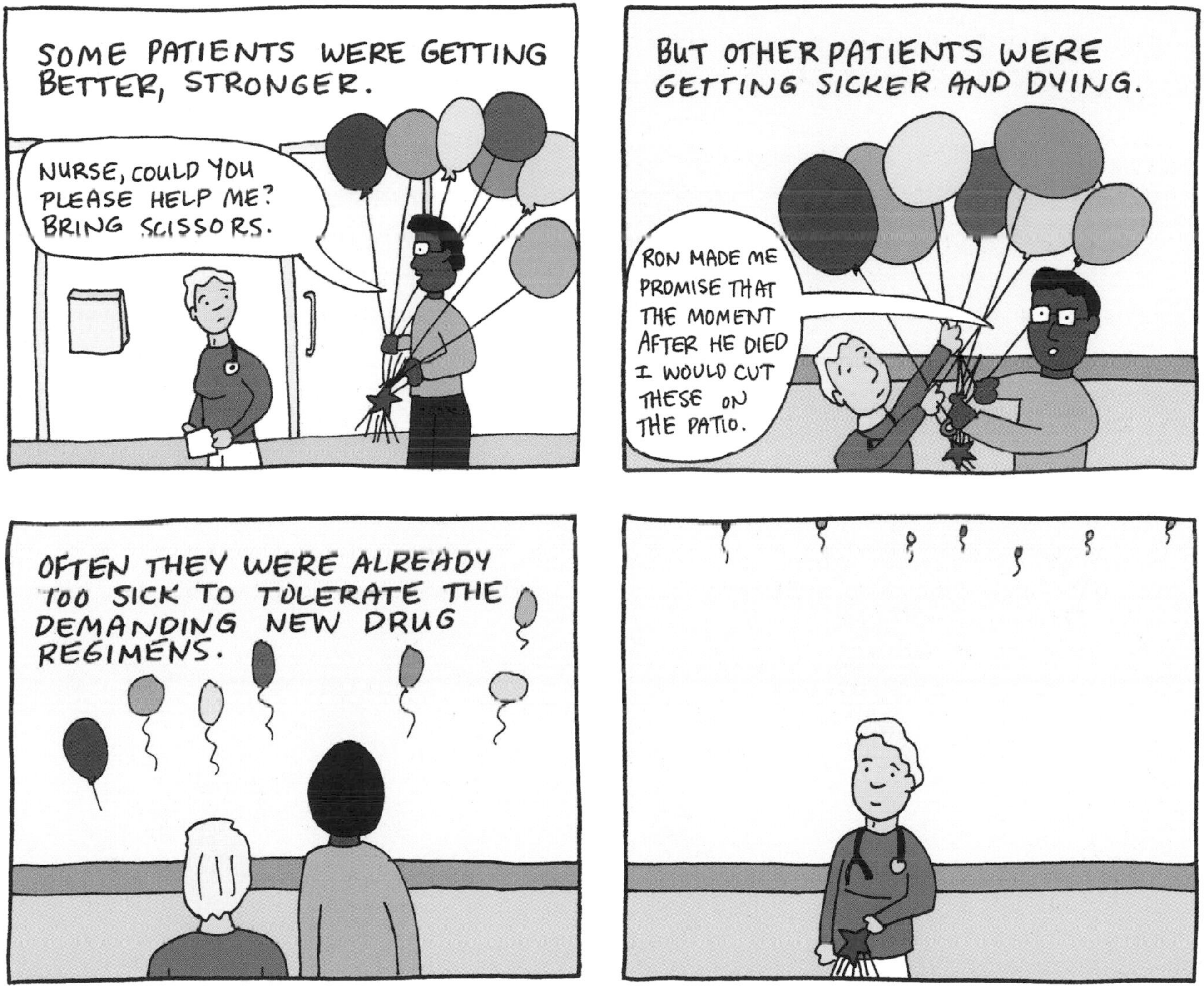

SOME PATIENTS WERE GETTING BETTER, STRONGER.
NURSE, COULD YOU PLEASE HELP ME? BRING SCISSORS.
BUT OTHER PATIENTS WERE GETTING SICKER AND DYING.
RON MADE ME PROMISE THAT THE MOMENT AFTER HE DIED I WOULD CUT THESE ON THE PATIO.
OFTEN THEY WERE ALREADY TOO SICK TO TOLERATE THE DEMANDING NEW DRUG REGIMENS.

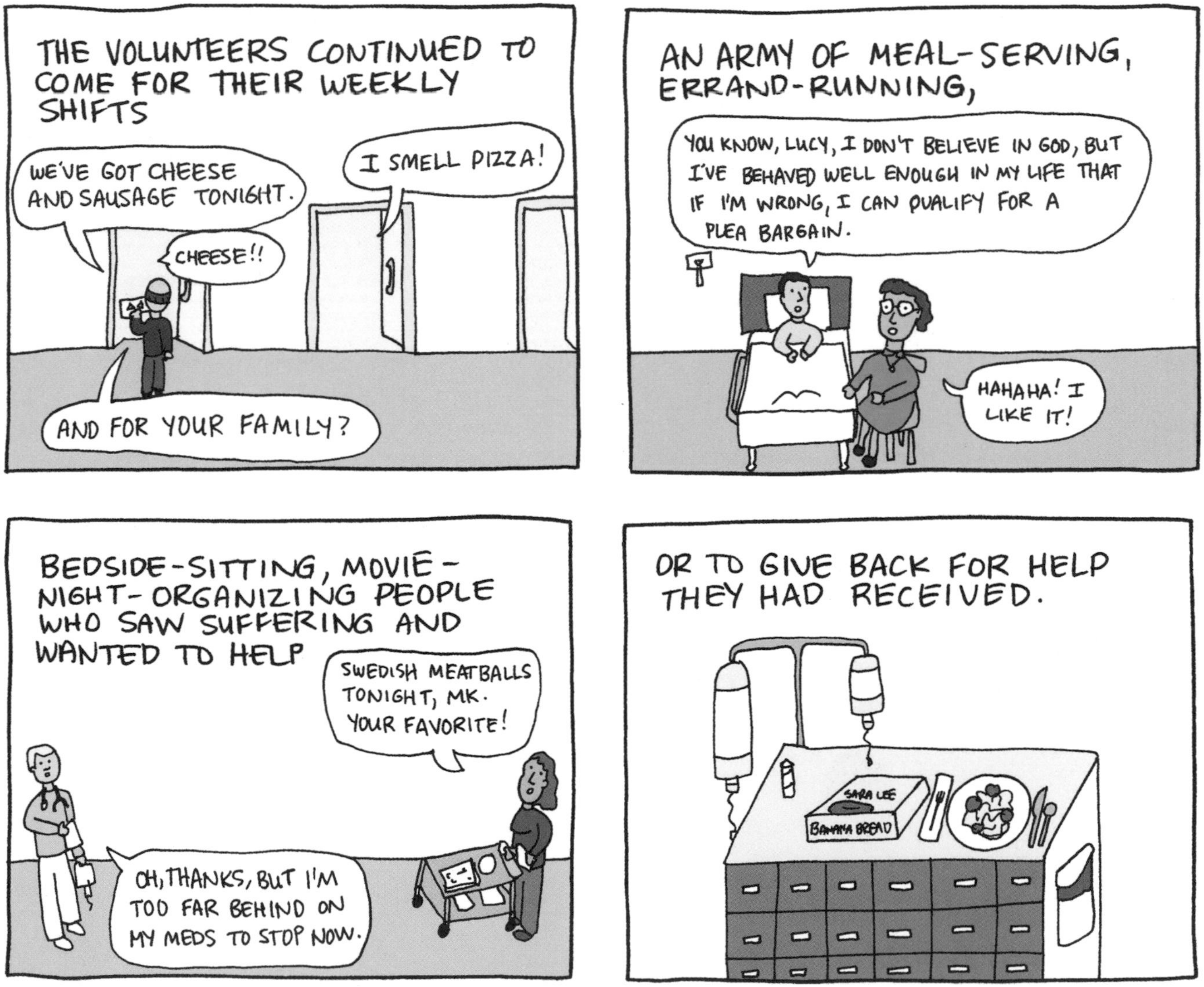
THE VOLUNTEERS CONTINUED TO COME FOR THEIR WEEKLY SHIFTS
WE'VE GOT CHEESE AND SAUSAGE TONIGHT.
I SMELL PIZZA!
CHEESE!!
AND FOR YOUR FAMILY?
AN ARMY OF MEAL-SERVING, ERRAND-RUNNING,
YOU KNOW, LUCY, I DON'T BELIEVE IN GOD, BUT I'VE BEHAVED WELL ENOUGH IN MY LIFE THAT IF I'M WRONG, I CAN QUALIFY FOR A PLEA BARGAIN.
HAHAHA! I LIKE IT!
BEDSIDE-SITTING, MOVIE-NIGHT-ORGANIZING PEOPLE WHO SAW SUFFERING AND WANTED TO HELP
SWEDISH MEATBALLS TONIGHT, MK. YOUR FAVORITE!
OH, THANKS, BUT I'M TOO FAR BEHIND ON MY MEDS TO STOP NOW.
OR TO GIVE BACK FOR HELP THEY HAD RECEIVED.
SARA LEE
BANANA BREAD

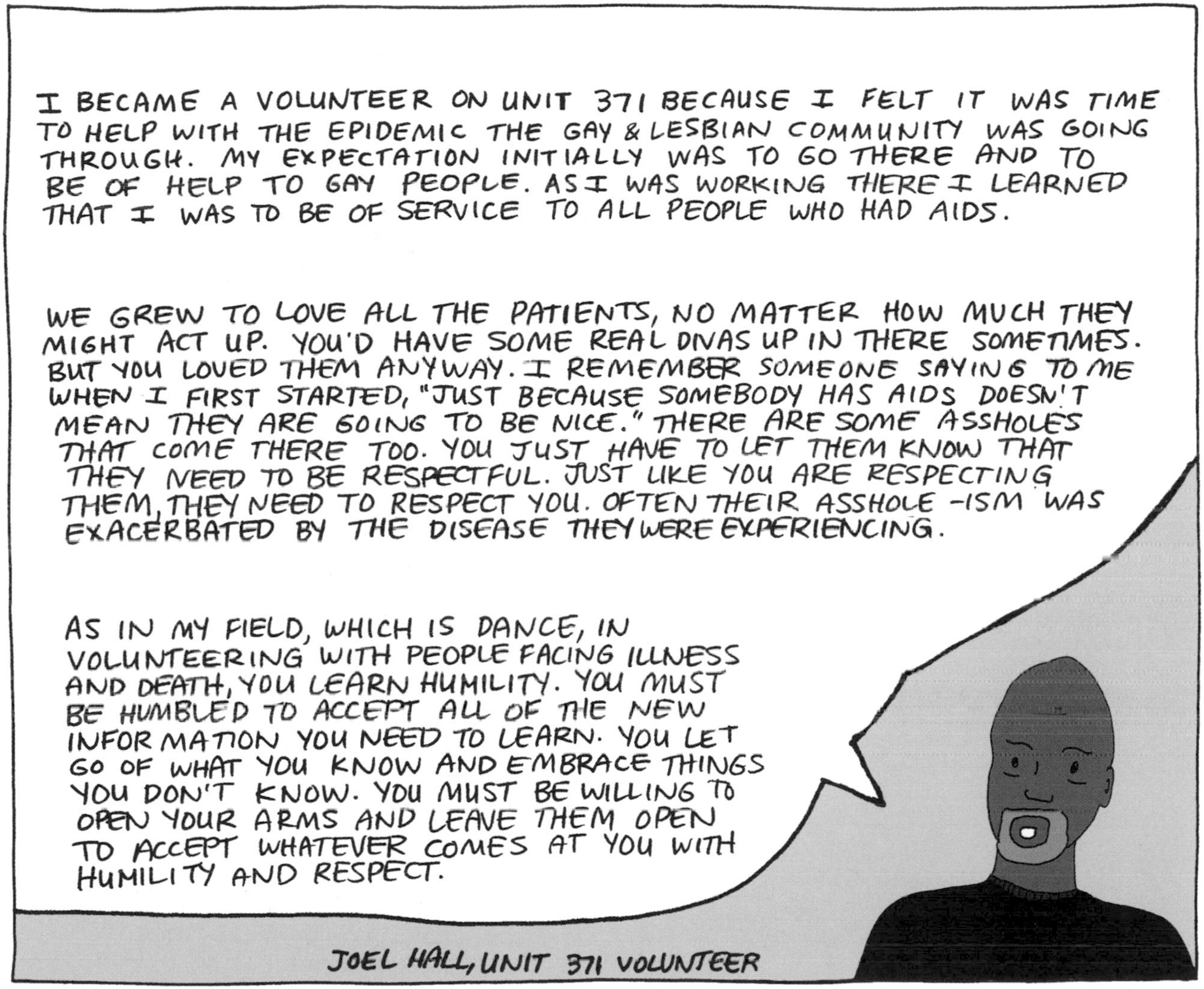
I BECAME A VOLUNTEER ON UNIT 371 BECAUSE I FELT IT WAS TIME TO HELP WITH THE EPIDEMIC THE GAY & LESBIAN COMMUNITY WAS GOING THROUGH. MY EXPECTATION INITIALLY WAS TO GO THERE AND TO BE OF HELP TO GAY PEOPLE. AS I WAS WORKING THERE I LEARNED THAT I WAS TO BE OF SERVICE TO ALL PEOPLE WHO HAD AIDS.
WE GREW TO LOVE ALL THE PATIENTS, NO MATTER HOW MUCH THEY MIGHT ACT UP. YOU'D HAVE SOME REAL DIVAS UP IN THERE SOMETIMES. BUT YOU LOVED THEM ANYWAY. I REMEMBER SOMEONE SAYING TO ME WHEN I FIRST STARTED, "JUST BECAUSE SOMEBODY HAS AIDS DOESN'T MEAN THEY ARE GOING TO BE NICE." THERE ARE SOME ASSHOLES THAT COME THERE TOO. YOU JUST HAVE TO LET THEM KNOW THAT THEY NEED TO BE RESPECTFUL. JUST LIKE YOU ARE RESPECTING THEM, THEY NEED TO RESPECT YOU. OFTEN THEIR ASSHOLE -ISM WAS EXACERBATED BY THE DISEASE THEY WERE EXPERIENCING.
AS IN MY FIELD, WHICH IS DANCE, IN VOLUNTEERING WITH PEOPLE FACING ILLNESS AND DEATH, YOU LEARN HUMILITY. YOU MUST BE HUMBLED TO ACCEPT ALL OF THE NEW INFORMATION YOU NEED TO LEARN. YOU LET GO OF WHAT YOU KNOW AND EMBRACE THINGS YOU DON'T KNOW. YOU MUST BE WILLING TO OPEN YOUR ARMS AND LEAVE THEM OPEN TO ACCEPT WHATEVER COMES AT YOU WITH HUMILITY AND RESPECT.
JOEL HALL, UNIT 371 VOLUNTEER

1998

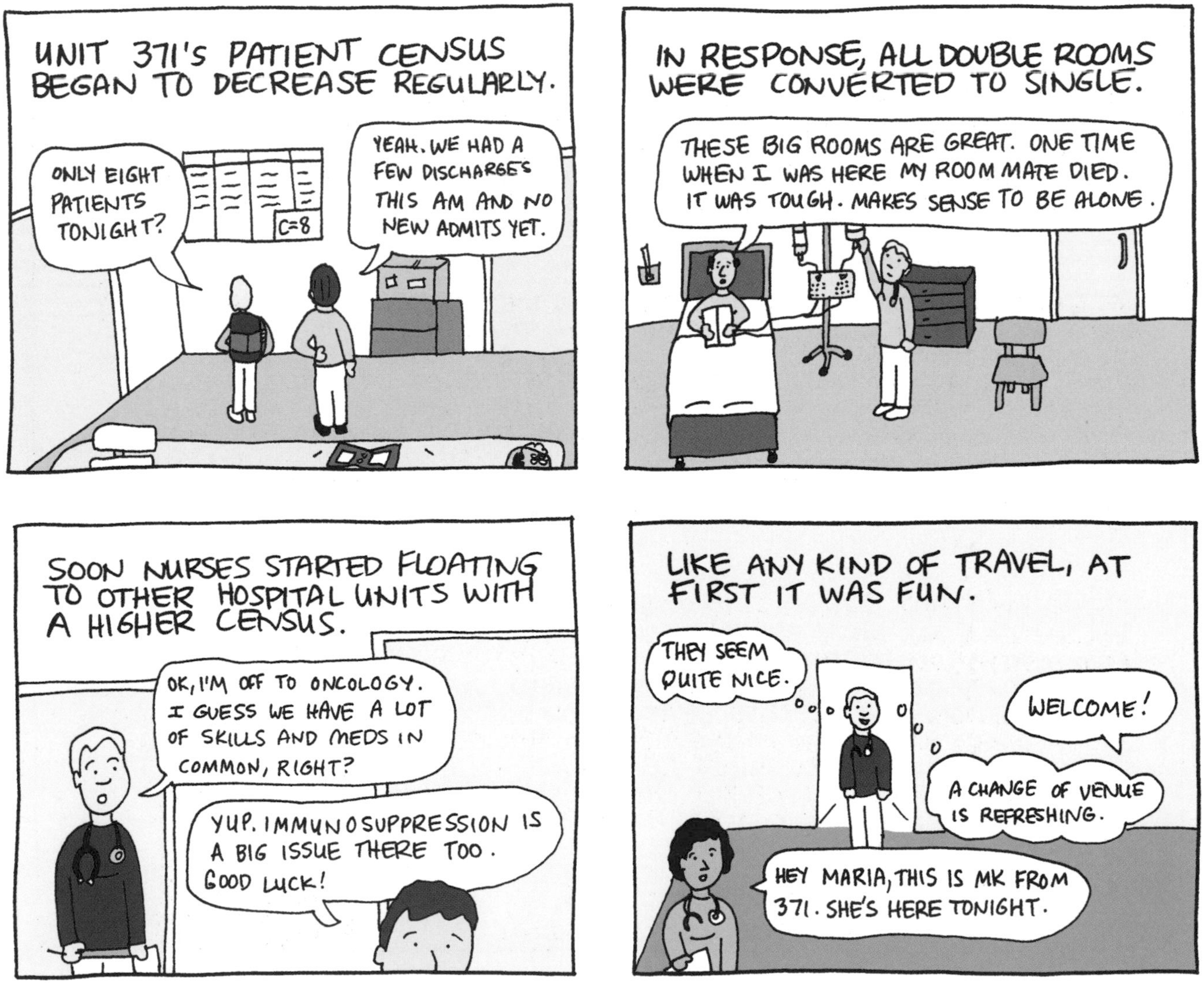
UNIT 371'S PATIENT CENSUS BEGAN TO DECREASE REGULARLY.
ONLY EIGHT PATIENTS TONIGHT?
C=8
YEAH. WE HAD A FEW DISCHARGES THIS AM AND NO NEW ADMITS YET.
IN RESPONSE, ALL DOUBLE ROOMS WERE CONVERTED TO SINGLE.
THESE BIG ROOMS ARE GREAT. ONE TIME WHEN I WAS HERE MY ROOMMATE DIED. IT WAS TOUGH. MAKES SENSE TO BE ALONE.
SOON NURSES STARTED FLOATING TO OTHER HOSPITAL UNITS WITH A HIGHER CENSUS.
OK, I'M OFF TO ONCOLOGY. I GUESS WE HAVE A LOT OF SKILLS AND MEDS IN COMMON, RIGHT?
YUP. IMMUNOSUPPRESSION IS A BIG ISSUE THERE TOO. GOOD LUCK!
LIKE ANY KIND OF TRAVEL, AT FIRST IT WAS FUN.
THEY SEEM QUITE NICE.
WELCOME!
A CHANGE OF VENUE IS REFRESHING.
HEY MARIA, THIS IS MK FROM 371. SHE'S HERE TONIGHT.

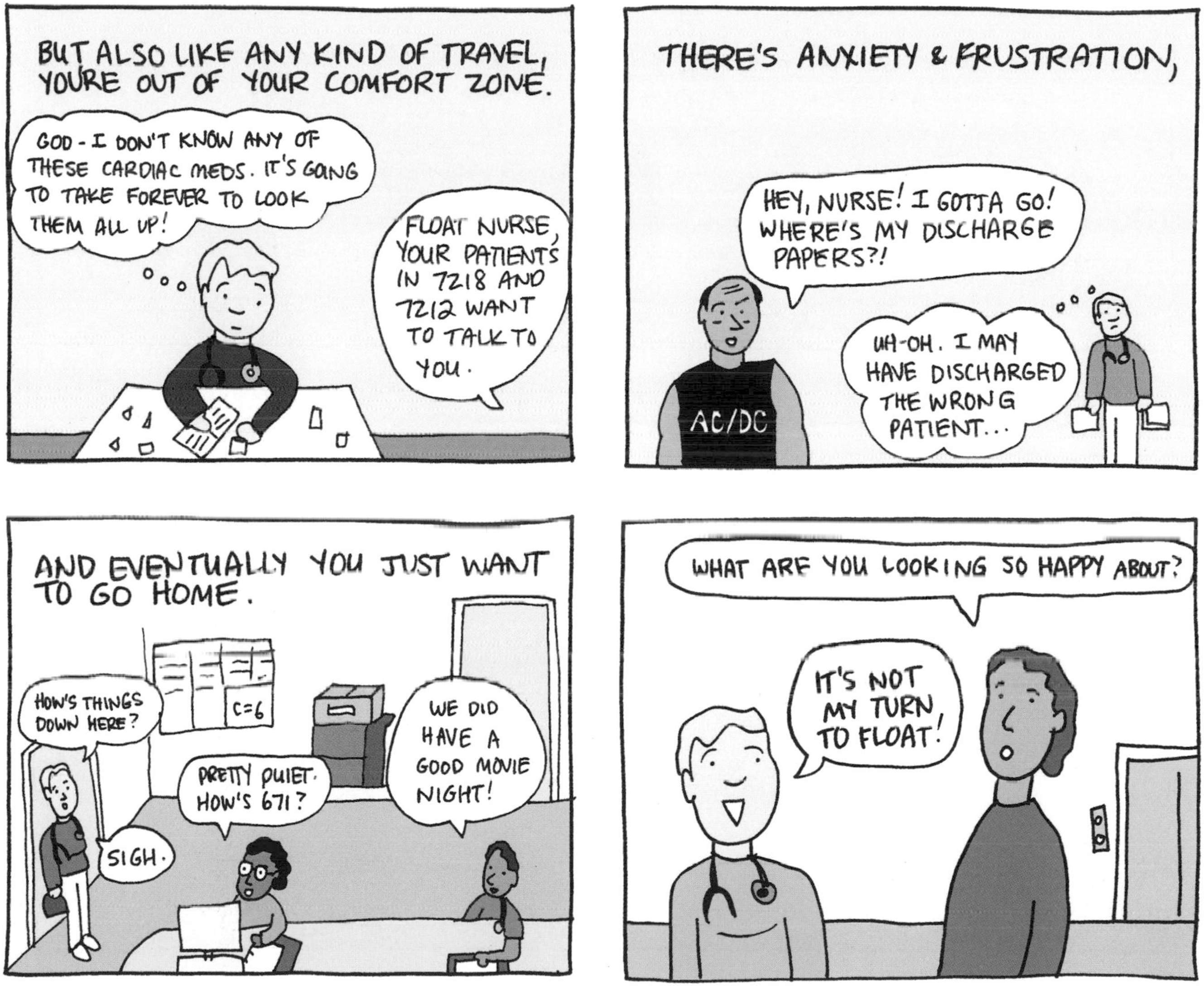
BUT ALSO LIKE ANY KIND OF TRAVEL, YOU'RE OUT OF YOUR COMFORT ZONE.
GOD - I DON'T KNOW ANY OF THESE CARDIAC MEDS. IT'S GOING TO TAKE FOREVER TO LOOK THEM ALL UP!
FLOAT NURSE, YOUR PATIENTS IN 7218 AND 7212 WANT TO TALK TO YOU.
THERE'S ANXIETY & FRUSTRATION,
HEY, NURSE! I GOTTA GO! WHERE'S MY DISCHARGE PAPERS?!
AC/DC
UH-OH. I MAY HAVE DISCHARGED THE WRONG PATIENT...
AND EVENTUALLY YOU JUST WANT TO GO HOME.
C=6
HOW'S THINGS DOWN HERE?
PRETTY QUIET. HOW'S 671?
WE DID HAVE A GOOD MOVIE NIGHT!
SIGH.
WHAT ARE YOU LOOKING SO HAPPY ABOUT?
IT'S NOT MY TURN TO FLOAT!

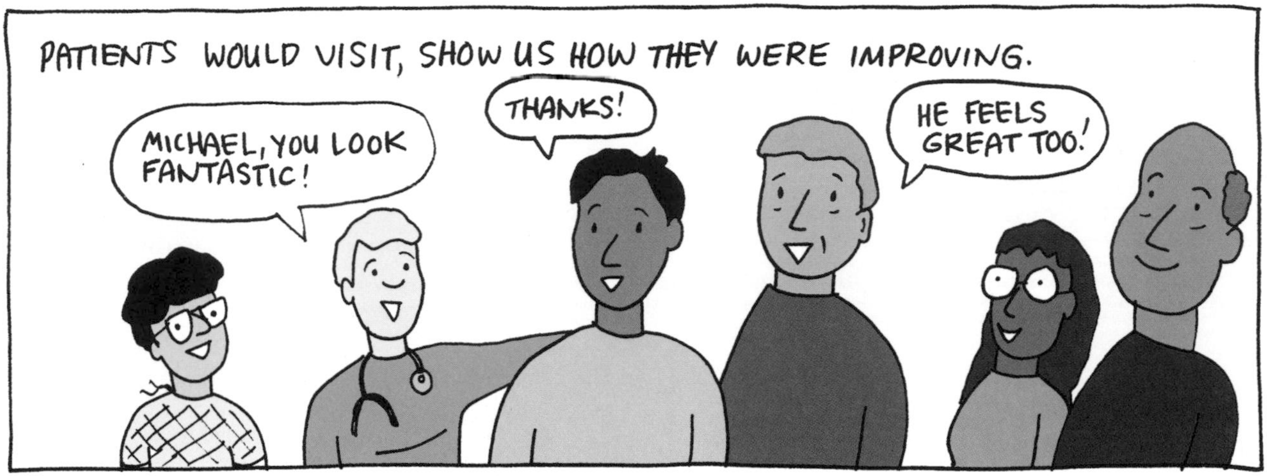
PATIENTS WOULD VISIT, SHOW US HOW THEY WERE IMPROVING.
MICHAEL, YOU LOOK FANTASTIC!
THANKS!
HE FEELS GREAT TOO!

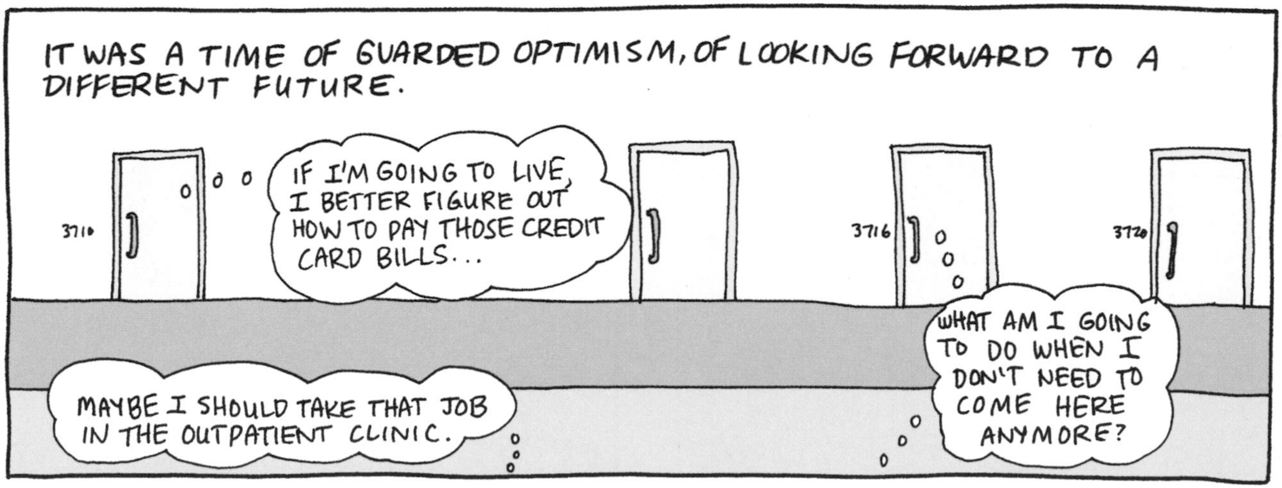
IT WAS A TIME OF GUARDED OPTIMISM, OF LOOKING FORWARD TO A DIFFERENT FUTURE.
3710
IF I'M GOING TO LIVE, I BETTER FIGURE OUT HOW TO PAY THOSE CREDIT CARD BILLS...
3716
3720
WHAT AM I GOING TO DO WHEN I DON'T NEED TO COME HERE ANYMORE?
MAYBE I SHOULD TAKE THAT JOB IN THE OUTPATIENT CLINIC.

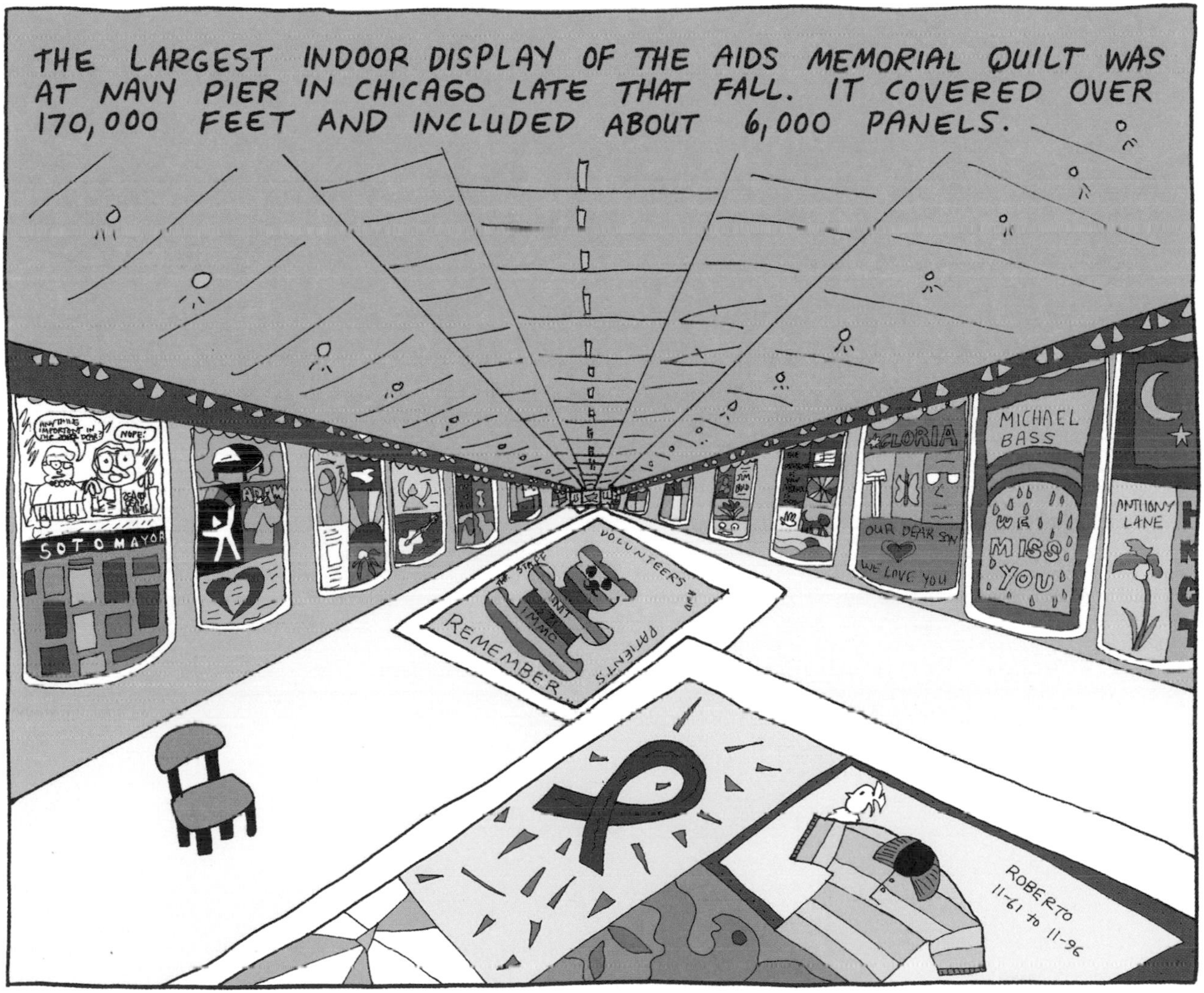
THE LARGEST INDOOR DISPLAY OF THE AIDS MEMORIAL QUILT WAS AT NAVY PIER IN CHICAGO LATE THAT FALL. IT COVERED OVER 170,000 FEET AND INCLUDED ABOUT 6,000 PANELS.
NOPE!
SOTOMAYOR
ADAM
GLORIA
OUR DEAR SON
WE LOVE YOU
MICHAEL BASS
WE MISS YOU
ANTHONY LANE
VOLUNTEERS AND PATIENTS
REMEMBER...
ROBERTO
11-61 to 11-96

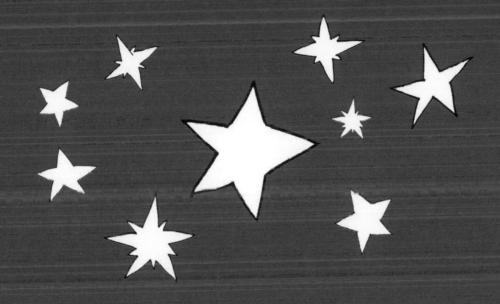

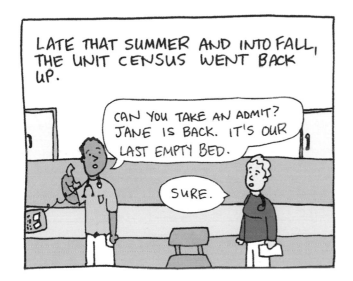

LATE THAT SUMMER AND INTO FALL, THE UNIT CENSUS WENT BACK UP.

CAN YOU TAKE AN ADMIT? JANE IS BACK. IT'S OUR LAST EMPTY BED.

SURE.

PATIENTS WHO HAD INITIALLY DONE WELL ON H.A.A.R.T. WERE STARTING TO GET SICK AGAIN.

JANE AND I WERE TWO MONTHS APART IN AGE. WE ENJOYED CHATTING ABOUT DATING AND I.V. POLE RACING IN THE HALLS. BUT BEYOND BEING LESBIANS CLOSE IN AGE, OUR LIVES WERE VERY DIFFERENT.

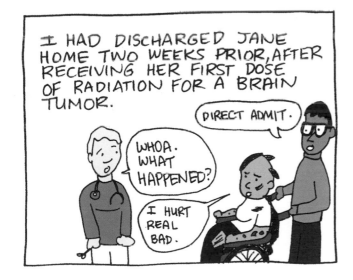

I HAD DISCHARGED JANE HOME TWO WEEKS PRIOR, AFTER RECEIVING HER FIRST DOSE OF RADIATION FOR A BRAIN TUMOR.

DIRECT ADMIT.

WHOA. WHAT HAPPENED?

I HURT REAL BAD.

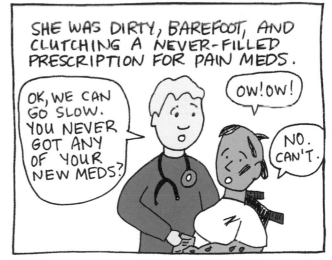

SHE WAS DIRTY, BAREFOOT, AND CLUTCHING A NEVER-FILLED PRESCRIPTION FOR PAIN MEDS.

OK, WE CAN GO SLOW. YOU NEVER GOT ANY OF YOUR NEW MEDS?

OW! OW!

NO. CAN'T.

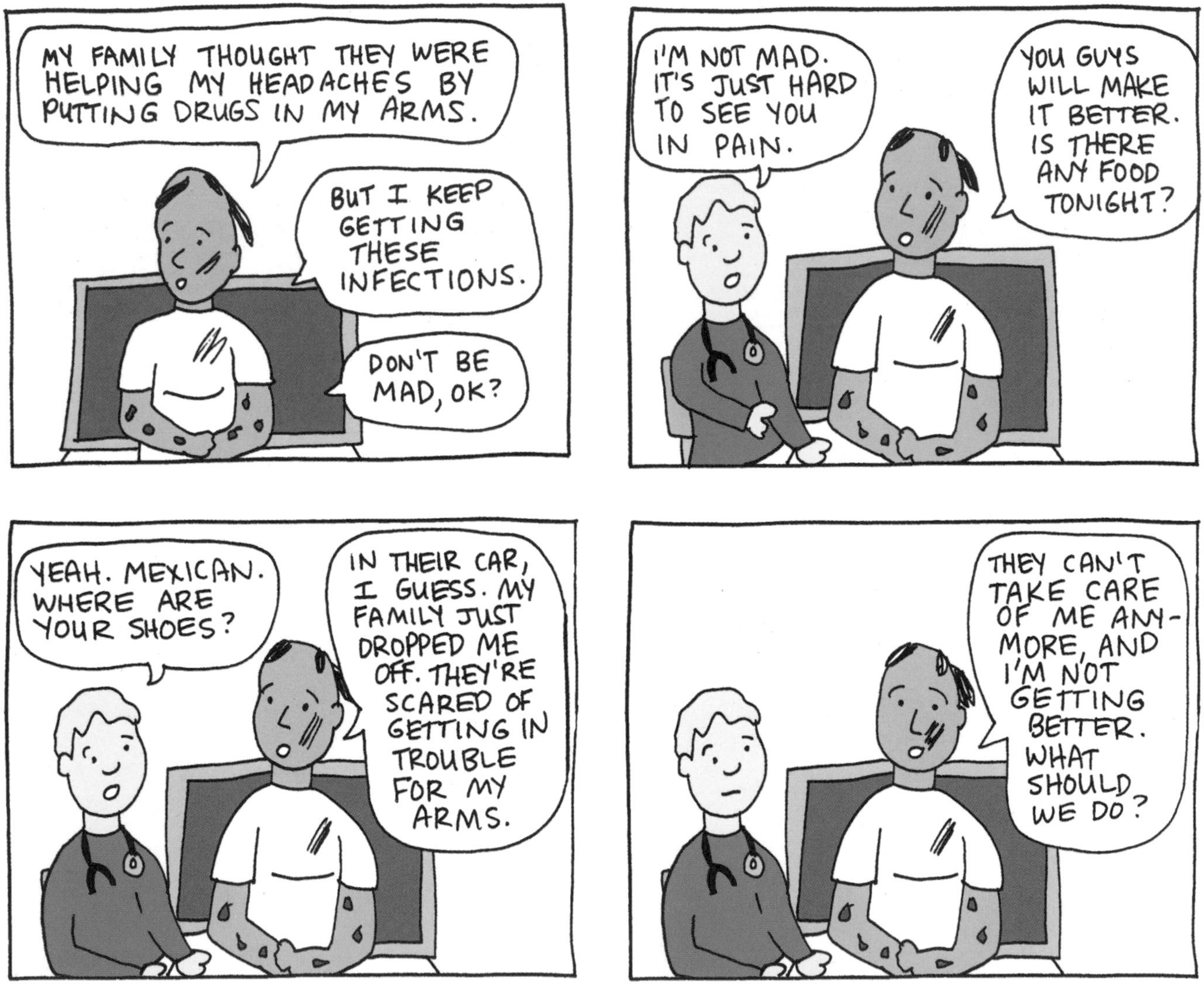
MY FAMILY THOUGHT THEY WERE HELPING MY HEADACHES BY PUTTING DRUGS IN MY ARMS.
BUT I KEEP GETTING THESE INFECTIONS.
DON'T BE MAD, OK?
I'M NOT MAD. IT'S JUST HARD TO SEE YOU IN PAIN.
YOU GUYS WILL MAKE IT BETTER. IS THERE ANY FOOD TONIGHT?
YEAH. MEXICAN. WHERE ARE YOUR SHOES?
IN THEIR CAR, I GUESS. MY FAMILY JUST DROPPED ME OFF. THEY'RE SCARED OF GETTING IN TROUBLE FOR MY ARMS.
THEY CAN'T TAKE CARE OF ME ANY-MORE, AND I'M NOT GETTING BETTER. WHAT SHOULD WE DO?

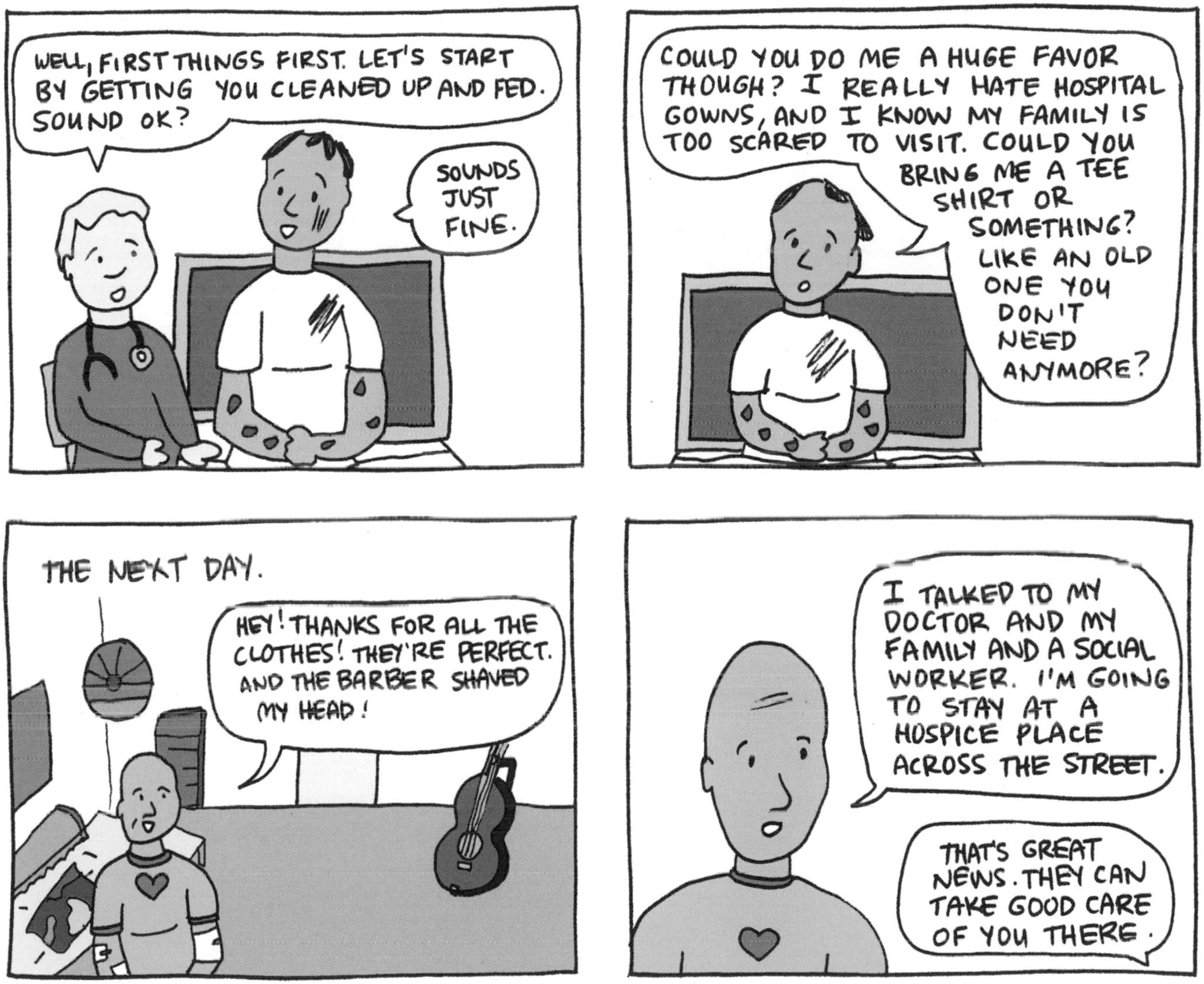
WELL, FIRST THINGS FIRST. LET'S START BY GETTING YOU CLEANED UP AND FED. SOUND OK?
SOUNDS JUST FINE.
COULD YOU DO ME A HUGE FAVOR THOUGH? I REALLY HATE HOSPITAL GOWNS, AND I KNOW MY FAMILY IS TOO SCARED TO VISIT. COULD YOU BRING ME A TEE SHIRT OR SOMETHING? LIKE AN OLD ONE YOU DON'T NEED ANYMORE?
THE NEXT DAY.
HEY! THANKS FOR ALL THE CLOTHES! THEY'RE PERFECT. AND THE BARBER SHAVED MY HEAD!
I TALKED TO MY DOCTOR AND MY FAMILY AND A SOCIAL WORKER. I'M GOING TO STAY AT A HOSPICE PLACE ACROSS THE STREET.
THAT'S GREAT NEWS. THEY CAN TAKE GOOD CARE OF YOU THERE.

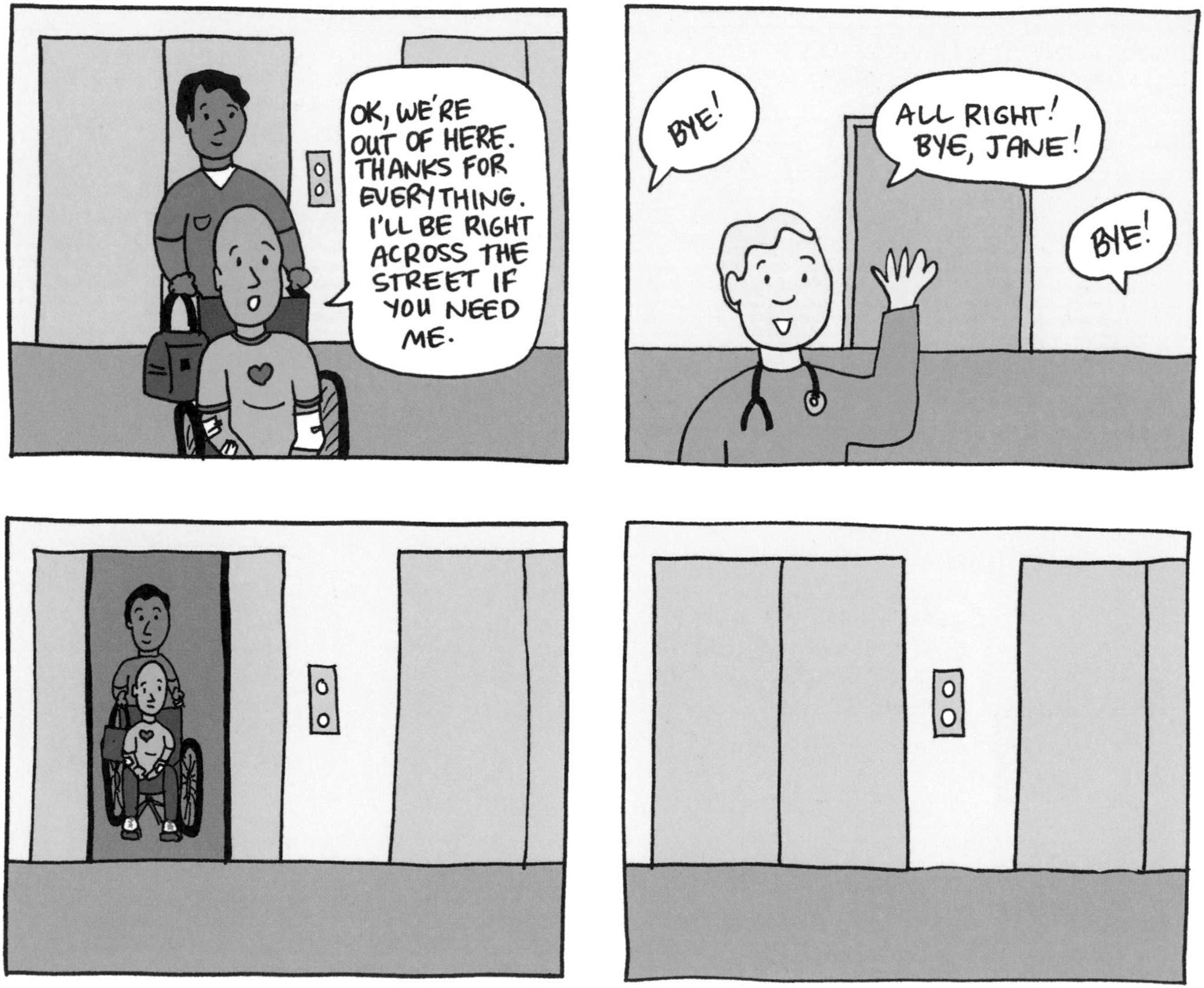
OK, WE'RE OUT OF HERE. THANKS FOR EVERYTHING. I'LL BE RIGHT ACROSS THE STREET IF YOU NEED ME.
BYE!
ALL RIGHT! BYE, JANE!
BYE!

1999

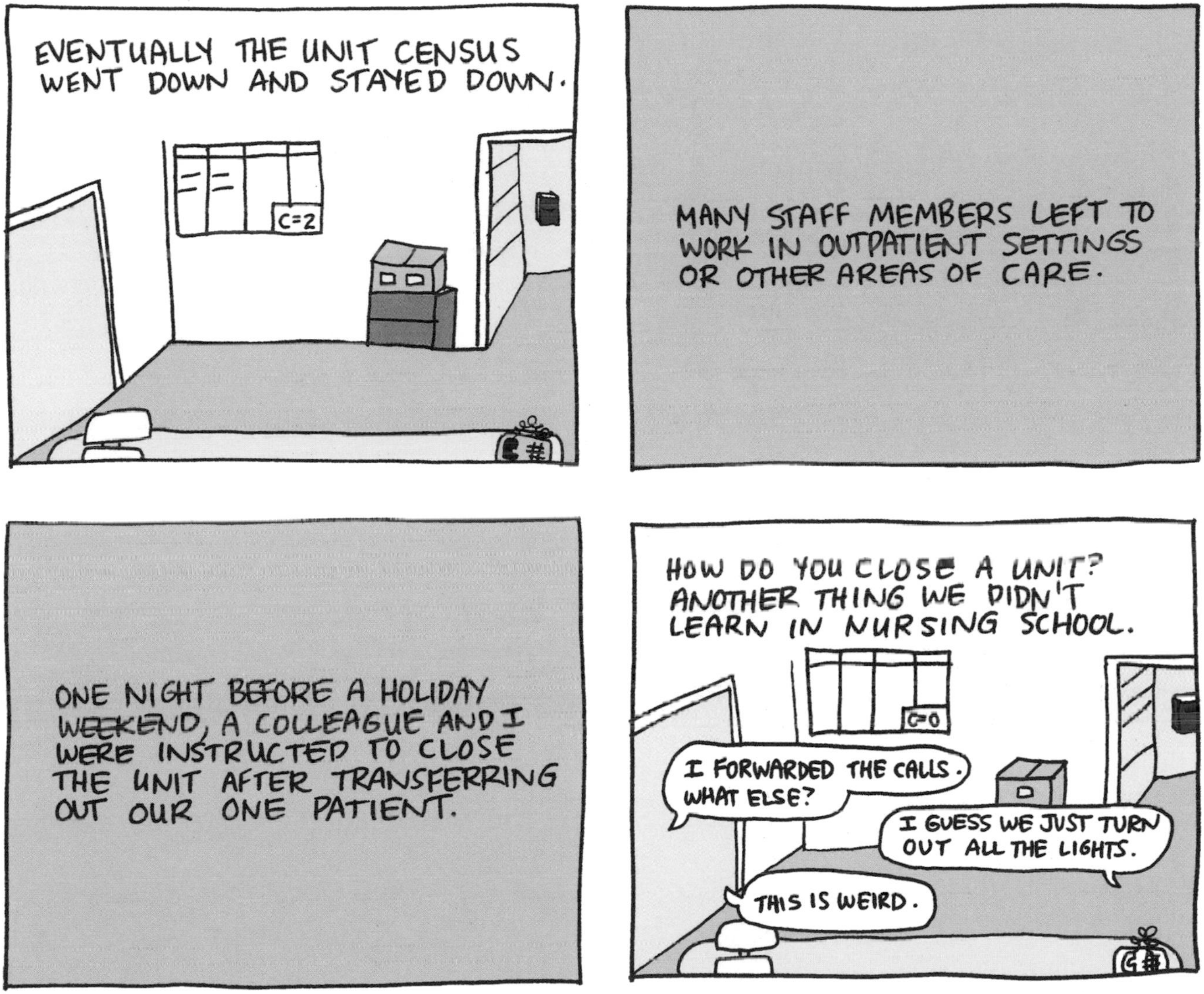
EVENTUALLY THE UNIT CENSUS WENT DOWN AND STAYED DOWN.
C=2
MANY STAFF MEMBERS LEFT TO WORK IN OUTPATIENT SETTINGS OR OTHER AREAS OF CARE.
ONE NIGHT BEFORE A HOLIDAY WEEKEND, A COLLEAGUE AND I WERE INSTRUCTED TO CLOSE THE UNIT AFTER TRANSFERRING OUT OUR ONE PATIENT.
HOW DO YOU CLOSE A UNIT? ANOTHER THING WE DIDN'T LEARN IN NURSING SCHOOL.
C=0
I FORWARDED THE CALLS. WHAT ELSE?
I GUESS WE JUST TURN OUT ALL THE LIGHTS.
THIS IS WEIRD.

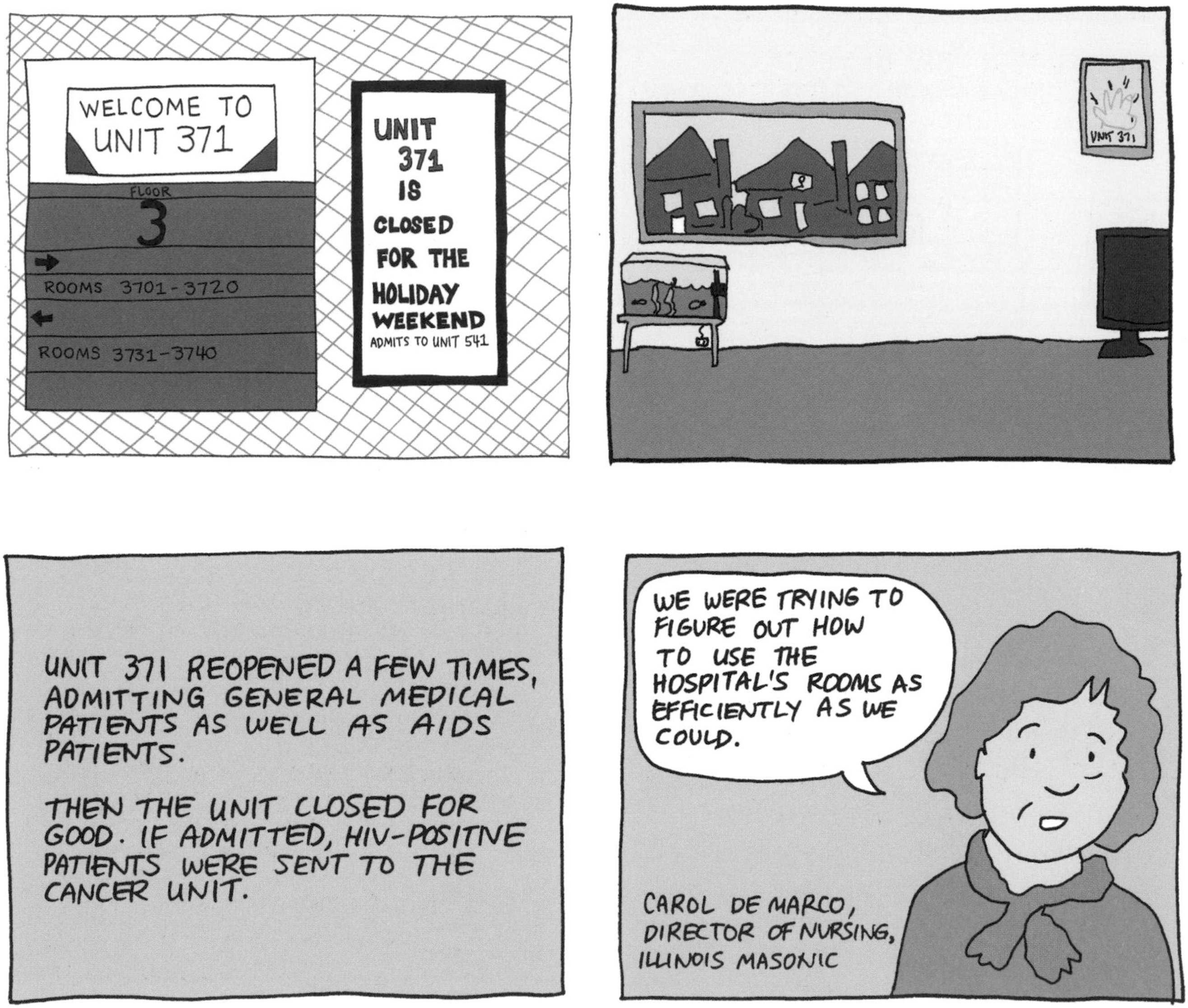
WELCOME TO UNIT 371
FLOOR 3
ROOMS 3701-3720
ROOMS 3731-3740
UNIT 371 IS CLOSED FOR THE HOLIDAY WEEKEND
ADMITS TO UNIT 541
UNIT 371
UNIT 371 REOPENED A FEW TIMES, ADMITTING GENERAL MEDICAL PATIENTS AS WELL AS AIDS PATIENTS.
THEN THE UNIT CLOSED FOR GOOD. IF ADMITTED, HIV-POSITIVE PATIENTS WERE SENT TO THE CANCER UNIT.
WE WERE TRYING TO FIGURE OUT HOW TO USE THE HOSPITAL'S ROOMS AS EFFICIENTLY AS WE COULD.
CAROL DE MARCO, DIRECTOR OF NURSING, ILLINOIS MASONIC

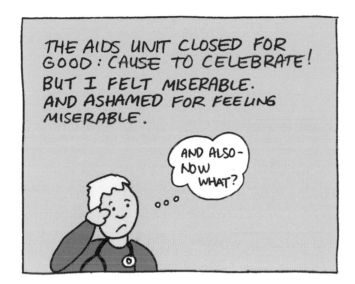

THE AIDS UNIT CLOSED FOR GOOD: CAUSE TO CELEBRATE! BUT I FELT MISERABLE. AND ASHAMED FOR FEELING MISERABLE.

AND ALSO— NOW WHAT?

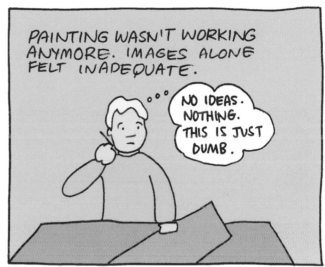

PAINTING WASN'T WORKING ANYMORE. IMAGES ALONE FELT INADEQUATE.

NO IDEAS. NOTHING. THIS IS JUST DUMB.

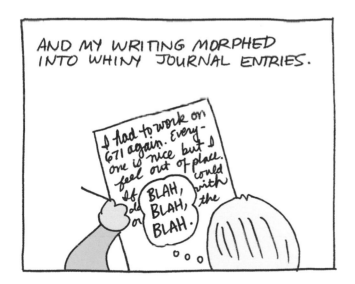

AND MY WRITING MORPHED INTO WHINY JOURNAL ENTRIES.

I had to work on 671 again. Everyone is nice but I feel out of place. If old ... could ... with the

BLAH, BLAH, BLAH.

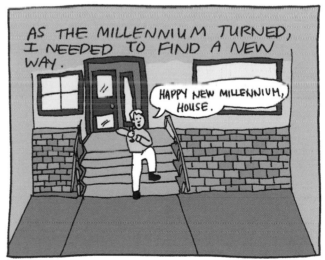

AS THE MILLENNIUM TURNED, I NEEDED TO FIND A NEW WAY.

HAPPY NEW MILLENNIUM, HOUSE.

OR PERHAPS I NEEDED TO LET A NEW WAY FIND ME.

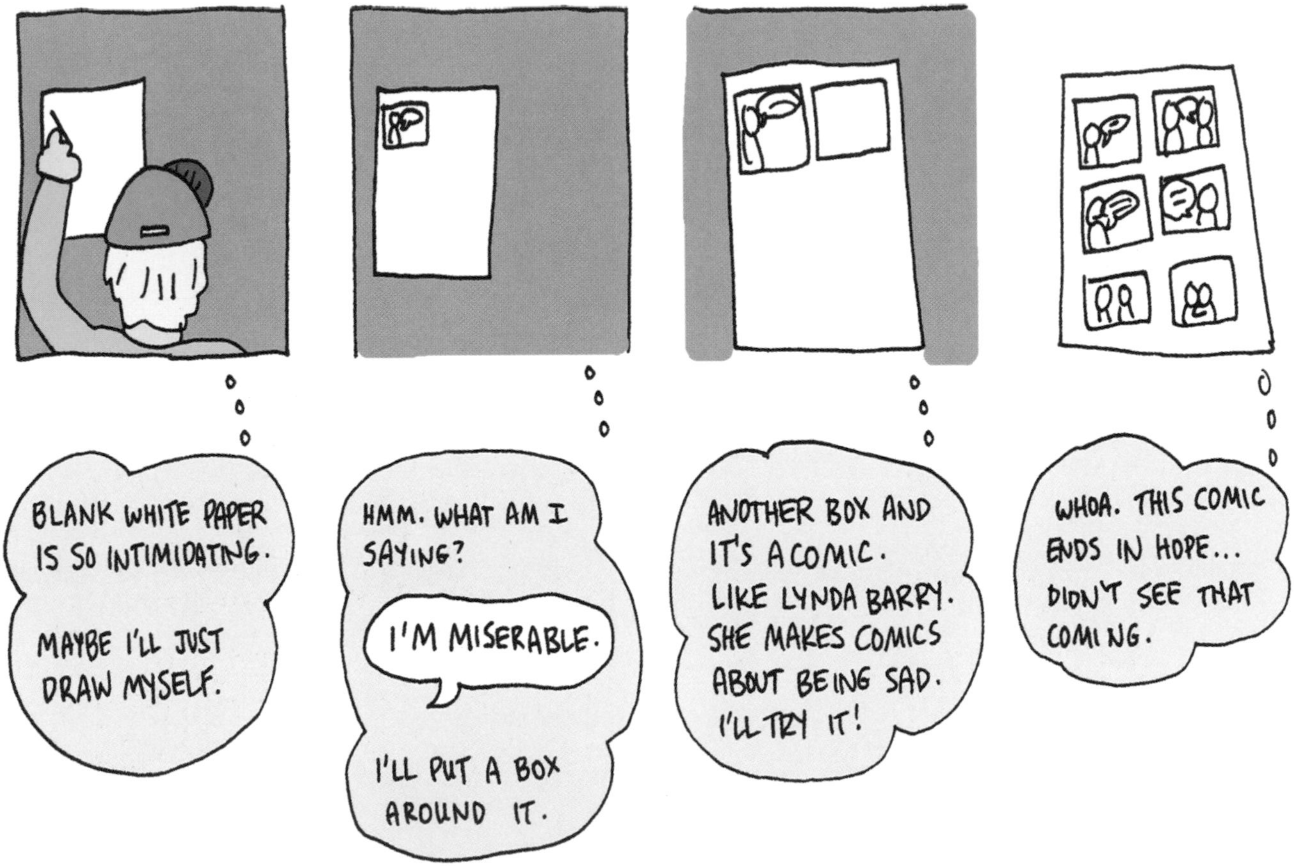
BLANK WHITE PAPER IS SO INTIMIDATING.
MAYBE I'LL JUST DRAW MYSELF.
HMM. WHAT AM I SAYING?
I'M MISERABLE.
I'LL PUT A BOX AROUND IT.
ANOTHER BOX AND IT'S A COMIC. LIKE LYNDA BARRY. SHE MAKES COMICS ABOUT BEING SAD. I'LL TRY IT!
WHOA. THIS COMIC ENDS IN HOPE... DIDN'T SEE THAT COMING.

2008

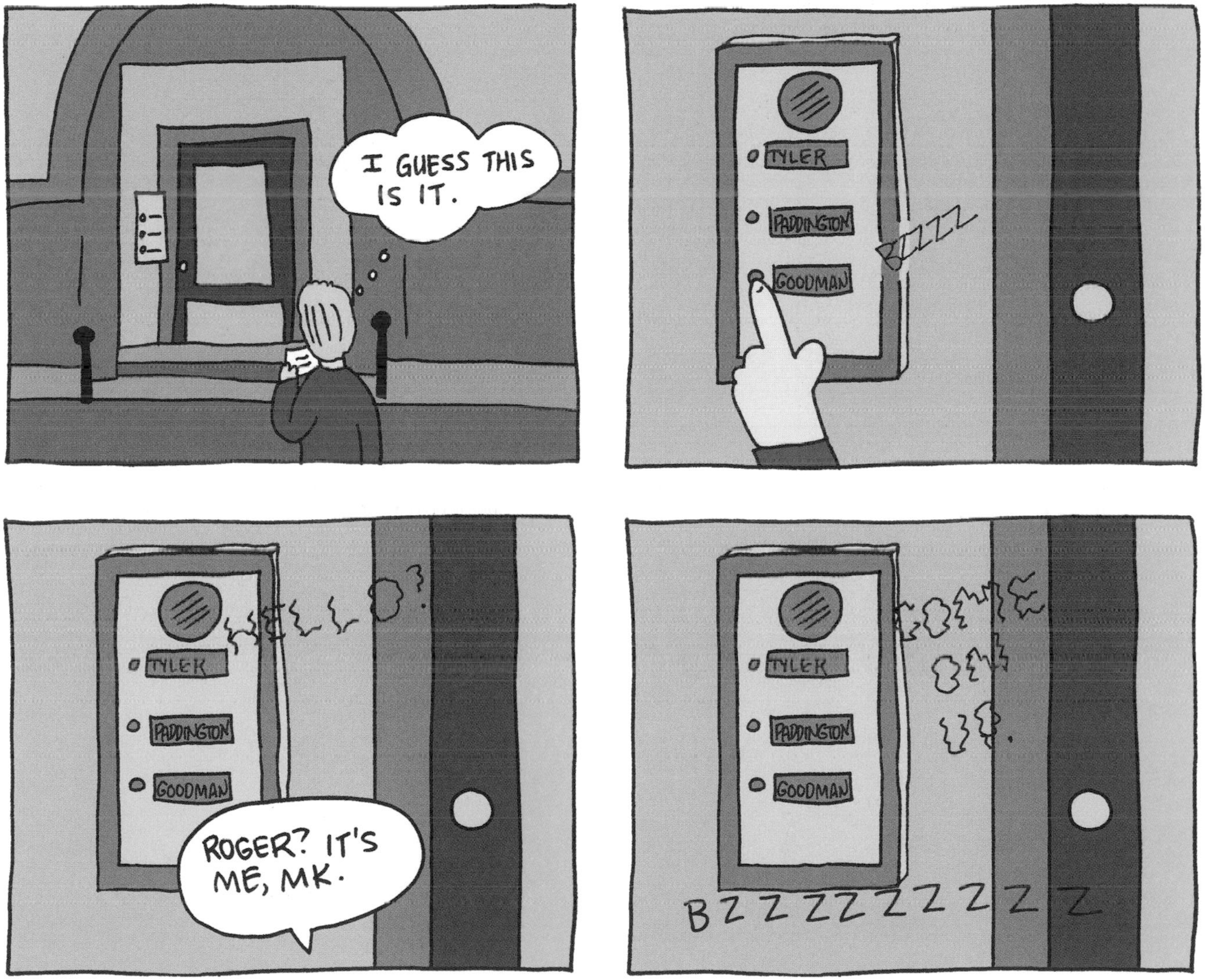
I GUESS THIS IS IT.
TYLER
PADDINGTON
GOODMAN
BZZZZ
ROGER? IT'S ME, MK.
BZZZZZZZZZ

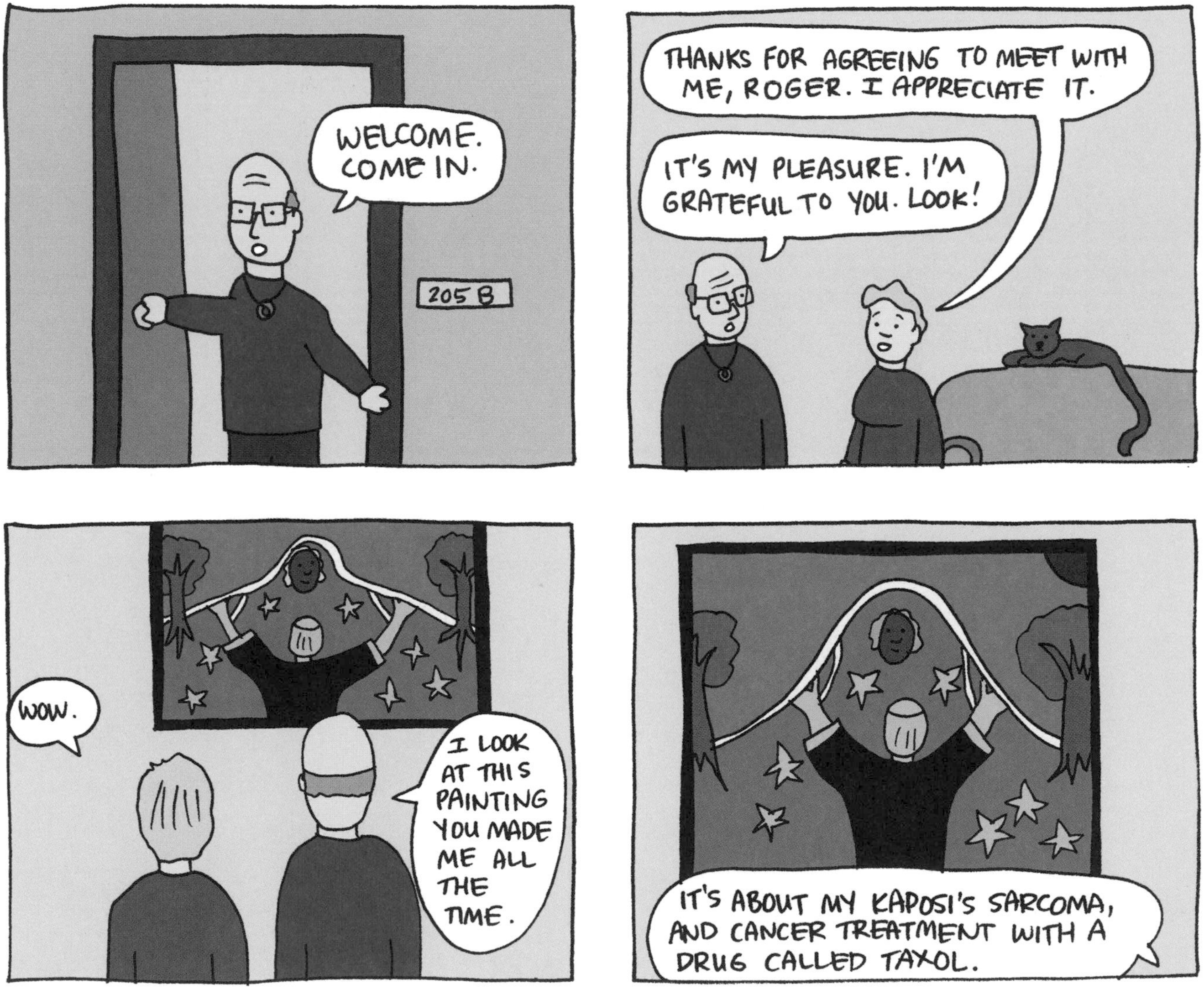
WELCOME. COME IN.
205 B
THANKS FOR AGREEING TO MEET WITH ME, ROGER. I APPRECIATE IT.
IT'S MY PLEASURE. I'M GRATEFUL TO YOU. LOOK!
WOW.
I LOOK AT THIS PAINTING YOU MADE ME ALL THE TIME.
IT'S ABOUT MY KAPOSI'S SARCOMA, AND CANCER TREATMENT WITH A DRUG CALLED TAXOL.

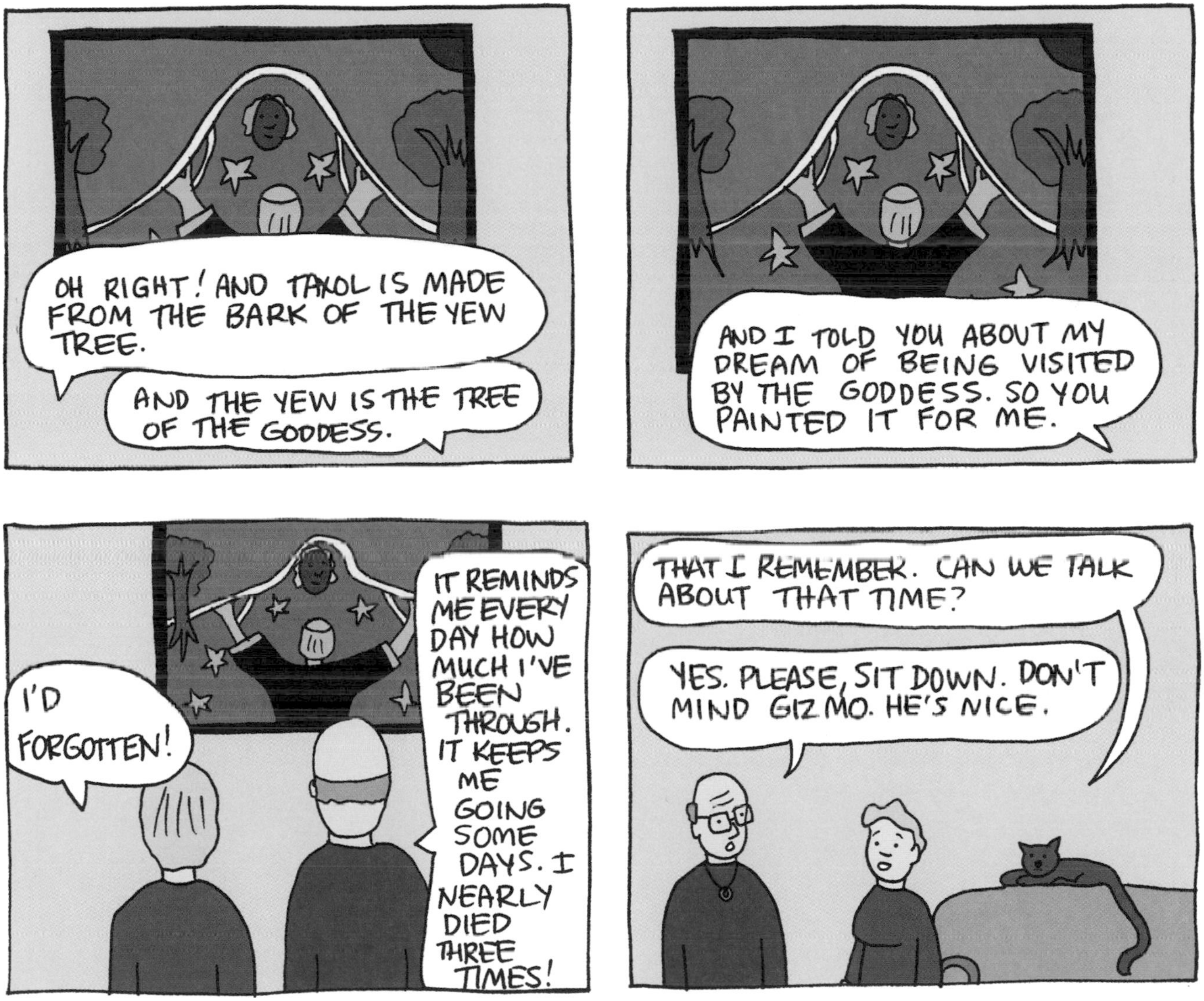
OH RIGHT! AND TAXOL IS MADE FROM THE BARK OF THE YEW TREE.
AND THE YEW IS THE TREE OF THE GODDESS.
AND I TOLD YOU ABOUT MY DREAM OF BEING VISITED BY THE GODDESS. SO YOU PAINTED IT FOR ME.
I'D FORGOTTEN!
IT REMINDS ME EVERY DAY HOW MUCH I'VE BEEN THROUGH. IT KEEPS ME GOING SOME DAYS. I NEARLY DIED THREE TIMES!
THAT I REMEMBER. CAN WE TALK ABOUT THAT TIME?
YES. PLEASE, SIT DOWN. DON'T MIND GIZMO. HE'S NICE.

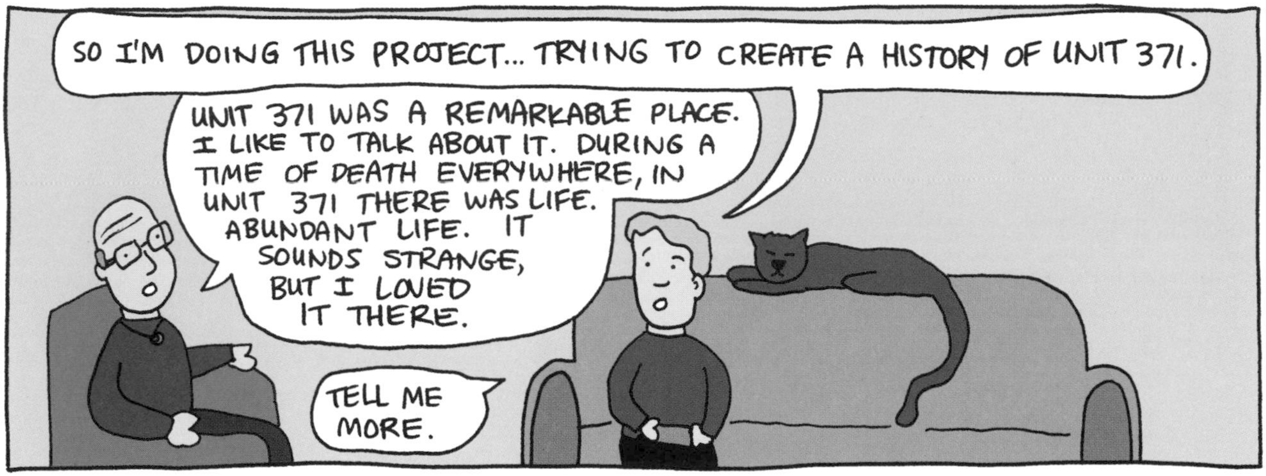
SO I'M DOING THIS PROJECT... TRYING TO CREATE A HISTORY OF UNIT 371.
UNIT 371 WAS A REMARKABLE PLACE. I LIKE TO TALK ABOUT IT. DURING A TIME OF DEATH EVERYWHERE, IN UNIT 371 THERE WAS LIFE. ABUNDANT LIFE. IT SOUNDS STRANGE, BUT I LOVED IT THERE.
TELL ME MORE.

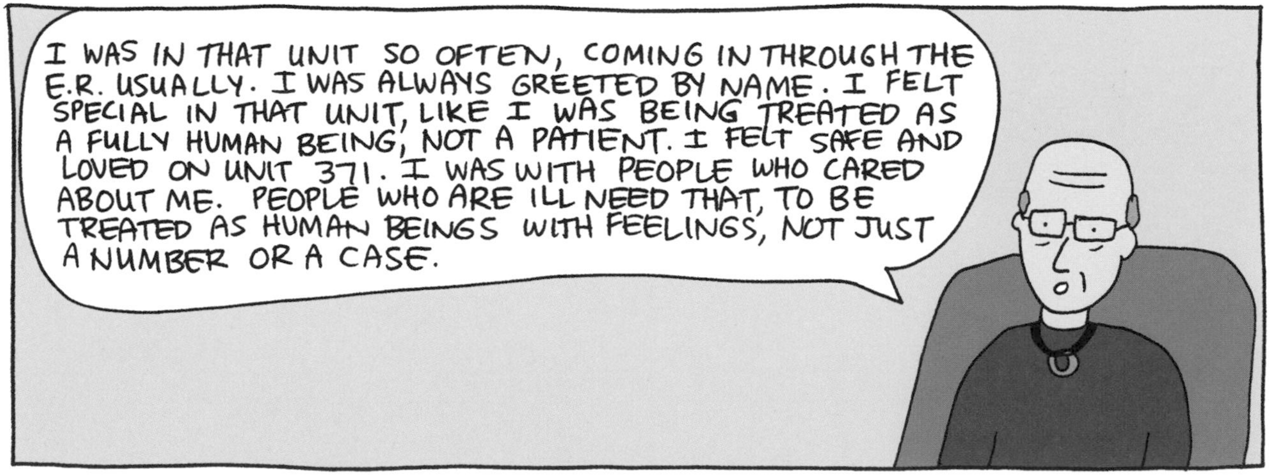
I WAS IN THAT UNIT SO OFTEN, COMING IN THROUGH THE E.R. USUALLY. I WAS ALWAYS GREETED BY NAME. I FELT SPECIAL IN THAT UNIT, LIKE I WAS BEING TREATED AS A FULLY HUMAN BEING, NOT A PATIENT. I FELT SAFE AND LOVED ON UNIT 371. I WAS WITH PEOPLE WHO CARED ABOUT ME. PEOPLE WHO ARE ILL NEED THAT, TO BE TREATED AS HUMAN BEINGS WITH FEELINGS, NOT JUST A NUMBER OR A CASE.

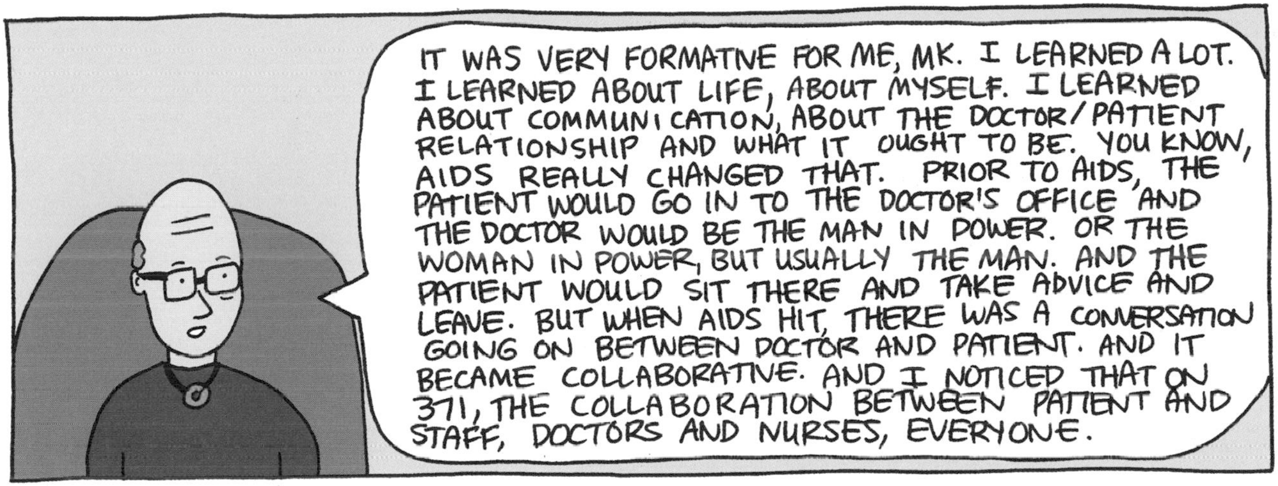
IT WAS VERY FORMATIVE FOR ME, MK. I LEARNED A LOT. I LEARNED ABOUT LIFE, ABOUT MYSELF. I LEARNED ABOUT COMMUNICATION, ABOUT THE DOCTOR/PATIENT RELATIONSHIP AND WHAT IT OUGHT TO BE. YOU KNOW, AIDS REALLY CHANGED THAT. PRIOR TO AIDS, THE PATIENT WOULD GO IN TO THE DOCTOR'S OFFICE AND THE DOCTOR WOULD BE THE MAN IN POWER. OR THE WOMAN IN POWER, BUT USUALLY THE MAN. AND THE PATIENT WOULD SIT THERE AND TAKE ADVICE AND LEAVE. BUT WHEN AIDS HIT, THERE WAS A CONVERSATION GOING ON BETWEEN DOCTOR AND PATIENT. AND IT BECAME COLLABORATIVE. AND I NOTICED THAT ON 371, THE COLLABORATION BETWEEN PATIENT AND STAFF, DOCTORS AND NURSES, EVERYONE.

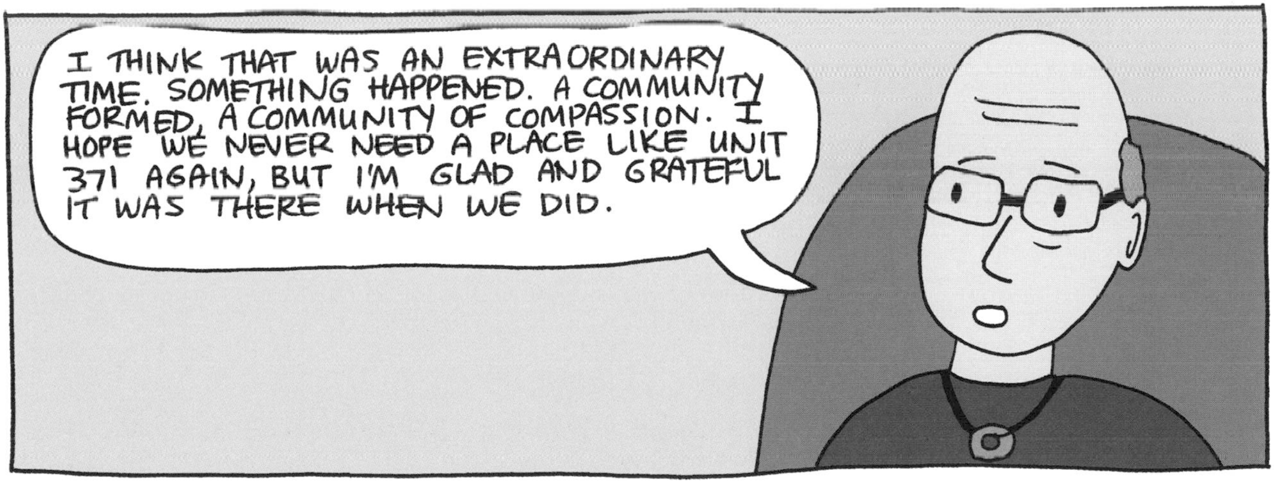
I THINK THAT WAS AN EXTRAORDINARY TIME. SOMETHING HAPPENED. A COMMUNITY FORMED, A COMMUNITY OF COMPASSION. I HOPE WE NEVER NEED A PLACE LIKE UNIT 371 AGAIN, BUT I'M GLAD AND GRATEFUL IT WAS THERE WHEN WE DID.

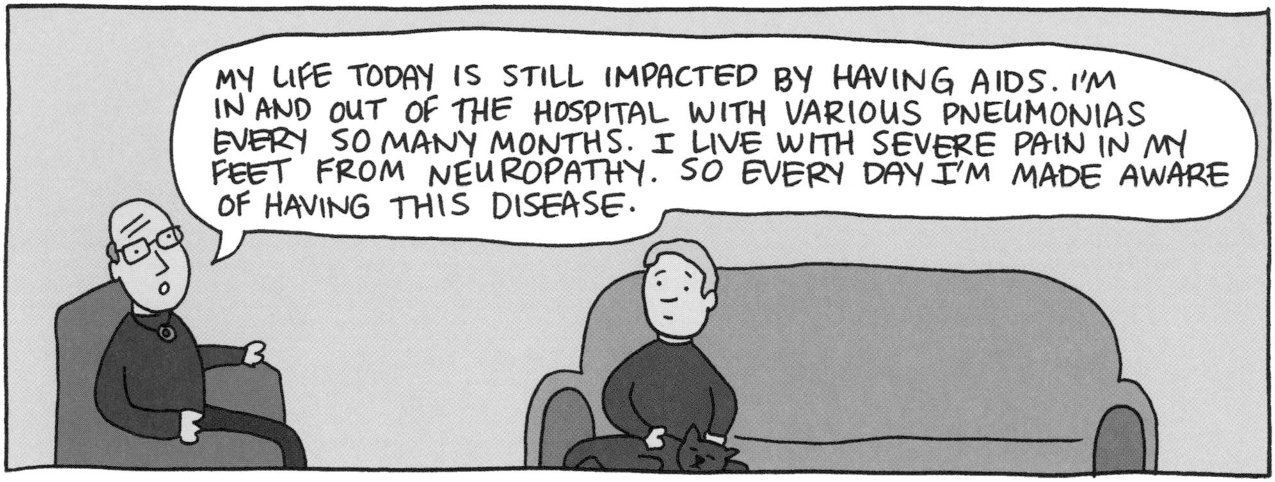
MY LIFE TODAY IS STILL IMPACTED BY HAVING AIDS. I'M IN AND OUT OF THE HOSPITAL WITH VARIOUS PNEUMONIAS EVERY SO MANY MONTHS. I LIVE WITH SEVERE PAIN IN MY FEET FROM NEUROPATHY. SO EVERY DAY I'M MADE AWARE OF HAVING THIS DISEASE.

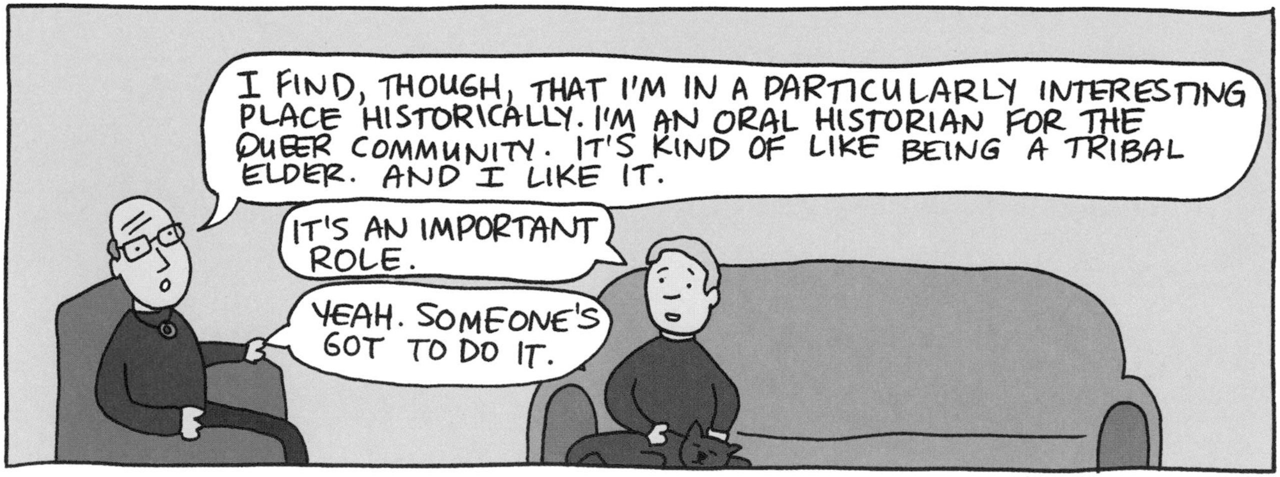
I FIND, THOUGH, THAT I'M IN A PARTICULARLY INTERESTING PLACE HISTORICALLY. I'M AN ORAL HISTORIAN FOR THE QUEER COMMUNITY. IT'S KIND OF LIKE BEING A TRIBAL ELDER. AND I LIKE IT.
IT'S AN IMPORTANT ROLE.
YEAH. SOMEONE'S GOT TO DO IT.

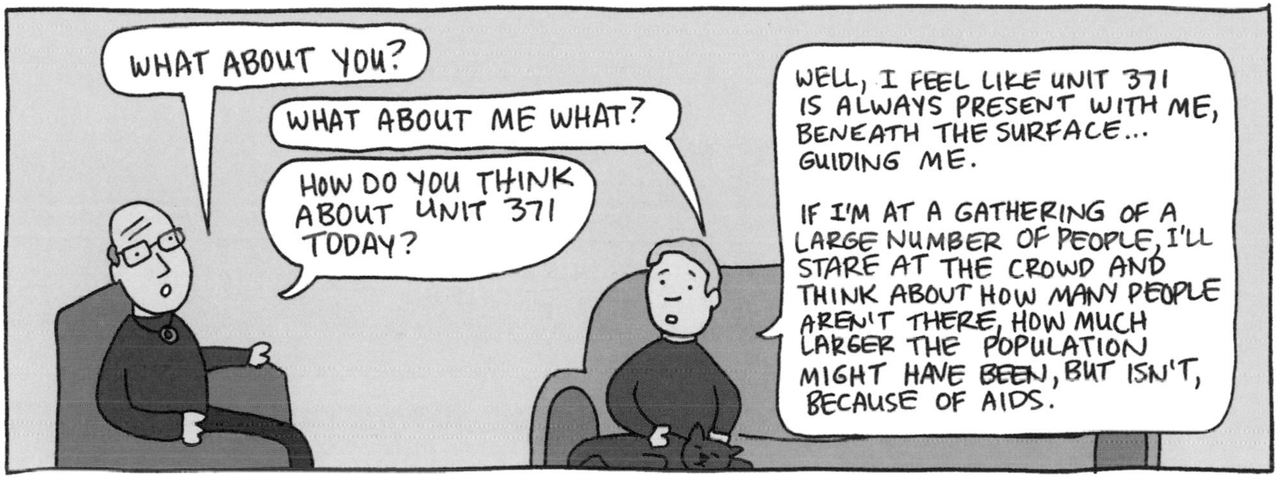
WHAT ABOUT YOU?
WHAT ABOUT ME WHAT?
HOW DO YOU THINK ABOUT UNIT 371 TODAY?
WELL, I FEEL LIKE UNIT 371 IS ALWAYS PRESENT WITH ME, BENEATH THE SURFACE... GUIDING ME.
IF I'M AT A GATHERING OF A LARGE NUMBER OF PEOPLE, I'LL STARE AT THE CROWD AND THINK ABOUT HOW MANY PEOPLE AREN'T THERE, HOW MUCH LARGER THE POPULATION MIGHT HAVE BEEN, BUT ISN'T, BECAUSE OF AIDS.

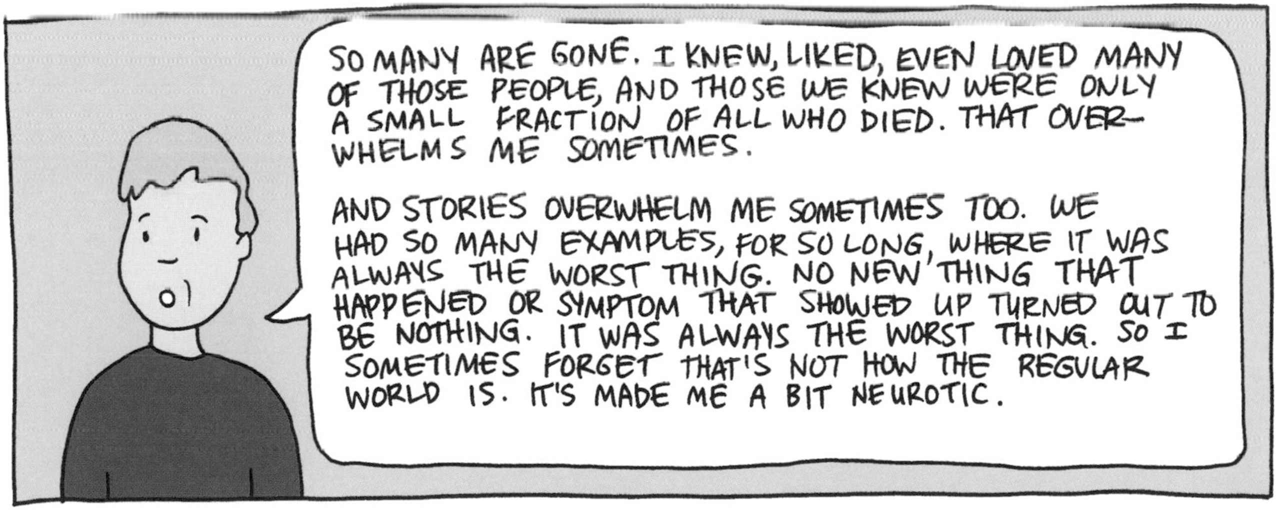
SO MANY ARE GONE. I KNEW, LIKED, EVEN LOVED MANY OF THOSE PEOPLE, AND THOSE WE KNEW WERE ONLY A SMALL FRACTION OF ALL WHO DIED. THAT OVER-WHELMS ME SOMETIMES.
AND STORIES OVERWHELM ME SOMETIMES TOO. WE HAD SO MANY EXAMPLES, FOR SO LONG, WHERE IT WAS ALWAYS THE WORST THING. NO NEW THING THAT HAPPENED OR SYMPTOM THAT SHOWED UP TURNED OUT TO BE NOTHING. IT WAS ALWAYS THE WORST THING. SO I SOMETIMES FORGET THAT'S NOT HOW THE REGULAR WORLD IS. IT'S MADE ME A BIT NEUROTIC.

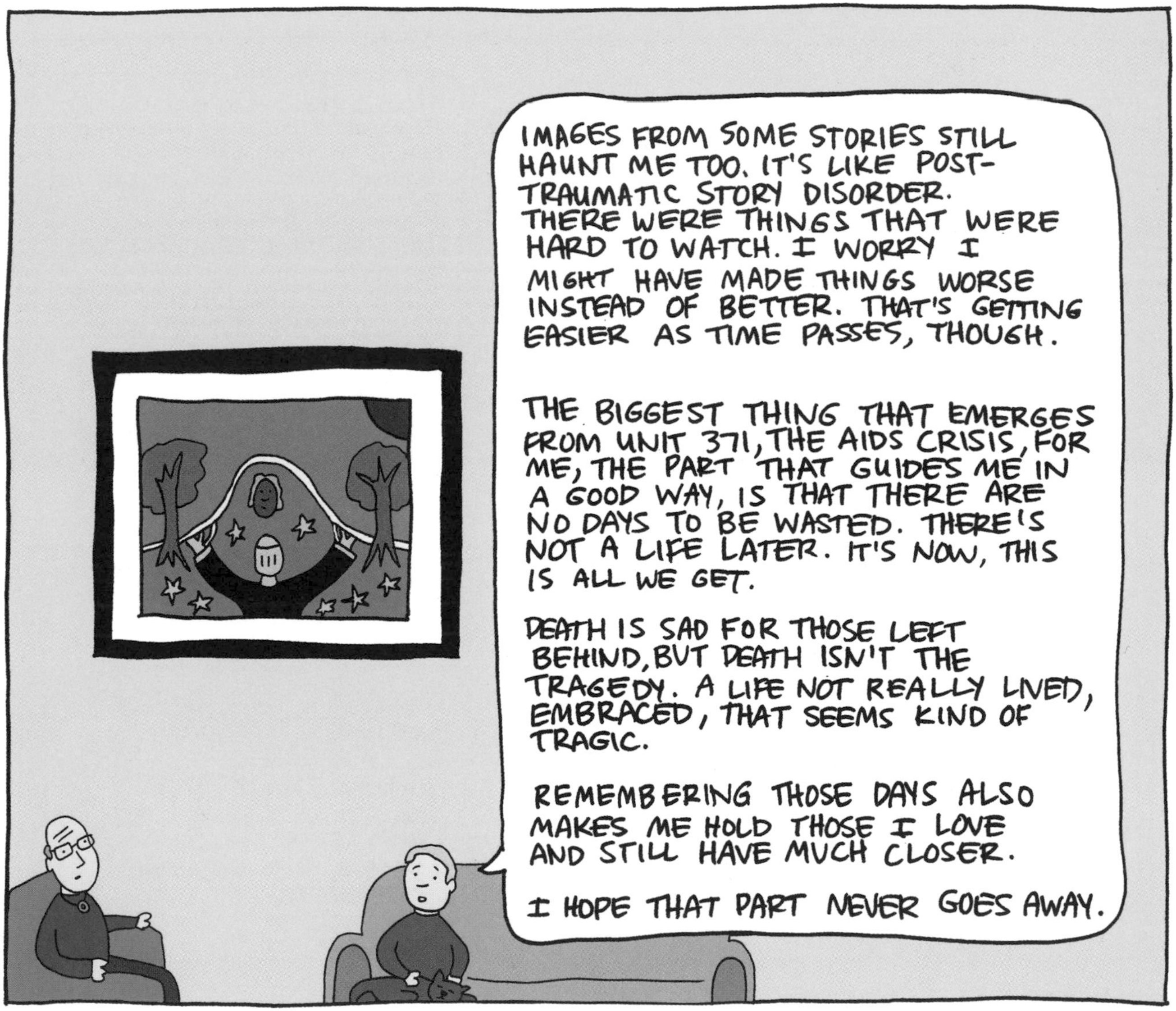
IMAGES FROM SOME STORIES STILL HAUNT ME TOO. IT'S LIKE POST-TRAUMATIC STORY DISORDER. THERE WERE THINGS THAT WERE HARD TO WATCH. I WORRY I MIGHT HAVE MADE THINGS WORSE INSTEAD OF BETTER. THAT'S GETTING EASIER AS TIME PASSES, THOUGH.
THE BIGGEST THING THAT EMERGES FROM UNIT 371, THE AIDS CRISIS, FOR ME, THE PART THAT GUIDES ME IN A GOOD WAY, IS THAT THERE ARE NO DAYS TO BE WASTED. THERE'S NOT A LIFE LATER. IT'S NOW, THIS IS ALL WE GET.
DEATH IS SAD FOR THOSE LEFT BEHIND, BUT DEATH ISN'T THE TRAGEDY. A LIFE NOT REALLY LIVED, EMBRACED, THAT SEEMS KIND OF TRAGIC.
REMEMBERING THOSE DAYS ALSO MAKES ME HOLD THOSE I LOVE AND STILL HAVE MUCH CLOSER.
I HOPE THAT PART NEVER GOES AWAY.

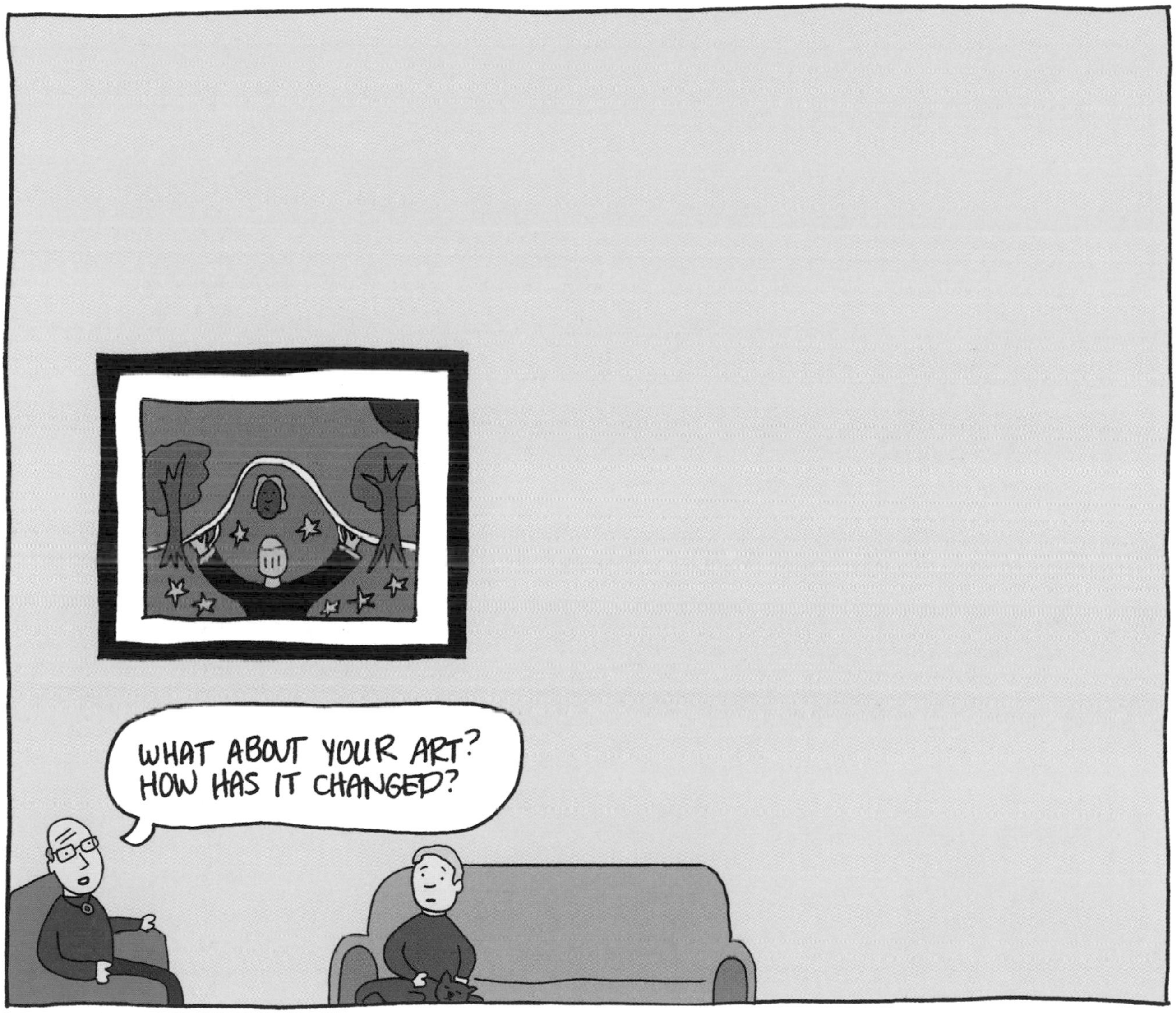
WHAT ABOUT YOUR ART? HOW HAS IT CHANGED?

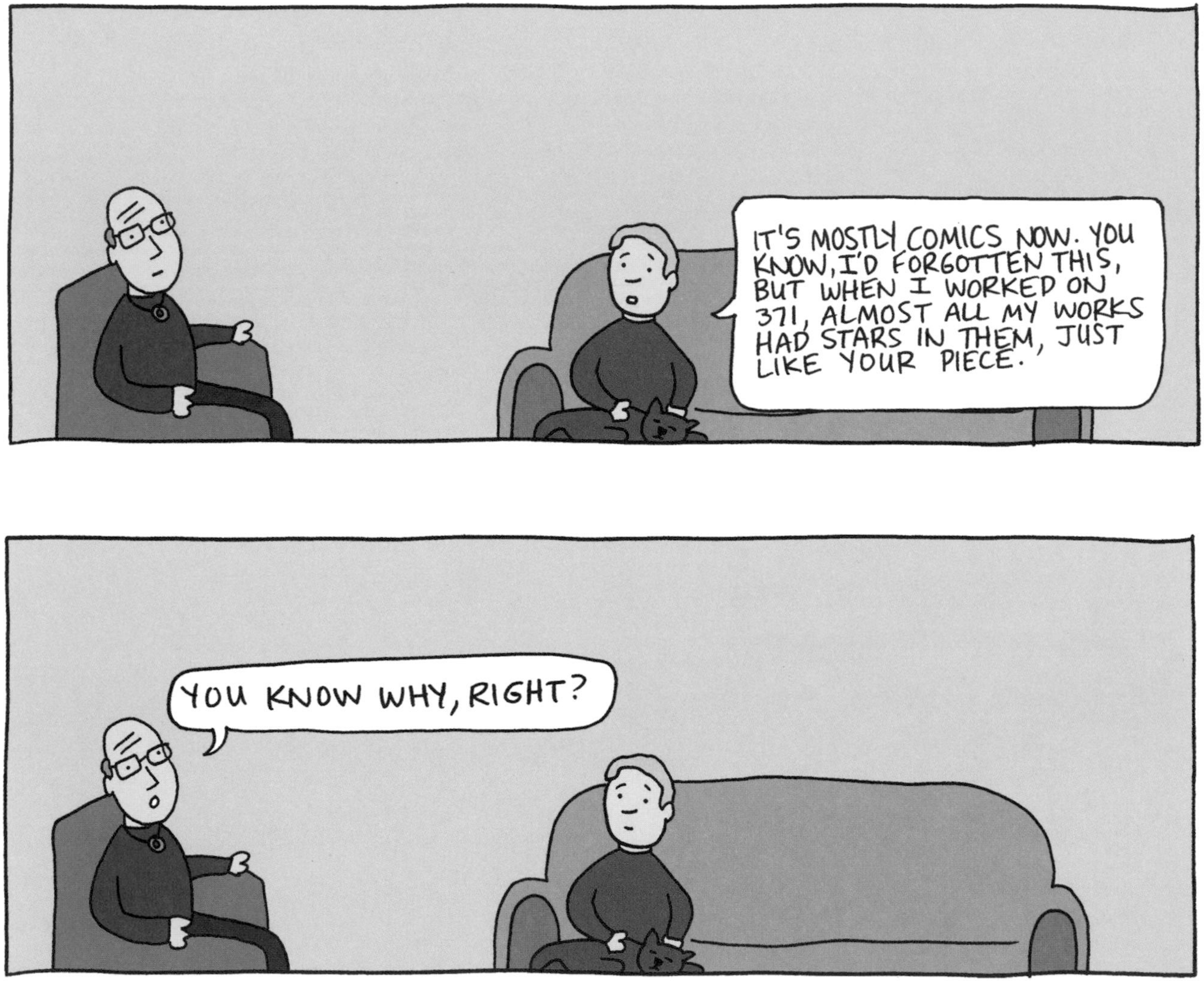
IT'S MOSTLY COMICS NOW. YOU KNOW, I'D FORGOTTEN THIS, BUT WHEN I WORKED ON 371, ALMOST ALL MY WORKS HAD STARS IN THEM, JUST LIKE YOUR PIECE.
YOU KNOW WHY, RIGHT?

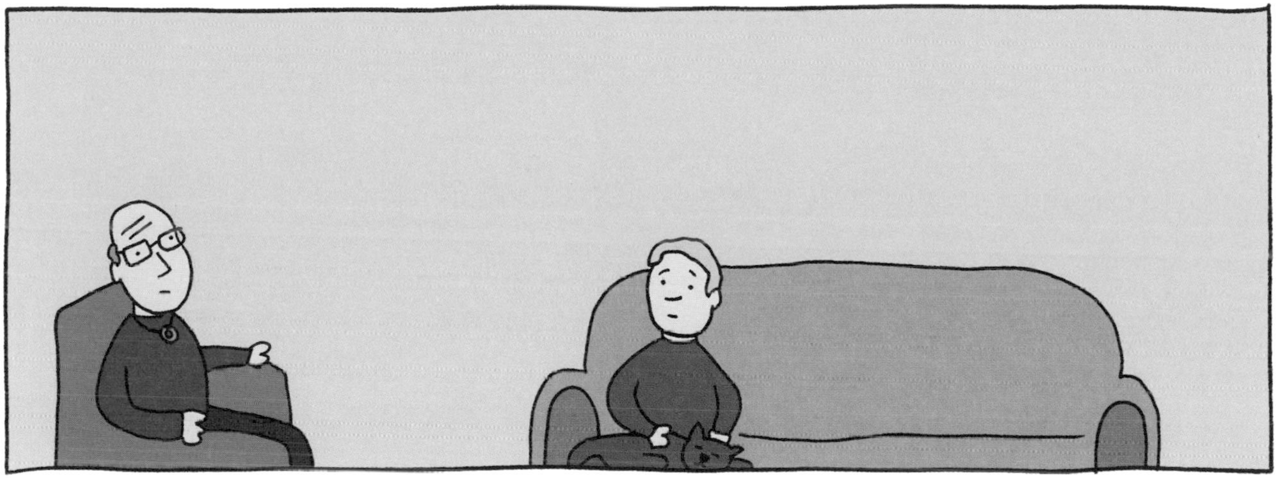

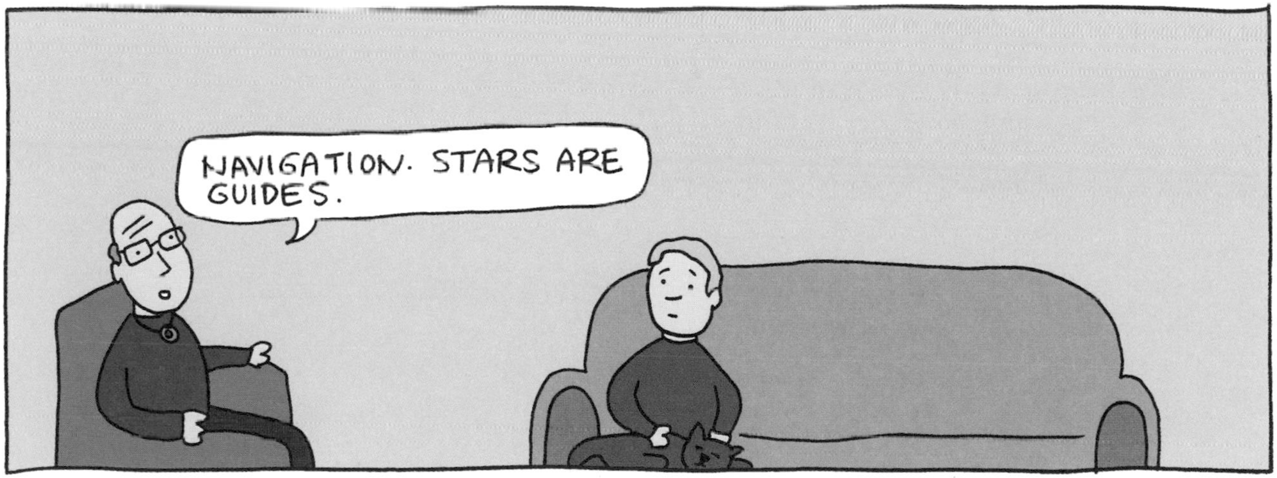
NAVIGATION. STARS ARE GUIDES.

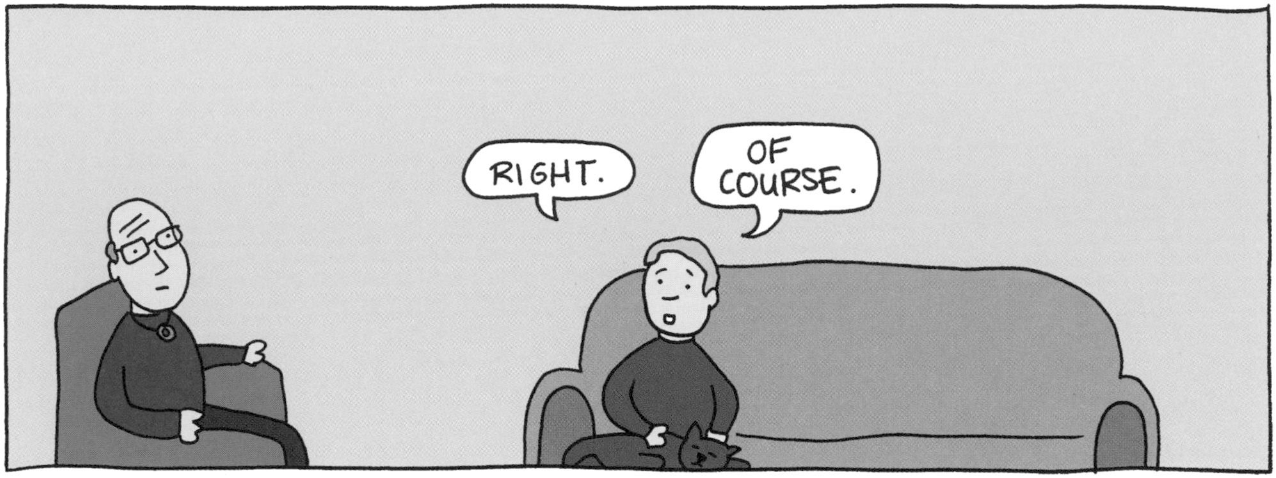
RIGHT.
OF COURSE.

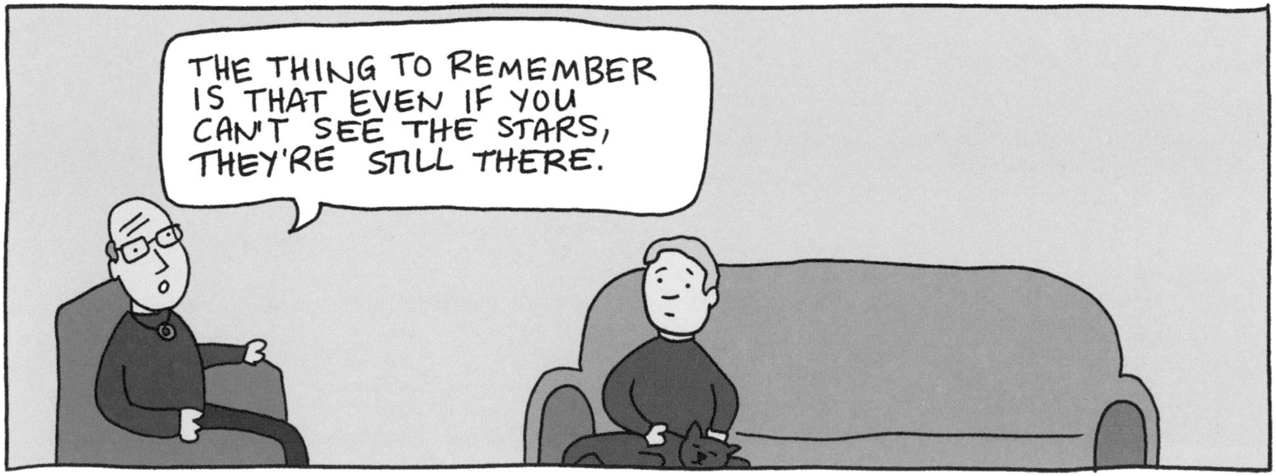
THE THING TO REMEMBER IS THAT EVEN IF YOU CAN'T SEE THE STARS, THEY'RE STILL THERE.

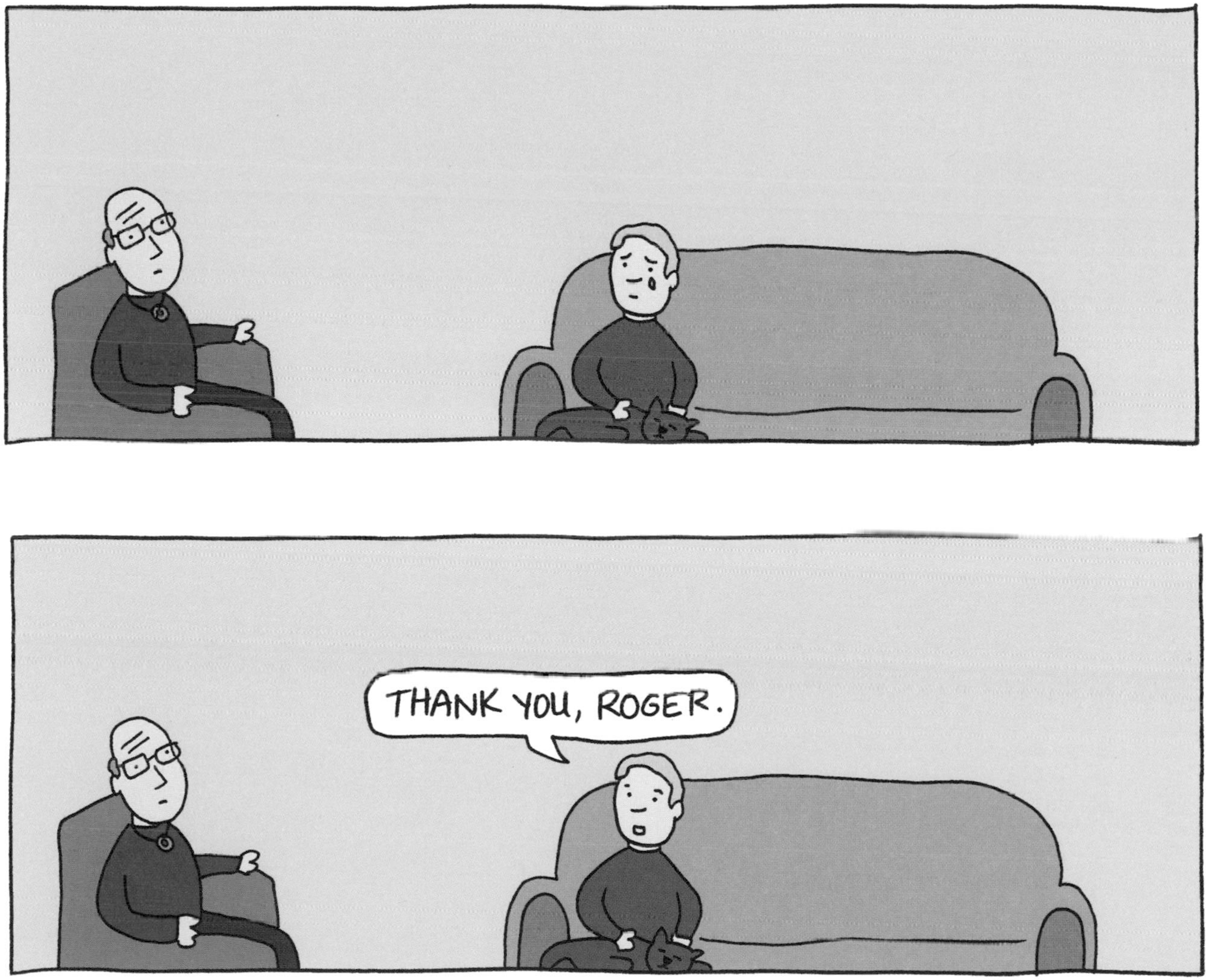
THANK YOU, ROGER.

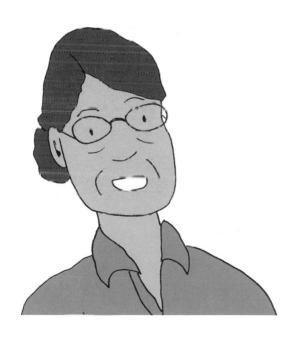

I THINK I DID MY BEST. I RECEIVED
A LOT. IT'S NOT WHAT I GAVE, IT'S
WHAT I RECEIVED.

— ROSA ORTIZ

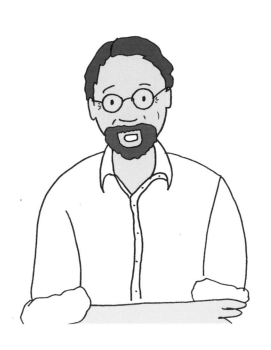

UP UNTIL THE AIDS EPIDEMIC, WE WERE TOLD THERE WAS GOING TO BE A SHOT OR A SURGICAL TREATMENT FOR JUST ABOUT EVERYTHING. AIDS CAUGHT THE MEDICAL COMMUNITY WITH ITS PANTS DOWN.

LUCKILY THERE WERE PEOPLE WHO WERE FORWARD THINKING ENOUGH TO SAY, "WE CAN'T DO THIS OURSELVES. MY REFLEX MALLET, MY BLOOD PRESSURE CUFF, MY THERMOMETER AREN'T GOING TO DO JACK SHIT HERE."

FOR ME, THE ULTIMATE MESSAGE, MEANING, GIFT, WHATEVER OF THIS EPIDEMIC IS THAT THERE ARE MANY DIFFERENT WAYS TO HEAL. AND IF YOU CAN'T HEAL OR CURE, THEN COMFORT. TRULY CARE FOR PEOPLE.

-RUSS LEANDER

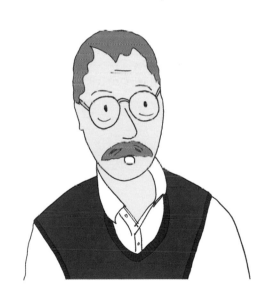

I FEEL LIKE WE WERE ABLE TO
PROVIDE SOMETHING OF VALUE—
NOT ONLY CAREGIVING BUT ALSO.
A COMMUNITY EXPERIENCE, A
PLACE WHERE THE COMMUNITY
COULD COME TO WITNESS WHAT
WAS HAPPENING, TO CONTRIBUTE
TO BE A PART OF IT. AND FOR THE
PATIENTS, WE WANTED THEM TO
FEEL SURROUNDED BY A SAFETY
NET OF THE FAMILIAR.

—DAVID MOORE

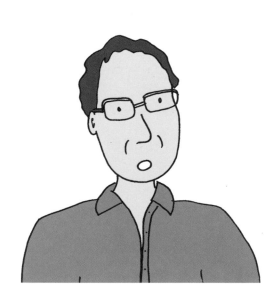

MY TIME ON 371 DEFINITELY
IMPACTED ME. I THINK I
TOOK FROM IT MORE OF
WHAT I BROUGHT TO IT, AN
APPRECIATION FOR HOW SHORT
LIFE IS. AND I'M SO SAD THAT
SO MANY COULDN'T LIVE A
LITTLE LONGER UNTIL THE
NEW DRUGS CAME.

—KAREN COLEMAN

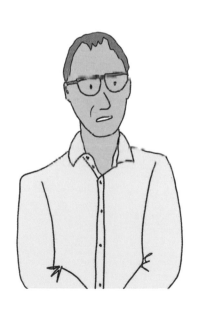

TO THIS DAY, I DON'T KNOW THAT
I'VE FULLY PROCESSED OR DEALT
WITH ALL THOSE EXPERIENCES
I HAD BACK THEN.

-CHRIS HAEN

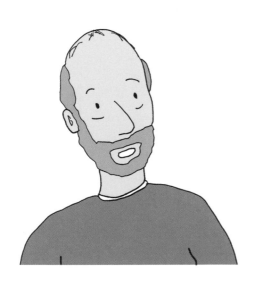

I THINK HIV AND THE EPIDEMIC INFORMED MY LIFE IN A BIG WAY. I JUST GOT LUCKY. NOT FOR ANY PURPOSE, BECAUSE ALL THOSE OTHER PEOPLE HAD PURPOSES. AFTER GOING THROUGH ALL THAT, MOST OF THE ORDINARY STUFF THAT WOULD BE ANNOYING IS STILL SORT OF ANNOYING BUT IT'S HARD TO TAKE IT SERIOUSLY BECAUSE I'M THE LUCKIEST GUY IN THE HISTORY OF THE WORLD.

—DAVID BLATT

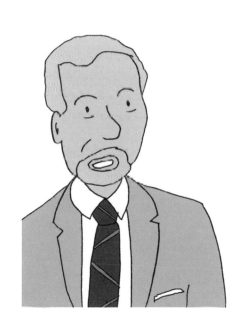

MOURNING IS A PROCESS. WHEN YOU ASK ME, IT'S ALL THERE, LIKE TOUCHSTONES. AND THERE ARE HUNDREDS.

I WAS IMMEASURABLY ENRICHED BY THE EXPERIENCE OF UNIT 371. IT'S HELPED ME BECOME WHO I AM. IT'S NEVER STOPPED.

-WALTER MILLER

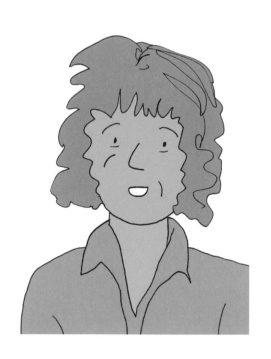

THIS WAS OUR PLAGUE. IT WAS DEVASTATION OF A GENERATION, A COUPLE OF GENERATIONS. WHO KNOWS WHAT WAS LOST IN THOSE GENERATIONS? ARTISTS, SCIENTISTS, WARM, LOVING PARENTS AND CHILDREN. AND SOME ASSHOLES TOO.

—JOYCE WEGMULLER

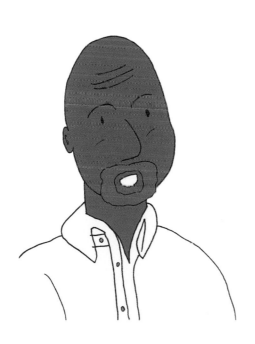

I'M STILL AFFECTED BY THAT EXPERIENCE. 371 IS SOMETHING THAT NEVER GOES AWAY. IT'S ALWAYS THERE.

371 IS A POINT OF REFERENCE, A RESOURCE IF YOU WILL, A RESOURCE FOR MY OWN PERSON.

LEARNING HOW TO DIE IS LEARNING HOW TO LIVE. YOU LEARN HOW TO LIVE FOR YOURSELF FROM SEEING PEOPLE DIE WITH DIGNITY.

AND I HAVE ROLE MODELS TO ASPIRE TO, TO LOOK TOWARDS. BOY, I'D LIKE TO BE THAT BRAVE WHEN IT'S TIME FOR ME NOT TO BE ON THE PLANET.

—JOEL HALL

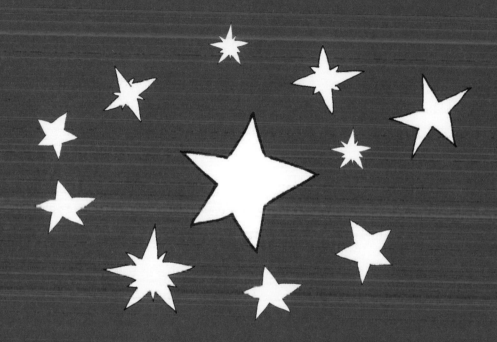

2016

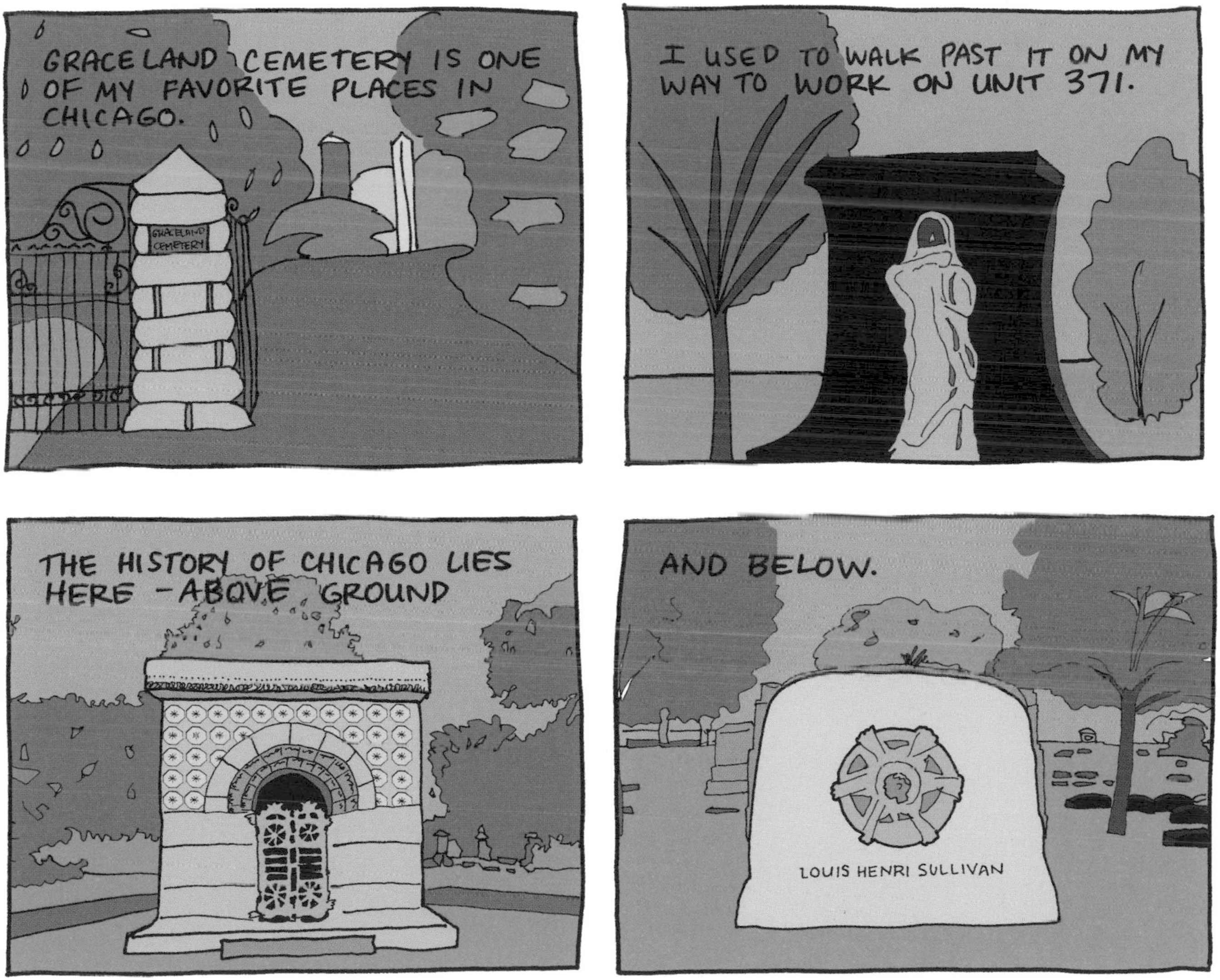
GRACELAND CEMETERY IS ONE OF MY FAVORITE PLACES IN CHICAGO.
GRACELAND CEMETERY
I USED TO WALK PAST IT ON MY WAY TO WORK ON UNIT 371.
THE HISTORY OF CHICAGO LIES HERE - ABOVE GROUND
AND BELOW.
LOUIS HENRI SULLIVAN

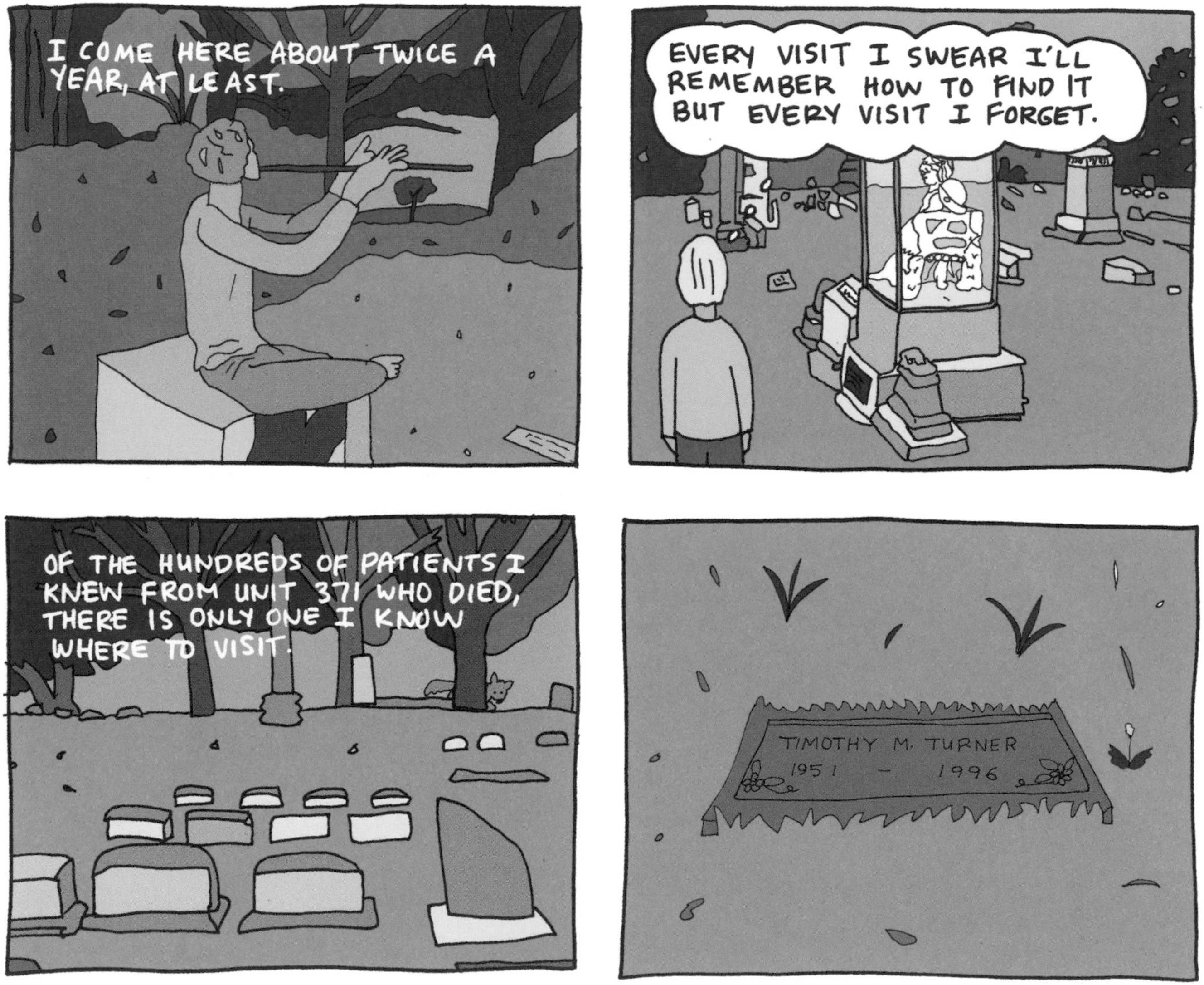
I COME HERE ABOUT TWICE A YEAR, AT LEAST.
EVERY VISIT I SWEAR I'LL REMEMBER HOW TO FIND IT BUT EVERY VISIT I FORGET.
OF THE HUNDREDS OF PATIENTS I KNEW FROM UNIT 371 WHO DIED, THERE IS ONLY ONE I KNOW WHERE TO VISIT.
TIMOTHY M. TURNER
1951 - 1996

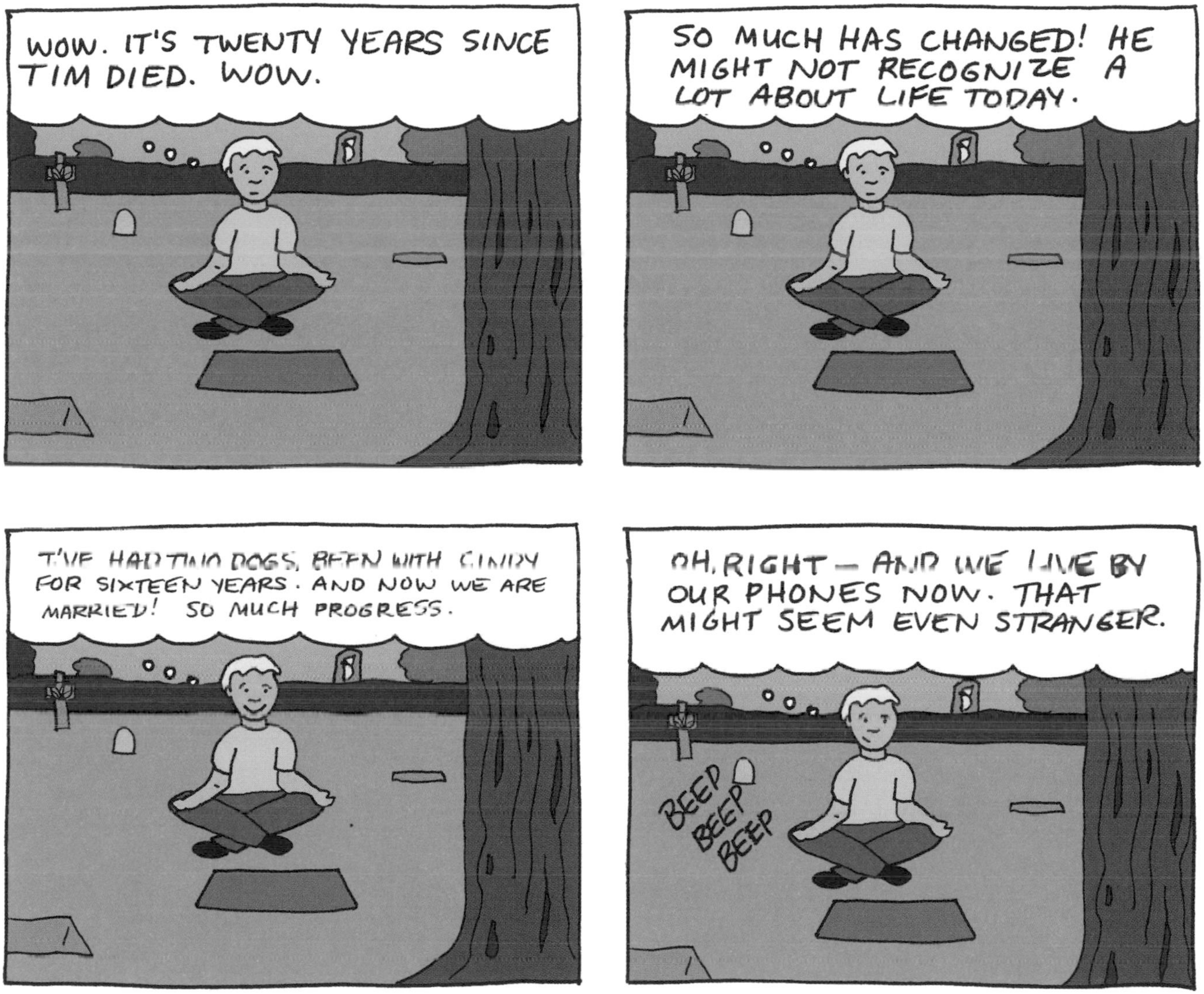
WOW. IT'S TWENTY YEARS SINCE TIM DIED. WOW.
SO MUCH HAS CHANGED! HE MIGHT NOT RECOGNIZE A LOT ABOUT LIFE TODAY.
I'VE HAD TWO DOGS, BEEN WITH CINDY FOR SIXTEEN YEARS. AND NOW WE ARE MARRIED! SO MUCH PROGRESS.
OH, RIGHT — AND WE LIVE BY OUR PHONES NOW. THAT MIGHT SEEM EVEN STRANGER.
BEEP BEEP BEEP

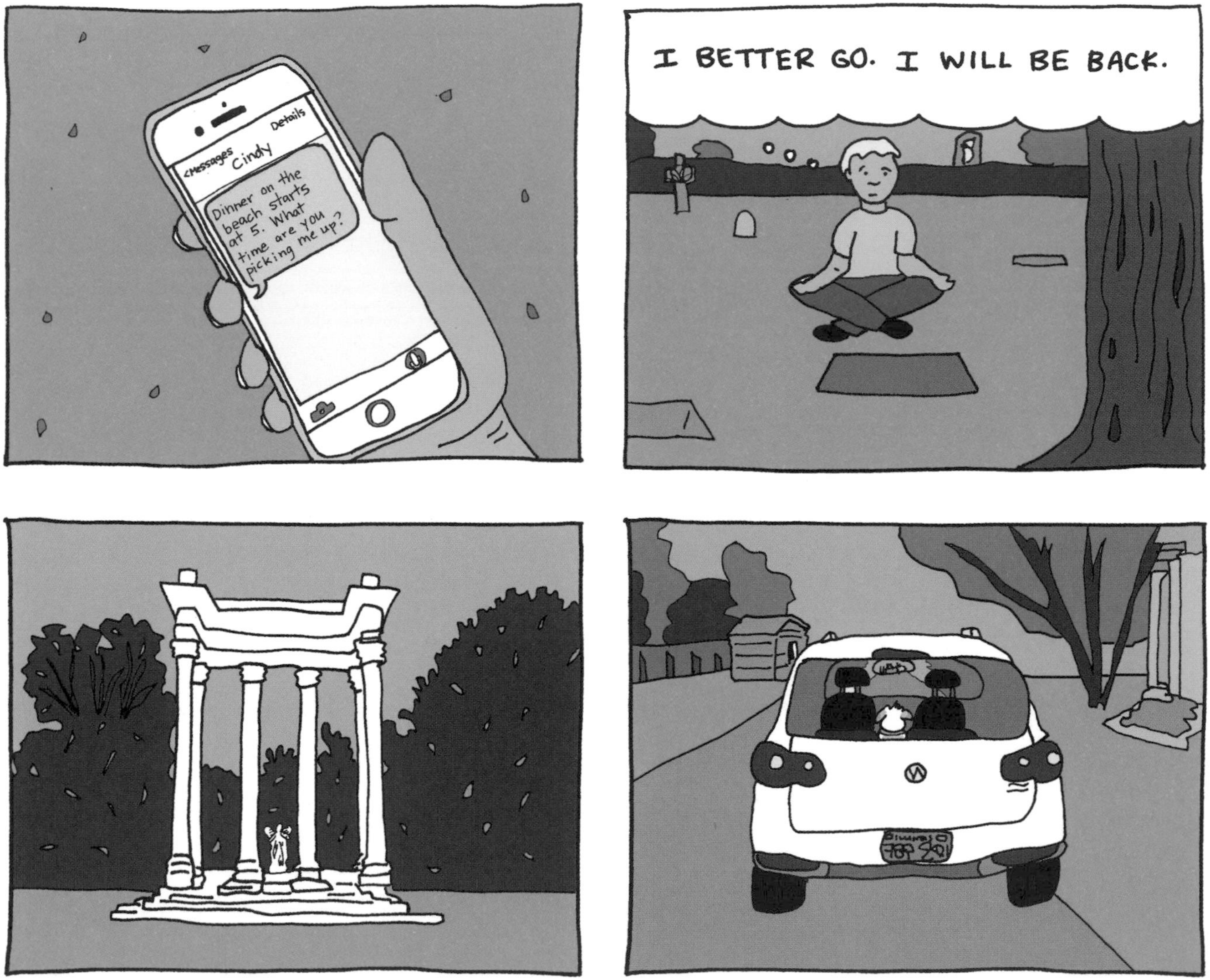
<Messages
Cindy
Details
Dinner on the beach starts at 5. What time are you picking me up?
I BETTER GO. I WILL BE BACK.

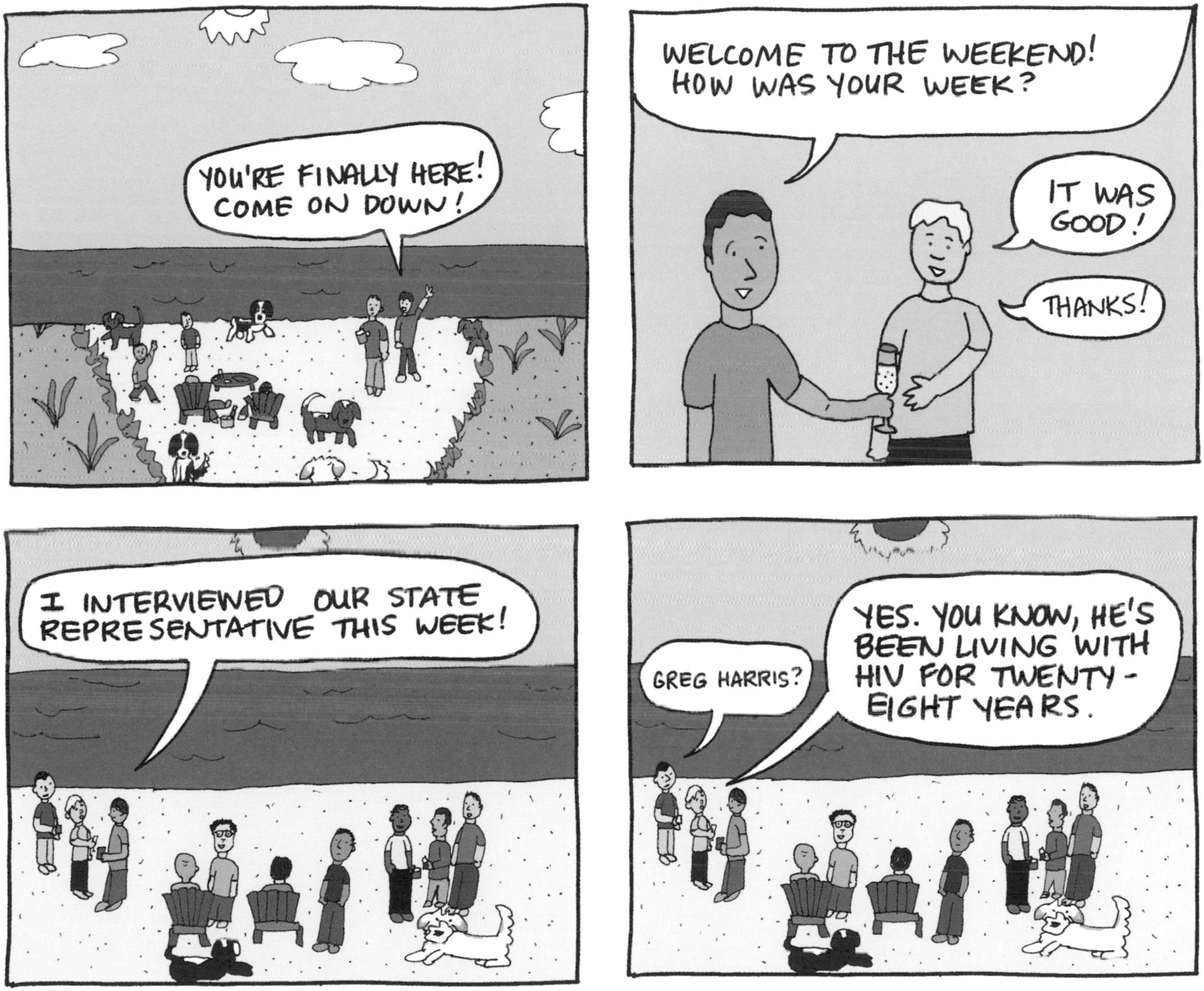
YOU'RE FINALLY HERE! COME ON DOWN!
WELCOME TO THE WEEKEND! HOW WAS YOUR WEEK?
IT WAS GOOD!
THANKS!
I INTERVIEWED OUR STATE REPRESENTATIVE THIS WEEK!
GREG HARRIS?
YES. YOU KNOW, HE'S BEEN LIVING WITH HIV FOR TWENTY-EIGHT YEARS.

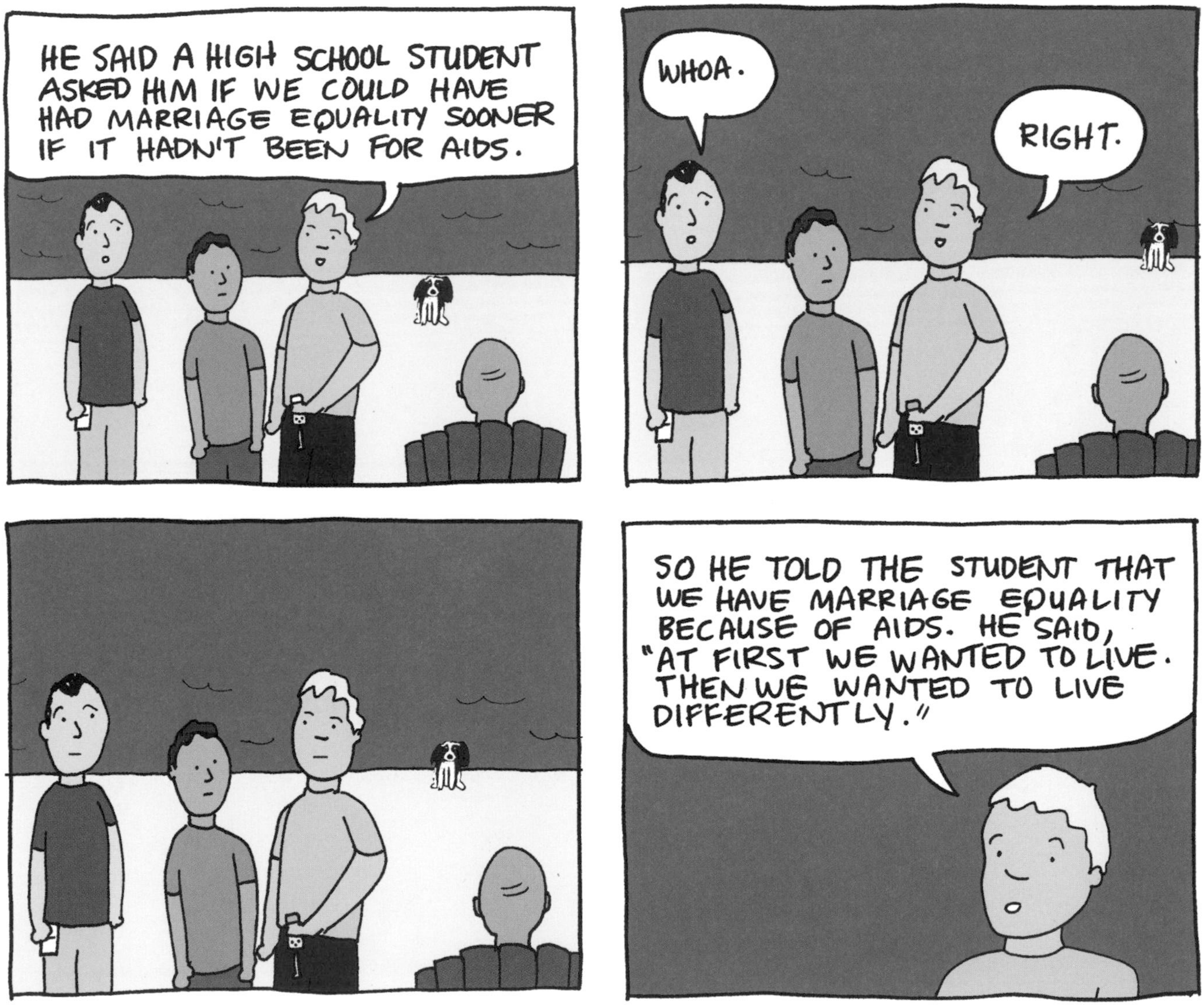
HE SAID A HIGH SCHOOL STUDENT ASKED HIM IF WE COULD HAVE HAD MARRIAGE EQUALITY SOONER IF IT HADN'T BEEN FOR AIDS.
WHOA.
RIGHT.
SO HE TOLD THE STUDENT THAT WE HAVE MARRIAGE EQUALITY BECAUSE OF AIDS. HE SAID, "AT FIRST WE WANTED TO LIVE. THEN WE WANTED TO LIVE DIFFERENTLY."

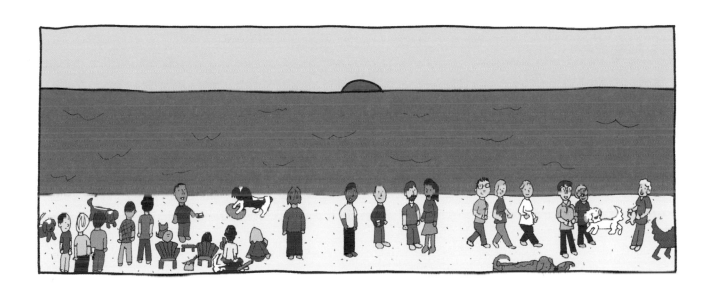

FIN

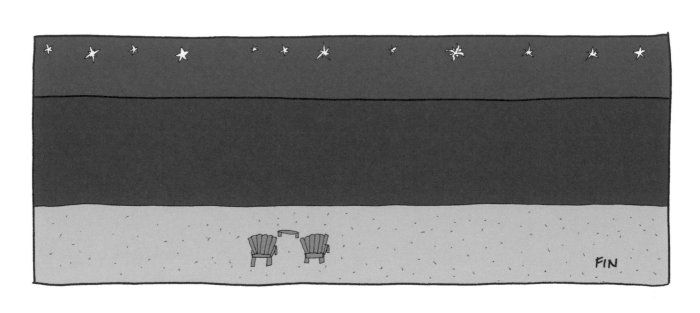

This is one story. What are more stories? What are more stories from this time, from this era? Maybe stories that haven't been heard yet?

—LIN-MANUEL MIRANDA

p. xv Poet Marie Howe's quote arises from an interview with Krista Tippet for an episode of *On Being*, aired August 28, 2014. Full interview and transcript are available at http://www.onbeing.org/program/the-poetry-of-ordinary -time-with-marie-howe/5301.

p. 1 The instructor at Rush University School of Nursing depicted here is Beth-Anne Christopher.

p. 5 AIDS data statistic citations in this book are from the Centers for Disease Control, http://www.cdc.org; Illinois Department of Health, http://www.idph.org; and the AIDS Foundation of Chicago, http://www.aidschicago.org.

p. 6 My watercolor painting on this page is based on an online image from Institut Cochin. It is actually a T-cell (blue) and a dendritic cell (yellow). Reference photo was accessed via http://www.wired.com/2008/04/a-new -tactic-ag/.

p. 11 Citation for the study I did with George Fitchett is "When a Loved One Is Dying: Families Talk About Nursing Care," *American Journal of Nursing* 96, no. 5 (May 1996).

p. 17 Citation for the history of Illinois Masonic Medical Center is Harold Blake Walker, *Caring Community: A History of Illinois Masonic Medical Center* (Illinois Masonic Medical Center, 1987). For information about the history of AIDS in Chicago, we are all indebted to journalist, author, and historian Tracy Baim for *Windy City Times*, *Outlines*, and *Out and Proud in Chicago: An Overview of the City's Gay Community* (Surrey Books, 2008). Also see her oral history website, http://www.chicagogayhistory.com.

p. 19 The oral history interviews that appear in this book were conducted between September 2008 and October 2016. All narrators have approved of their representations here with the exception of Roger Goodman, who passed away in June 2015, before he was able to see this work. Gretchen Case taught me to conduct an oral history, and I was influenced by the work of Studs Terkel, Alessandro Portelli, Dave Isay, Sayantani DasGupta, and Valerie Yow.

p. 29 Other hospital units in Chicago provided care for HIV/AIDS patients, including St. Joseph's Hospital, Rush Medical Center, and Cook County Hospital. Unit 371's distinction was to be the first dedicated HIV/AIDS inpatient care unit in the Midwest. By "dedicated" I mean that the unit was intentionally opened to care exclusively for AIDS patients, and it was the preferred placement for all HIV+ patients admitted outside the intensive care unit. Unit 371 had its own medical, nursing, social service, chaplaincy, and volunteer staff tailored to the unique needs of this patient population. Eventually an HIV/AIDS medical education rotation was also established on Unit 371.

p. 31 Other physicians joined Dr. Blatt and Dr. Moore's HIV/AIDS practice in the 1990s, including Dr. Malte Schutz.

p. 32 In case you are wondering, the five rights of medication administration are: right medication, right patient, right dose, right route, and right time.

p. 34 Unit 371 was founded as a 23-bed inpatient unit. At first, "the back" (rooms 3731–3740, on the left of the map) was dedicated to patients in hospice. But by the time I arrived in 1994, room demand and patient acuity had forced this plan to be abandoned. Private rooms were reserved for dying or infectious patients. After 1998, all double rooms were converted to single rooms and the unit capacity was lowered to 17.

p. 44 All patients represented in this book are fictional. They are composite characters, containing a mix of elements inspired by real people whom I remember fondly. The stories represented in this book are based on real events.

p. 48 The piece referenced on the right in the first panel is by Danny Sotomayor. See http://www.nytimes.com/1992/02/16/obituaries/daniel-sotomayor-cartoonist-33.html and http://www.windycitymediagroup.com/lgbt/AIDS-One-of-a-kind-Danny-Sotomayor-acted-up-and-fought-back-/31467.html.

p. 62 Annie Dillard, *Pilgrim at Tinker Creek* (Harper Perennial, 1974), 270.

p. 64 "A great man is gone," from e. e. cummings, *73 Poems* (W. W. Norton, 2003).

p.69 Cryptosporidium is a parasitic infection of the gastrointestinal tract that causes an abundant, watery diarrhea common in AIDS patients at this time. The smell of crypto to which Rosa refers is quite distinct, more sweet than foul.

p.85 I did this watercolor painting based on photographs of this actual object. Despite much effort, I was unable to uncover the name of the original artist of this piece. Per the hospital chaplain Reverend Dee (via Esther Bloch, LBD Fine Art, Inc.), this piece was a reproduction of a Chagall window commissioned by a physician, donated to the hospital chapel in memory of his wife.

p. 110 The pulmonary lab was the closest neighbor of Unit 371, and very much a part of the unit's community. Several of the hospital's departments responded exceptionally to the needs of AIDS patients and their caregivers, including the GI lab, the blood bank, the pharmacy, radiology, and the emergency room. In exploring this, I'm very influenced by Annemarie Mol's extraordinary "ethnography of an ordinary disease" in *The Body Multiple: Ontology in Medical Practice* (Duke University Press, 2002).

p. 150 The volunteers served food delivered three times weekly by community restaurants. Monday was Pete's Pizza, Wednesday was El Jardin, and Thursday was Ann Sather. The volunteers would call the restaurant with the evening's patient census and the number of staff and visitors who needed to be fed that evening. Every week, for nearly fifteen years, the restaurants would deliver more than enough food for everyone at no cost to the unit. Nearly all narrators in the oral history I conducted mentioned this donated food as an important part of the unit's culture.

p. 155 Data citation: http://articles.chicagotribune.com/1998-11-27/news/9811270194_1_aids-memorial-quilt-aids-treatment-world-aidsday.

p. 195 Panel 2: *Eternal Silence*, sculpted by Lorado Taft. It marks the burial plot of Dexter Graves and his family, among the first settlers of Chicago. Panel 3: The Getty Tomb, designed by Louis Sullivan, stands on its own triangle of land. It was built in 1890. In 1971, it was formally designated a city landmark. It is considered the birthplace of modern architecture in America. Panel 4: Louis Sullivan's grave. Five years after Sullivan's death in 1924, Thomas Tallmadge designed this monument.

p. 196 Panel 1: Grave of Christopher Manuel, M.D., 1964–2005. See http://chicago-architecture-jyoti.blogspot.com/2009/11/tomb-of-drchristopher-d-manuel.html. Panel 2: Grave of six-year-old Inez Clark. See http://www.cemeteryguide.com/inezclarke.html.

p. 198 Grave of the Kimball family. Monument designed by McKim, Mead & White, a firm that also designed buildings for the 1893 White City.

p. 211 Rebecca Garden, "Who Speaks for Whom? Health Humanities and the Ethics of Representation," *Medical Humanities* 41 (2015): 77–80.

Additional Bibliography

I believe that whatever we receive we must share. When I endure an experience, the experience cannot stay with me alone. It must be opened, it must become an offering, it must be deepened and given and shared. Without memory, there is no culture. Without memory, there would be no civilization, no society, no future.

—ELIE WIESEL

Armstrong, W. "St. Vincent's Remembered." OUT Magazine, September 2010.

Bayer, Ronald, and Gerald M. Oppenheimer. AIDS Doctors: Voices from the Epidemic; An Oral History. New York: Oxford University Press, 2000.

Canning, Richard. "The Epidemic That Barely Was." Gay & Lesbian Review, March–April 2011.

Garb, Maggie. "Physicians Fight Burnout in the Battle Against AIDS." Chicago Sun-Times, February 27, 1990.

Harfmann, Barbara. "At the Heart of HIV Care." Caring: A Publication of Illinois Masonic Medical Center, Winter 1999.

Howe, Marie. What the Living Do. New York: W. W. Norton, 1999.

Lanctot, Barbara. A Walk Through Graceland Cemetery: A Chicago Architecture Foundation Walking Tour. Chicago: Chicago Architecture Foundation, 1988.

Pogash, C. As Real as It Gets: The Life of a Hospital at the Center of the AIDS Epidemic. New York: Penguin, 1992.

Saltmarsh, S. "A Tale of Two Healers." Positively Aware: The HIV Treatment Journal of Test Positive Aware Network, May/June 2011. http://www.positivelyaware.com/archives/2011/11_03/two_healers.shtml.

Sontag, Susan. "Illness and Metaphor" and "AIDS and Its Metaphors." New York: Picador, 1990.

Sullivan, Andrew. "When Plagues End: Note on the Twilight of an Epidemic." New York Times Magazine, November 10, 1996.

AIDS Resources

This disease will be the end of many of us, but not nearly all, and the dead will be commemorated and we will struggle on with the living. We are not going away. We won't die secret deaths anymore. The world only spins forward. We will be citizens. The time has come.

—TONY KUSHNER, *ANGELS IN AMERICA*

Brandt, A. "AIDS in Historical Perspective: Four Lessons from the History of Sexually Transmitted Diseases." In *Sickness and Health in America*, ed. K. Leavitt and R. Numbers. Madison: University of Wisconsin Press, 1997.

Fanning, David, executive producer. "Frontline: The Age of AIDS." Public Broadcasting Service. First aired May 30, 2006.

Geidner, Chris. "13 Times the Reagan White House Press Briefing Erupted with Laughter over AIDS." *Buzz-Feed News*, December 2, 2013. https://www.buzz-feed.com/chrisgeidner/times-the-reagan-white-house-press-briefing-erupted-with?utm_term=.jx8llXjB0p#.toVbbRA308.

Gould, Deborah. *Moving Politics: Emotion and ACT-UP's Fight Against AIDS*. Chicago: University of Chicago Press, 2009.

Hoffman, Amy. *Hospital Time*. Durham: Duke University Press, 1997.

How to Survive a Plague. Documentary by David France. 2012.

Jones, Carolyn. *Living Proof: Courage in the Face of AIDS*. New York: Abbeville Press, 1994.

Kramer, Larry. *The Normal Heart*. New York: Penguin Books, 1985.

Kushner, Tony. *Angels in America*. New York: Theater Communications Group, 1992.

Lewis, Sydney. *Hospital: An Oral History of Cook County Hospital*. New York: The New Press, 1994.

Longtime Companion. Film directed by Norman René, 1990.

Mustich, Emma. "A History of AIDS Hysteria." *Salon*, Sunday, June 5, 2011. http://www.salon.com/2011/06/05/aids_hysteria/.

The Recollectors. "Remembering Parents Lost to AIDS." http://therecollectors.com; http://www.nytimes.com/2015/03/22/style/adult-children-of-aids-victims-take-their-memories-out-of-the-shadows.html.

Robbins, Trina, et al., eds. *Strip AIDS U.S.A.: A Collection of Cartoon Art to Benefit People with AIDS*. San Francisco: Last Gasp, 1988.

Shilts, Randy. *And the Band Played On: Politics, People, and the AIDS Epidemic*. New York: Macmillan, 2000.

Silverlake Life: The View from Here. Film directed by Tom Joslin and Peter Friedman, 1993.

Specter, Michael. "Hillary Clinton, Nancy Reagan, and AIDS." *The New Yorker*, March 11, 2016. http://www.newyorker.com/news/dailycomment/hillary-clinton-nancy-reagan-and-aids.

Terkel, Studs. *Will the Circle Be Unbroken: Reflections on Death, Rebirth, and a Hunger for a Faith*. New York: The New Press, 2001.

We Were Here: The AIDS Years in San Francisco. Documentary directed by David Weissman, 2001.

Wilson, Terry. "Volunteers Help Patients Who Have HIV, AIDS to Cope." *Chicago Tribune*, January 22, 1995.

Wojnarowicz, David. *7 Miles a Second*. Seattle: Fantagraphics, 2012.

Resources on Compassion Fatigue and Caregiving

The expectation that we can be immersed in suffering and loss daily and not be touched by it is as unrealistic as expecting to be able to walk through water without getting wet.

— RACHEL NAOMI REMEN

Professional Quality of Life Elements and Theory Measurement
  http://www.proqol.org
Rosalynn Carter Institute for Caregiving
  http://www.rosalynncarter.org
The Schwartz Center for Compassionate Healthcare
  http://www.theschwartzcenter.org

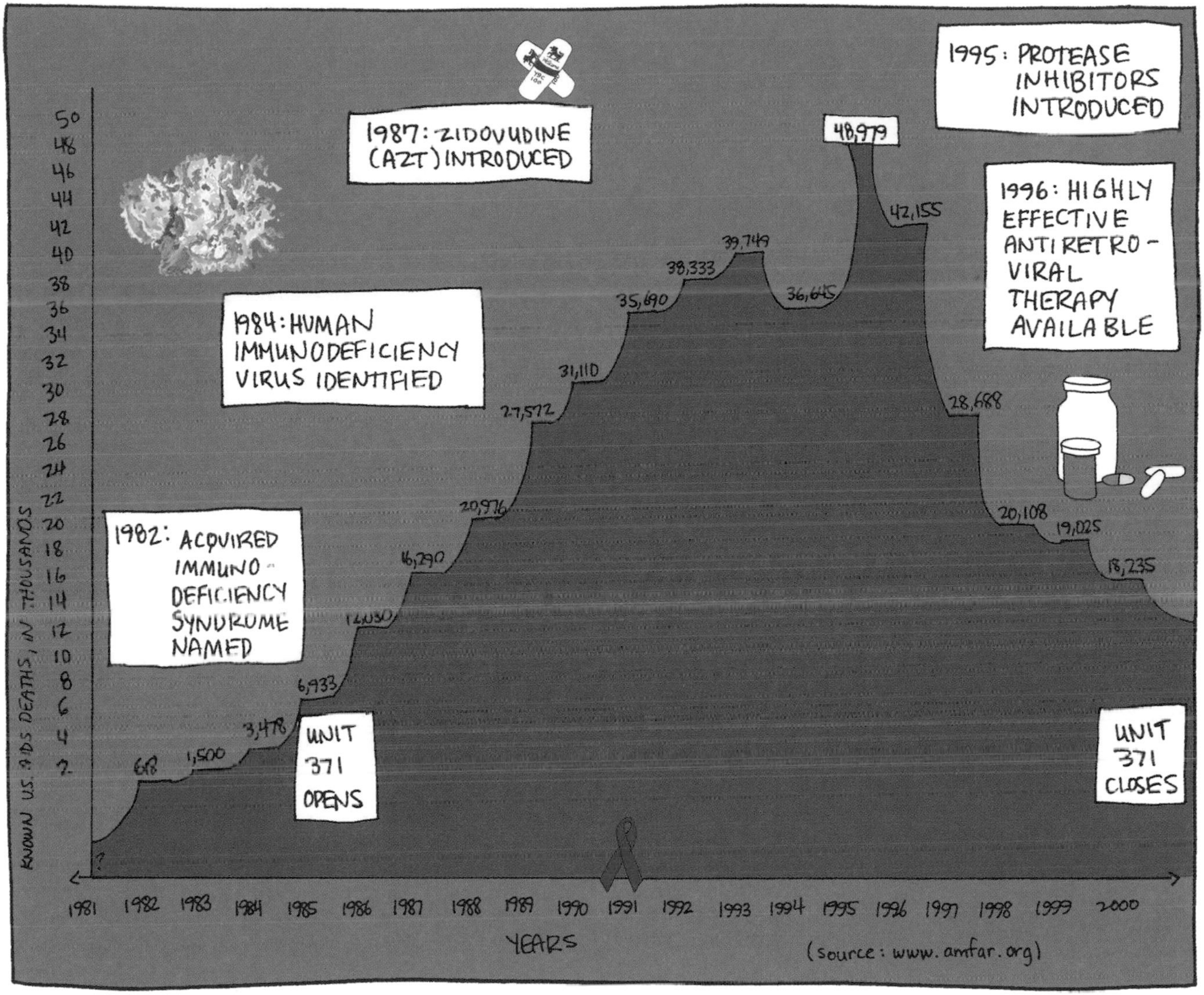
1987: ZIDOVUDINE (AZT) INTRODUCED
1995: PROTEASE INHIBITORS INTRODUCED
1996: HIGHLY EFFECTIVE ANTIRETRO-VIRAL THERAPY AVAILABLE
1984: HUMAN IMMUNODEFICIENCY VIRUS IDENTIFIED
1982: ACQUIRED IMMUNO-DEFICIENCY SYNDROME NAMED
UNIT 371 OPENS
UNIT 371 CLOSES
50
48
46
44
42
40
38
36
34
32
30
28
26
24
22
20
18
16
14
12
10
8
6
4
2
618
1,500
3,478
6,933
12,030
16,290
20,976
27,572
31,110
35,690
38,333
39,749
36,645
48,979
42,155
28,688
20,108
19,025
18,235
KNOWN U.S. AIDS DEATHS, IN THOUSANDS
1981
1982
1983
1984
1985
1986
1987
1988
1989
1990
1991
1992
1993
1994
1995
1996
1997
1998
1999
2000
YEARS
(source: www.amfar.org)

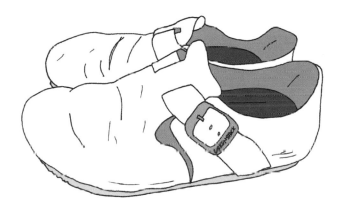

Library of Congress Cataloging-in-Publication Data

Names: Czerwiec, MK (MaryKay), 1967– author, artist.
Title: Taking turns : stories from HIV/AIDS care unit 371 / MK Czerwiec.
Description: University Park, Pennsylvania : Graphic Mundi, [2021] | Includes bibliographical references.
Summary: "A graphic memoir and adapted oral history of Unit 371, an inpatient AIDS care hospital unit in Chicago that was in existence from 1985 to 2000. Examines the human costs of caregiving and the role art can play in the grieving process"—Provided by publisher.
Identifiers: LCCN 2021030148 | ISBN 9781637790076 (paperback)
Subjects: MESH: Illinois Masonic Medical Center. Unit 371. | Acquired Immunodeficiency Syndrome—nursing | HIV Infections—nursing | Art Therapy | Hospital Units | Nurse-Patient Relations | Nurses—psychology | Chicago | Graphic Novel | Personal Narrative
Classification: LCC RC606.6 | NLM WY 17 | DDC 362.19697/92—dc23
LC record available at https://lccn.loc.gov/2021030148

Printed in Lithuania
Published by The Pennsylvania State University Press,
University Park, PA 16802–1003

graphic mundi
drawing our worlds together

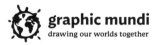

Graphic Mundi is an imprint of The Pennsylvania State University Press.

The Pennsylvania State University Press is a member of the Association of University Presses.

It is the policy of The Pennsylvania State University Press to use acid-free paper. Publications on uncoated stock satisfy the minimum requirements of American National Standard for Information Sciences—Permanence of Paper for Printed Library Material, ANSI Z39.48–1992.